Atlas of Touch Preparation Cytopathology

Atlas of Touch Preparation Cytopathology

Liron Pantanowitz, MD
Professor of Pathology and Biomedical Informatics
Director of Cytopathology
UPMC Shadyside
Director of Pathology Informatics Fellowship Program
Director of the Pathology Informatics Division
University of Pittsburgh Medical Center
Pittsburgh, Pennsylvania

Juan Xing, MD
Assistant Professor of Pathology
University of Pittsburgh Medical Center
Pittsburgh, Pennsylvania

Sara E. Monaco, MD
Associate Professor of Pathology
Director of Cytopathology Fellowship Program
Director of Fine Needle Aspiration Clinic
University of Pittsburgh Medical Center
Pittsburgh, Pennsylvania

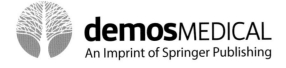

demosMEDICAL
An Imprint of Springer Publishing

Visit our website at www.demosmedical.com

ISBN: 9781620700686
ebook ISBN: 9781617052378

Acquisitions Editor: David D'Addona
Compositor: diacriTech

Medicine is an ever-changing science. Research and clinical experience are continually expanding our knowledge, in particular our understanding of proper treatment and drug therapy. The authors, editors, and publisher have made every effort to ensure that all information in this book is in accordance with the state of knowledge at the time of production of the book. Nevertheless, the authors, editors, and publisher are not responsible for errors or omissions or for any consequences from application of the information in this book and make no warranty, expressed or implied, with respect to the contents of the publication. Every reader should examine carefully the package inserts accompanying each drug and should carefully check whether the dosage schedules mentioned therein or the contraindications stated by the manufacturer differ from the statements made in this book. Such examination is particularly important with drugs that are either rarely used or have been newly released on the market.

Library of Congress Cataloging-in-Publication Data
Names: Pantanowitz, Liron, author. | Xing, Juan (Of University of Pittsburgh
  Medical Center (2003-)), author. | Monaco, Sara E., author.s
Title: Atlas of touch preparation cytopathology / Liron Pantanowitz, Juan Xing, Sara E. Monaco.
Description: New York : Demos, [2018] | Includes bibliographical references and index.
Identifiers: LCCN 2017017714| ISBN 9781620700686 | ISBN 9781617052378 (e-book)
Subjects: | MESH: Cytodiagnosis–methods | Histocytological Preparation
  Techniques–methods | Atlases
Classification: LCC RB43 | NLM QY 17 | DDC 616.07/582—dc23 LC record available at https://lccn.loc.gov/2017017714

Contact us to receive discount rates on bulk purchases.
We can also customize our books to meet your needs.
For more information please contact: sales@springerpub.com

Printed in the United States of America by Bang Printing.
17 18 19 20 21 / 5 4 3 2 1

To Heidi, Joshua & Maya for their support and giving me the time to write this book.
Liron Pantanowitz

To my lovely husband Guodong and our two amazing daughters, Catherine and Sarah, for their unconditional love and support.
Juan Xing

To my parents, husband, and children (Eddie, Julia, and Nicholas) for their endless support and love.
Sara E. Monaco

Contents

Contributors

Deborah J. Chute, MD
Staff Pathologist
Assistant Professor of Pathology
RJ-Tomsich Institute of Pathology and
    Laboratory Medicine
Cleveland Clinic
Cleveland, Ohio

Julia Kofler, MD
Assistant Professor of Pathology
University of Pittsburgh Medical Center
Pittsburgh, Pennsylvania

Zaibo Li, MD, PhD
Assistant Professor of Pathology
The Ohio State University Wexner Medical Center
Columbus, Ohio

Reetesh K. Pai, MD
Associate Professor of Pathology
Director of the Gastrointestinal Pathology
    Center of Excellence
Director of the Gastrointestinal Pathology Fellowship
University of Pittsburgh Medical Center
Pittsburgh, Pennsylvania

Anil V. Parwani, MD, PhD
Professor of Pathology
Vice Chair of Anatomic Pathology
Director of Pathology Informatics
The Ohio State University Wexner Medical Center
Columbus, Ohio

Chengquan Zhao, MD
Professor of Pathology
Codirector of Cytopathology and Director of Fine
    Needle Aspiration at Magee-Women's Hospital,
    and Chief of Pathology, UPMC-China Enterprise
University of Pittsburgh Medical Center
Pittsburgh, Pennsylvania

Preface

The touch preparation technique was officially introduced in the medical literature back in 1927. However, I hardly recall seeing a touch preparation cytology slide during my pathology residency training in the early 2000s. Even during my cytopathology fellowship, touch preparations were an infrequent occurrence. The only instance when I encountered an occasional imprint during my training years was when one was performed during a frozen section, or when it accompanied a hematopathology case work-up. Since then, the popularity of touch preparations has steadily increased in cytopathology practice. Today, I am regularly called upon several times a day to provide rapid onsite evaluations of core needle biopsies by employing touch preps.

The method of performing and interpreting a touch preparation or imprint is relatively unique from other cytology preparations such as fine needle aspirations. The sample cellularity, cytological patterns, and artifacts of these preparations may differ considerably from those described in direct smears or liquid based specimens. A poorly prepared touch may even damage tissue samples and result in loss of valuable cells, hindering the ability to perform subsequent ancillary testing. Most cytopathology textbooks today do not discuss touch preparations nor do they address some of these important differences. Therefore, I have invited several cytopathology colleagues who have accrued years of practical experience in handling touch preparations, imprints, and/or squash preparations to help me write this unique textbook and atlas, which fills an emerging gap in cytopathology.

Liron Pantanowitz, MD

CHAPTER 1

Introduction

Sara E. Monaco and Liron Pantanowitz

BACKGROUND

Touch preparations (TPs) (Figure 1.1) and cytology imprints are important techniques encountered in the practice of cytopathology. Table 1.1 defines the subtle differences between TPs, imprints, smears, and scrapes. In 1927, Dudgeon and Patrick from London developed a simple method to obtain rapid cytological diagnoses of freshly cut specimens. They demonstrated that their findings in 200 consecutive specimens had reliable accuracy rates when compared to control examination of paraffin embedded and fixed tissue sections prepared from the same tissue (1). Since then, touch imprint cytology has been commonly utilized for intraoperative evaluations of tumors to complement frozen section evaluation in order to reach a more definitive diagnosis, or for examination of tissue prior to processing for guiding specimen triage (e.g., lymphoma work-up). Previously, obtaining an imprint cytology sample of gastric mucosa to rapidly diagnose *Helicobacter pylori* infection was popular (2). In the current era of personalized medicine, the use of TPs is increasing as a stand-alone preparation to evaluate small tissue samples for adequacy, rapid onsite diagnosis, and triage for ancillary studies while minimizing tissue loss

and destruction (3–5). This trend is partially explained by the fact that image-guided small core needle biopsies (CNBs) offer an accurate, minimally invasive mechanism to procure tumor tissue for molecular testing or other theranostic testing. Evaluation of histological architecture in core biopsies can help diagnose certain entities that would otherwise be difficult or impossible to make by fine needle aspiration (FNA) alone. When aspirates are scant in cellularity or nondiagnostic, a CNB along with TP offers an alternative to obtain more diagnostic tissue that can still be utilized for rapid onsite cytological evaluation (Figure 1.2). Another reason supporting the use of CNB is that many new ancillary studies are validated primarily on histological material.

TPs have been reported to be helpful in unique scenarios such as postmortem examination, testis biopsy in the work-up of male fertility, and to evaluate mucocutaneous ulcers (e.g., Tzanck test). In the setting of autopsies, particularly those carried out in a medical examiners' office where routine histology may not be performed, TPs provide a cost-effective way to rapidly assess postmortem tissues (Figures 1.3 and 1.4) (6,7). Despite the increasing trend to obtain CNBs for many superficial- and deep-seated lesions, some tissue types have not seen this dramatic

---

TABLE 1.1 Definition of Different Cytologic Preparations

- **Touch imprint:** Cytology slide prepared by pressing a glass slide on to a large tissue or organ specimen that is freshly cut for evaluation.
  - a. Example: Touch imprint performed at the time of frozen section of a large tumor resection.
  - b. Usually supplements a concurrent H&E-stained frozen section for immediate evaluation.
- **TP:** Cytology slide prepared by touching a small tissue biopsy on to a glass slide and at times moving or dragging the tissue along the surface of the slide.
  - a. Example: TP of an image-guided core needle biopsy of a tumor for rapid onsite cytologic evaluation.
  - b. Usually unaccompanied by a frozen section and reviewed at the time of immediate evaluation.
- **Smear preparation:** Cytology slide prepared from a small tissue sample that is crushed or smeared between two glass slides.
  - a. Example: Smear preparation prepared for neuropathology intraoperative evaluation of a brain lesion.
  - b. Usually avoids the need to also perform a frozen section. This form of preparation is also used for FNA samples.
- **Scrape preparation:** Cytology slide prepared by scraping the lesional surface of a tissue sample with a scalpel blade, or the edge of a slide, and then smearing the scraped material on to a clean glass slide.
  - a. Example: Cytoscrape performed at the time of frozen section of a large tumor resection, or prepared at the bedside from a patient's skin lesion (e.g., Tzanck test).
  - b. Usually supplements a concurrent H&E-stained frozen section during intraoperative evaluation.

H&E, hematoxylin and eosin; TP, touch preparation.

increase. This has been the case for sampling lesions in the pancreatobiliary region, which is primarily sampled with FNA or slightly larger needles (e.g., Sharkcore and ProCore needles), given the need to use flexible needles during endoscopic procedures and to minimize complications such as postprocedure pancreatitis (8).

TPs have been widely employed in pathology for many years. Nevertheless, there is still a relative paucity of literature on how best to perform and interpret a TP and/or cytology imprint. Compared to the histological evaluation of hematoxylin and eosin (H&E)-stained core biopsies, TPs like FNA smears allow cellular material to be rapidly visualized with different stains (e.g., Papanicolaou and Diff-Quik [DQ] stains) and without fixation or frozen tissue artifacts. These cytology samples often provide a more tumor-rich sample with less background stroma, minimizing the need for microdissection prior to molecular testing. Although many morphological features seen on TP overlap with traditional cytomorphology seen on direct smears (Figure 1.5), there may be distinct differences, as outlined in Table 1.2. Compared to imprints, FNA smears more evenly disperse cells (Figure 1.6), permitting their cohesive or discohesive nature to become readily apparent. With TPs there may be more architectural clues present as the tissue imprint forms a replica on the glass slide with less smearing artifact (Figure 1.7). However, this can also result in thick areas and false clustering of cells (Figure 1.8), which makes cytologic evaluation difficult for those who are unfamiliar with TPs. Some tumors readily identified on FNA may show less characteristic features on TP as a result of forced discohesion of cells (Figure 1.9) and formation of stripped nuclei. Also, background material, which provides important diagnostic clues (e.g., lymphoglandular bodies due to disrupted cytoplasm that occurs with lymphoid lesions), may not always be distinctive in touch imprints.

Overall, when interpreted correctly, intraprocedural and intraoperative cytologic TPs and imprints are a powerful tool, which is increasingly being recognized. This book is intended to be a high-yield atlas of TP that will hopefully prove to be useful in the contemporary practice of cytopathology.

TABLE 1.2 Cytomorphological Differences Between Smears, Touch Preparations, and Histological Evaluation of Core Biopsies

Cytologic Features	Aspirate Smears	Touch Preparations	Biopsy Tissue Sections
Cellularity	Usually cellular	Variable	Variable
Heterogeneity	High, especially with multiple passes	Limited	Limited
Cohesive cell groups	Present without surrounding stroma	Present without surrounding stroma	Present with surrounding stroma
Discohesive cells	Present, including lymphocytes with lymphoglandular bodies	May show artifactual cell clustering, including lymphocytes with/without lymphoglandular bodies	Appear as infiltrative sheets of intact cells
Spindle cells	Easily appreciated if aspirated, cytoplasm may be stripped resulting in naked nuclei	Easily appreciated if present, cytoplasm may be stripped resulting in naked nuclei	Nuclei can vary from spindled to round or oval, and usually have intact cytoplasm
Stroma	Not present or scant	Not present or scant	Usually present
Cystic fluid	Easy to smear	Not feasible to perform	Typically not performed, but could identify lining
Background	Material (e.g., colloid, myxoid matrix) or disrupted cytoplasm (e.g., causing tigroid appearance) smears easily	Typically present and patchy	Material may not survive processing
Necrosis	Appears as granular debris aggregating in thick, curly lines	Appears as thick granular debris	May cause biopsy to fragment
Blood dilution	Often present	Limited	Usually absent
Overall architecture	Disrupted	Intact clues to architecture	Intact
Artifacts	Air-drying and crushed cells	Air-drying, thick groups, and stripped cells	Freeze artifact if frozen, formalin artifact if fixed (e.g., cellular contraction)

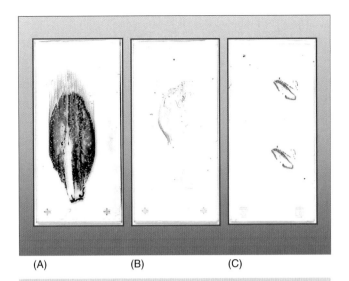

(A)   (B)   (C)

FIGURE 1.1 Cytology slides. Macroscopic slide comparison of a (A) DQ-stained FNA smear, (B) DQ-stained touch imprint of a core biopsy, and (C) core biopsy tissue sections (H&E stain) obtained from the same tumor. The cytomorphological features may differ for each of these preparations. DQ, Diff-Quik; FNA, fine needle aspiration; H&E, hematoxylin and eosin.

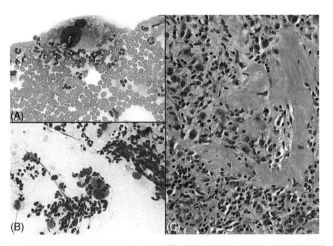

FIGURE 1.2 Classical Hodgkin lymphoma. (A) FNA aspirates in this case were bloody and had limited cellularity with only rare scattered large Reed–Sternberg cells. Thus, (C) a core biopsy was performed along with (B) a TP that shows quantitatively more Reed–Sternberg cells, leading to a more definitive and specific diagnosis. ((A) DQ-stained smear, high power; (B) DQ-stained TP, high power; (C) H&E-stained core biopsy, high power.) DQ, Diff-Quik; FNA, fine needle aspiration; H&E, hematoxylin and eosin; TP, touch preparation.

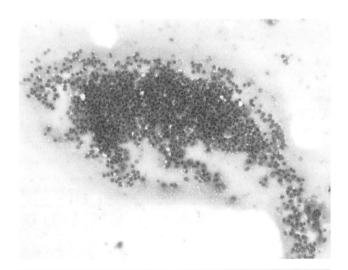

FIGURE 1.3 Acute pneumonia (postmortem). TP of a consolidated lung during autopsy shows abundant acute inflammatory cells (H&E-stained TP, low power). H&E, hematoxylin and eosin; TP, touch preparation.

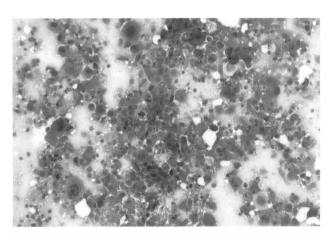

FIGURE 1.4 Pancreatic adenocarcinoma (postmortem). Imprint cytology of a pancreas mass during autopsy shows a poorly differentiated carcinoma. Poor cell preservation is related to postmortem change (H&E-stained TP, high power). H&E, hematoxylin and eosin; TP, touch preparation.

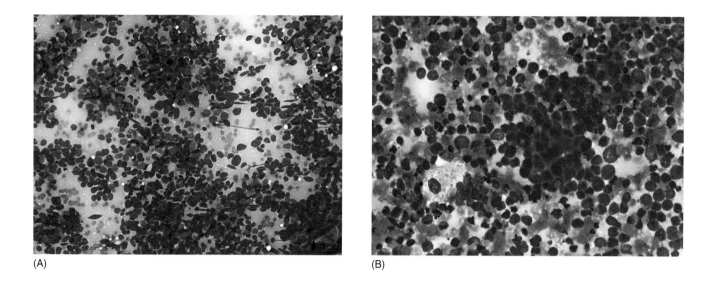

(A)   (B)

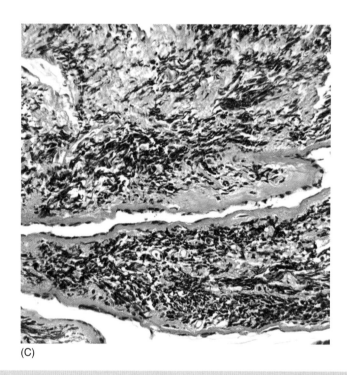

(C)

FIGURE 1.5 Small cell carcinoma. An aspiration smear (A) and TP (B) of small cell carcinoma show overlapping cytological features with high nuclear:cytoplasmic (N:C) ratio, nuclear hyperchromasia, and inconspicuous nucleoli associated with apoptosis. However, nuclear molding and crush or smear artifact are less conspicuous in the TP. Also, focal cell clustering on the TP may mimic basaloid squamous cell carcinoma. The core biopsy shown of small cell carcinoma (C) suffers from the worst crush artifact of the three preparations, damaging the cells beyond recognition. ((A) DQ-stained FNA smear, medium power; (B) DQ-stained TP, medium power; (C) H&E-stained core biopsy, medium power.) DQ, Diff-Quik; FNA, fine needle aspiration; H&E, hematoxylin and eosin; TP, touch preparation.

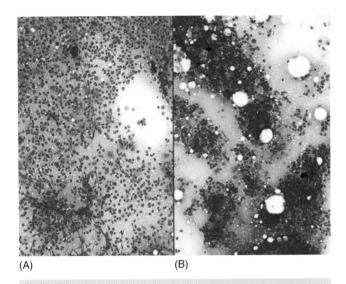

(A)   (B)

FIGURE 1.6 Non-Hodgkin B-cell lymphoma. (A) The aspirate is hypercellular and shows a uniform population of discohesive cells. Note that some areas have smearing or crush artifact. (B) A TP of the corresponding core biopsy shows geographic clustering of lymphoid cells where the tissue touched the slide. ((A) DQ-stained smear, low power; (B) DQ-stained TP, low power.) DQ, Diff-Quik; TP, touch preparation.

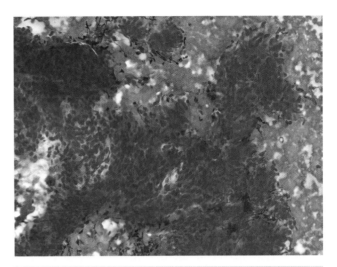

FIGURE 1.7 Spindle cell (Type A) thymoma. Touch imprint showing large, thick cohesive sheets of spindled cells that stuck to the glass slide during preparation (DQ-stained TP, low power). DQ, Diff-Quik; TP, touch preparation.

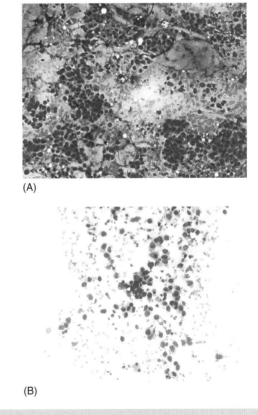

(A)

(B)

FIGURE 1.9 Colon adenocarcinoma. (A) The FNA smear shows high cellularity with characteristic cohesive clusters of tumor cells with columnar features and background mucin with dirty necrosis. (B) The TP of the same tumor shows more discohesive cells, stripped nuclei, and a clean background displaying less characteristic features of a colorectal adenocarcinoma. ((A) DQ-stained aspirate smear, low power; (B) DQ-stained TP, low power.) FNA, fine needle aspiration; TP, touch preparation.

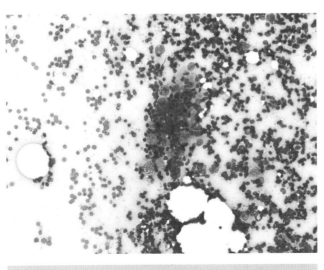

FIGURE 1.8 Nodal classical Hodgkin lymphoma. TP showing aggregation of many Reed–Sternberg cells that may mimic metastatic carcinoma (DQ-stained TP, high power). DQ, Diff-Quik; TP, touch preparation.

ACCURACY AND PERFORMANCE

Anecdotally, many of the early studies investigating the utility of TP looked at this procedure as an adjunct to frozen sections with immediate histological correlation. However, now that TPs are being commonly evaluated without concomitant frozen sections in many scenarios, they are being compared to traditional FNA. The pattern of practice varies at different medical centers, making it difficult to sometimes extrapolate research findings. Some institutions use both FNA and CNB with TP, others rely only on CNBs with TP, whereas others perform imprints in conjunction with frozen section (9,10). TP findings may also vary according to the number of passes, gauge and type of biopsy needle used, proceduralist, and type of tissue being biopsied.

In general, the accuracy of TP has been reported to be high at about 78% to 96%, showing concordance with CNB histopathology diagnoses in 80% to 92% of cases (11–17). In one study where TPs were prepared from 90 CT-guided core needle lung biopsies the sensitivity, specificity, positive predictive value, and negative predictive value were 89%, 100%, 100%, and 68%, respectively (18). Onsite touch imprint cytology has also been shown to reduce the number of cores required for adequate diagnostic material (19). The combination of FNA with TP of CNBs maximizes the diagnostic yield with about 95% accuracy. In a study where 622 patients with thoracic lesions underwent CT-guided biopsy, imprint cytology plus histology showed an improved diagnostic accuracy of 96.4% compared with that of imprint cytology alone (92.3%) or histopathology alone (93.0%) (20). The use of TP with frozen section has similarly been shown to maximize results with about 99% diagnostic accuracy.

The performance of both FNA and TP with CNB is high for malignant lesions, particularly epithelial type malignancies. Moreover, compared to FNA alone, the performance of TP with CNB appears to be superior and more specific for benign entities and nonepithelial malignant lesions (e.g., lymphoma, sarcoma) (12,13).

In addition to being used for morphological evaluation, TP slides can be used for ancillary studies. With sentinel lymph node evaluation for metastatic breast carcinoma, employing immunostains on touch imprints can improve diagnostic sensitivity (21). Cytology imprints can also be used for fluorescence in situ hybridization (FISH) and molecular studies, particularly since these preparations lack the nuclear truncation artifacts seen with histological sections. This has been shown to be advantageous for several cancer specimens (22–24). TP has been shown to provide tumor-enriched samples that are an excellent source of high-quality tumor DNA for molecular analysis (25,26). Furthermore, TP slides are a valuable reserve of cells that can provide critical back up to avoid repeat testing in some patients.

ADVANTAGES AND DISADVANTAGES

Table 1.3 summarizes some of the advantages and disadvantages of touch imprint cytology. TPs have increased in popularity for small tissue sample evaluation due to the many advantages they offer over frozen section and FNA evaluation. These advantages maximize the benefits of FNA (Safe, Accurate, Fast, and Economical; i.e., SAFE mnemonic) with those provided by tissue CNB (increased tissue procurement and examination of architecture). Touch imprints of CNBs have been shown to provide

TABLE 1.3 Advantages and Disadvantages of TPs

Advantages	Disadvantages
• Rapid, easy to perform, and minimally invasive • Requires minimal and inexpensive equipment • Adjunct to frozen section during intraoperative consultation • Less dependent on operator skill than FNA • Permits rapid onsite evaluation (ROSE) for CNB • Permits immediate evaluation of specimens for triage and diagnosis • Niche applications (e.g., fatty or hard bone tissue that is difficult to perform frozen sections on, testis biopsy for male fertility) • Complements routine processing of tissue specimens, providing an additional cytology preparation to examine cellular details with different stains • Less artifacts caused by freezing, formalin, and smearing • Offers cytomorphology not visualized on tissue sections (e.g., lymphoglandular bodies, tigroid background) • Conserves material by minimizing tissue destruction • Touch imprint slides can be used for ancillary studies such as immunostains, FISH, and molecular testing	• Unfamiliarity with preparing and evaluating cytology imprint slides • Greater risk of complications with core biopsy than with FNA, particularly for vascular lesions • Limited utility with fibrous lesions that do not release cells easily • Damage to cells when forcefully imprinting tissue that may impact morphology • Loss of tissue in remaining core biopsy, that may limit ancillary testing • Limited evaluation, compared to evaluating architecture in tissue sections • Challenging cytomorphologic differences compared to traditional aspirate smears • Absence of morphological clues, such as nuclear halos caused by tissue fixation

CNB, core needle biopsies; FISH, fluorescence in situ hybridization; FNA fine needle aspiration; TP, touch preparation.

higher diagnostic sensitivity than histologic evaluation alone, because cells can be collected from the entire surface of the core compared to just a longitudinal section through the middle of the core biopsy (27). TPs are relatively easy to perform, compared to frozen section, and offer the pathologist an additional method with which to visualize cells. However, there are some drawbacks. Touch imprints may be difficult to interpret, particularly if pathologists are unfamiliar with their presentation or falsely assume that they are analogous to cytology aspirates. These preparations are subject to different procedural artifacts, as well as tissue loss or damage. Loss of tissue from delicate core biopsies is more likely to follow vigorous TP (28). Hence, poor slide preparation technique can impact not only cytomorphology, but subsequent ancillary testing of specimens.

BILLING

Performing TPs is a billable service. In the USA, billing for TP uses current procedural terminology (CPT) codes 88333/88334 for immediate evaluation and the 88305/ 88307 (depending on the anatomic site) code for the final diagnosis (Table 1.4). If multiple core biopsies with TP are performed during the same event on the same tissue, then 88333 is billed for the first TP, followed by 88334 for additional TPs evaluated from additional sites from the same targeted lesion. When using 88333/88334, the core biopsies must be submitted separately such that the number of formalin containers equals the number of TP, and it should be documented clearly that the initial core biopsy was insufficient or suboptimal for diagnosis and/or ancillary studies, necessitating additional core biopsies.

One important caveat to remember is that billing differs in the intraoperative setting where a TP may be performed to complement a frozen section. In this scenario, the initial frozen section evaluation code 88331 is used, followed by 88334 (not 88333) for the intraoperative TP. In addition, if an FNA is performed with a TP, then the FNA codes, including 88172/88177 would apply, in addition to the core biopsy and TP codes. However, one caveat is that Medicare and some other payors may not see the utility of both a touch preparation and frozen section on the same tissue, as they view them as redundant, and thus, reimbursement for all these codes may not happen in every scenario. Reimbursement for TP tends to be less than that for a frozen section evaluation, leading some institutions to not provide onsite evaluation. However, given that the use of TP evaluation does improve diagnostic yield and decreases the need for a repeat biopsy, this procedure can save money for the global health care system.

CONCLUSION

TP is an important addition to the armamentarium of cytopathology and intraoperative consultation. Given the increasing use of this cytology technique in clinical practice, it has become important for pathologists and cytologists to be adept with these preparations. This textbook, dedicated solely to TP, provides one of the most comprehensive collections of images in an atlas format. The goal of this book is to provide readers with a high-yield reference so that they can familiarize themselves with TP technique and findings they may encounter in a variety of settings and that are prepared from various tissue types. Each chapter approaches TP by comparing the findings in normal tissue to benign and malignant neoplasms. Having this atlas on hand in the frozen section area or when evaluating small biopsies onsite will hopefully maximize the utility of TP, improve concordance of intraprocedural diagnoses with final results, and better conserve tissue to be triaged for ancillary testing.

ACKNOWLEDGMENT

We would like to thank Dr. Jeffrey Nine for supplying us with postmortem touch preparations.

TABLE 1.4 Billing Codes for Intraprocedural Preparations

FNA Intraprocedural Codes

88172 (cytopathology, evaluation of FNA; immediate cytohistologic study to determine adequacy for diagnosis, first evaluation episode, each site)

88177 (immediate cytohistologic study to determine adequacy for diagnosis, each additional evaluation episode, same site)

Intraprocedural codes for TPs and other cytological preparations from tissue specimens

88333 (pathology consultation during surgery; cytologic examination [e.g., touch prep, squash prep], initial site)

88334 (pathology consultation during surgery; cytologic examination [e.g., touch prep, squash prep], each additional site)

FNA, fine needle aspiration; TP, touch preparation.

REFERENCES

1. Dudgeon LS, Patrick CV. A new method for the rapid microscopical diagnosis of tumours, with an account of 200 cases so examined. *Br J Surg.* 1927;15:250-261.
2. Misra SP, Misra V, Dwivedi M, Singh PA, Gupta SC. Diagnosing *Helicobacter pylori* by imprint cytology: can the same biopsy specimen be used for histology? Diagn Cytopathol. 1998;18:330-332.
3. Gupta NJ, Wang HH. Increase of core biopsies in visceral organs—experience at one institution. *Diagn Cytopathol.* 2011;39:791-795.
4. Lindeman NI, Cagle PT, Beasley MB, et al. Molecular testing guideline for selection of lung cancer patients for EGFR and ALK tyrosine kinase inhibitors: guideline from the College of American Pathologists, International Association for the Study of Lung Cancer, and Association for Molecular Pathology. *J Thorac Oncol.* 2013;8:823-859.

5. Tong LC, Rudomina D, Rekhtman N, Lin O. Impact of touch preparations on core needle biopsies. *Cancer Cytopathol*. 2014;122: 851-854.

6. Suen KC, Yermakov V, Raudales O. The use of imprint technic for rapid diagnosis in postmortem examinations. A diagnostically rewarding procedure. *Am J Clin Pathol*. 1976;65:291-300.

7. Shirley S, Escoffery C. Usefulness of touch preparation cytology in postmortem diagnosis: a study from The University Hospital of the West Indies. *Int J Pathol*. 2004;3(2).

8. Dwyer J, Pantanowitz L, Ohori NP, et al. Endoscopic ultrasound-guided FNA and ProCore biopsy in sampling pancreatic and intra-abdominal masses. *Cancer Cytopathol*. 2016;124:110-121.

9. Fischer AH, Cibas ES, Howell LP, et al. Role of cytology in the management of non-small cell lung cancer. *J Clin Oncol*. 2011;29:3331-3332.

10. Griffin AC, Schwartz LE, Baloch ZW. Utility of onsite evaluation of endobronchial ultrasound-guided transbronchial needle aspiration specimens. *Cytojournal*. 2011;8:20.

11. Thomas SV, Lagana A, Dittmar KM, Wakely PE. Imprint cytopathology of core needle biopsies: a "first responder" role for cytotechnologists. *J Am Soc Cytopathol*. 2015;4:16-24.

12. Aviram G, Greif J, Man A, et al. Diagnosis of intrathoracic lesions: are sequential fine-needle aspiration (FNA) and core needle biopsy (CNB) combined better than either investigation alone? *Clin Radiol*. 2007;62:221-226.

13. Green RS, Matthew S. The contribution of cytologic imprints of stereotactically guided core needle biopsies of the breast in the management of patients with mammographic abnormalities. *Breast J*. 2001;7:214-218.

14. Gong Y, Sneige N, Guo M, Hicks ME, Moran CA. Transthoracic fine-needle aspiration vs concurrent core needle biopsy in diagnosis of intrathoracic lesions. *Am J Clin Pathol*. 2006;125:438-444.

15. Kubik MJ, Mohammadi A, Rosa M. Diagnostic benefits and cost-effectiveness of onsite imprint cytology adequacy evaluation of core needle biopsies of bone lesions. *Diagn Cytopathol*. 2014;42:506-513.

16. Azabdaftari G, Goldberg SN, Wang HH. Efficacy of onsite specimen adequacy evaluation of image-guided fine and core needle biopsies. *Acta Cytol*. 2010;54:132-137.

17. Liao WY, Jerng JS, Chen KY, Chang YL, Yang PC, Kuo SH. Value of imprint cytology for ultrasound-guided transthoracic core biopsy. *Eur Respir J*. 2004;24:905-909.

18. Paulose RR, Shee CD, Abdelhadi IA, Khan MK. Accuracy of touch imprint cytology in diagnosing lung cancer. *Cytopathology*. 2004;15:109-112.

19. Li Z, Tonkovich D, Shen R. Impact of touch imprint cytology on imaging-guided core needle biopsies: an experience from a large academic medical center laboratory. *Diagn Cytopathol*. 2016;44:87-90.

20. Chang YC, Yu CJ, Lee WJ, et al. Imprint cytology improves accuracy of computed tomography-guided percutaneous transthoracic needle biopsy. *Eur Respir J*. 2008;31:54-61.

21. Aihara T, Munakata S, Morino H, Takatsuka Y. Touch imprint cytology and immunohistochemistry for the assessment of sentinel lymph nodes in patients with breast cancer. *EJSO*. 2003;29: 845-848.

22. Moore JG, To V, Patel SJ, Sneige N. Her2/neu gene amplification in breast imprint cytology analyzed by fluorescence in situ hybridization: direct comparison with companion tissue sections. *Diagn Cytopathol*. 2000;23:299-302.

23. Gong X, Lu X, Wu X, et al. Role of bone marrow imprints in haematological diagnosis: a detailed study of 3781 cases. *Cytopathology*. 2012;23:86-95.

24. Amemiya K, Hirotsu Y, Goto T, et al. Touch imprint cytology with massively parallel sequencing (TIC-seq): a simple and rapid method to snapshot genetic alterations in tumors. *Cancer Med*. 2016;5:3426-3436.

25. Dogan S, Becker JC, Rekhtman N, et al. Use of touch imprint cytology as a simple method to enrich tumor cells for molecular analysis. Cancer Cytopathol. 2013;121:354-360.

26. Rekhtman N, Roy-Chowdhuri S. Cytology specimens: a goldmine for molecular testing. *Arch Pathol Lab Med*. 2016;140:1189-1190.

27. Mannweiler S, Pummer K, Auprich M, et al. Diagnostic yield of touch imprint cytology of prostate core needle biopsies. Pathol Oncol Res. 2009;15:97-101.

28. Rekhtman N, Kazi S, Yao J, et al. Depletion of core needle biopsy cellularity and DNA content as a result of vigorous touch preparations. *Arch Pathol Lab Med*. 2015;139:907-912.

CHAPTER 2

Preparation Techniques

Liron Pantanowitz

INTRODUCTION

The goal of touch/imprint cytology is to produce an impression of cells shed from tissue on a glass slide that displays correlative cytomorphology, and possibly architecture, to the corresponding tissue while still preserving individual cell cytology and without introducing artifacts. Different techniques are available whereby tissue can be touched to a glass slide or the slide is brought into contact with the tissue. These different cytologic preparations were defined in Chapter 1 (Table 1.1). Various preparations may be better suited for different scenarios and specimen types. Direct smears, for example, are best made when dealing with fine needle aspiration (FNA) samples. Touch preparations (TPs) are ideal to perform with a core needle biopsy (CNB), and imprints are best for intraoperative evaluation of large resected specimens. Sometimes these methods can be combined. For example, an initial imprint can subsequently be smeared, especially if all or a portion of the material on the slide is very thick. Also, a smear can be prepared from a TP where there is an accompanying cystic component. Cytoscrape preparations combine scraping tissue and subsequently making smears with the collected cellular material.

TPs and imprints will yield helpful slides for evaluation if performed on very cellular, nonsclerotic lesions that have many discohesive cells present, such as lymph nodes. Gently touching lymphoid tissue to a glass slide will easily yield diagnostic cells. However, with fibrotic tissues and/or cohesive lesions the cells remain more tightly bound to their stroma. A lesion that refuses to yield a cellular TP is still informative, indicating that this may be a sclerotic or desmoplastic process. Different slide preparation techniques each have their pros and cons. TPs are very helpful when trying to evaluate specimens that may be too small to scrape or smear. Smears tend to produce slides with more single cells and widely scattered small cell clusters whereas touch or imprint slides usually contain larger and more cohesive cell groups, therefore revealing more architectural detail (1). Unfortunately, handling delicate specimens and transferring cellular material on to a glass slide by touch or imprint preparation may damage core biopsies

and possibly result in fewer cells to examine on the permanent sections, cause cellular artifacts like streaking, and even mask the typical cytomorphologic features seen with FNA smears. Therefore, care when performing these techniques is paramount to yield optimal diagnostic slides while minimizing artifacts.

In a survey sent to laboratories participating in the College of American Pathologists (CAP) nongynecologic cytology education program, respondents indicated that the preparation of touch imprints was performed by pathologists, cytotechnologists, and less often by laboratory aides (2). Intraoperative imprints can be expected to also be prepared by noncytologists including surgical pathologists, pathology residents and trainees, as well as pathology assistants. In general, surgical pathologists are more likely to be comfortable with preparing and interpreting touch imprints than smears. According to the aforementioned CAP survey, techniques used to prepare a TP included touching the CNB on the slide, rolling the CNB on a slide, and rarely a crush preparation. The most common stain used with TPs by these laboratories was a modified Romanowsky stain (Diff-Quik [DQ]) on air-dried slides (2).

TPs of CNBs are increasingly being used for rapid onsite evaluation (ROSE). The questions asked during ROSE when evaluating TPs are similar to those with FNA, which are to determine specimen adequacy, render an immediate diagnosis, and consequently triage material for ancillary studies. A definitive cytologic diagnosis is not usually the goal of ROSE, but is necessary for an intraoperative consultation. It is feasible to remotely interpret TPs via telepathology (3). A true positive TP of a CNB onsite signifies that adequate cellular material is retrieved, which may obviate the need for unnecessary extra passes. At some institutions a CNB is often received along with an FNA. While laboratories may opt to separate their CNB and cytology material (TP and/or FNA), it is probably best to keep them together and issue a combined report that includes the immediate evaluation interpretation. Moreover, given that either the touch prep or CNB may lack diagnostic cells, an independent report of these preparations may lead to a discrepant diagnosis in a subset of cases (4).

SLIDE PREPARATION

Touch Preparation

A TP refers to a cytology slide prepared by touching a small tissue biopsy (e.g., image-guided CNB) on to a glass slide and at times moving or dragging the tissue along the surface of the slide. This can be performed using the "Drag," "Roll," or "Touch and Pick" method (Figures 2.1 and 2.2) (5). With the "Drag" method the piece of tissue or core is placed on a glass slide and gently dragged along the surface of the slide (Figure 2.3). Similarly, the specimen can be pushed along the glass slide for a short distance. With the core roll preparation (CRP) a tissue core is lightly rolled on a glass slide. A solid, firm core (e.g., bone biopsy) is easy to roll (Figure 2.4). However, for a soft core the tissue can be stabilized and protected by sticking it to a plastic needle cover and then rolling it gently on the slide (Figure 2.5). In a study that evaluated 25 CNB (20-gauge) neoplastic pulmonary specimens prepared with the CRP, investigators found that this technique did not alter the histopathology of any of the cases (6). However, 25% of their cases did show poor cell morphology compared with FNA smears. With the "Touch and Pick" method the tissue/core is gently touched on to the surface of a clean glass slide and then picked up again without dragging it (Figure 2.6). This can be repeated multiple times. However, for most cases touching the core only once or twice should suffice. The tissue/core will adhere to the slide, and can be lifted from the slide using a needle or plastic stick, but ideally not forceps, which can crush cells, except when dealing with larger pieces of tissue (Figures 2.7 and 2.8). In some situations, if tissue fragments or a CNB are received stuck to a nonadherent pad/cloth then a slide can be gently pressed against the specimen without having to remove and damage it (Figure 2.9). It is best to prepare a touch imprint along the short axis of a slide, which creates less drag and tumor shedding on the slide (2). Minimal tissue manipulation is desirable, especially if a core is thin and friable. For delicate cores that may easily fragment the touch and pick method is probably best. To avoid damaging a tissue core it can be kept within the well of the biopsy needle while pressing it to the slide. Depending on the type of needle used, however, if the walls of the needle prevent good contact between the CNB and slide surface, an adequate TP will not be obtained. Also, this should only be performed if the needle does not need to remain sterile for re-use. If another CNB will be performed, some proceduralists prefer to keep the needle sterile and avoid touching the slide, in order to use the same needle for another pass, as opposed to opening a new needle and incurring extra cost.

Imprint

An imprint refers to a cytology slide prepared by pressing a glass slide on to a large tissue specimen or resected organ

that is freshly cut for evaluation (Figures 2.10 and 2.11). This is typically performed at the time of frozen section of a large tumor resection. However, it can be performed with any tissue or organ including those at the grossing bench or during autopsy. An imprint should be obtained before the specimen is fixed. The surface of freshly cut tissue must be well exposed. Excess blood should be dabbed as this will reduce the surface tension with the slide surface and diminish cell transfer (Figure 2.12). A clean, dry glass slide should be gently and evenly pressed against the tissue surface only for a few seconds to obtain an imprint. Too much pressure can damage cells and lateral movement will cause cell streaking. Alternatively, for smaller specimens tissue can be touched to the slide instead of the slide being brought into contact with the specimen (Figure 2.9).

Cytoscrape

A cytoscrape refers to a cytology slide prepared by combining scraping tissue and making smears. This has also been called the "scrimp" technique (7). To do this, the cut surface of a specimen is scraped with a scalpel blade or the edge of a glass slide. The scraped cellular material collected is then immediately smeared onto a clean glass slide and spread with a second slide held at right angles to the first. The cytoscrape may produce a more concentrated cellular sample than an imprint due to forceful disruption of lesional tissue (Figure 2.13). This technique is good for fibrotic tumors that are unlikely to yield many cells by imprint.

Imprint cytology has been used to evaluate skin lesions such as ulcers and neoplasms (8,9). The Tzanck test (or Tzanck smear) is used to evaluate skin vesicles. This involves scraping a cutaneous ulcer base to look for Tzanck cells. These are large hyperchromatic epithelial cells found within vesicles formed as a result of acantholysis in the epithelium. They may be seen with herpes infection (Herpes simplex virus or Varicella). To perform this procedure a vesicle needs to be unroofed, the base scraped with a sterile scalpel blade, and cells smeared onto a clean glass slide. A slit skin smear is also valuable in the management of patients with leprosy. These smears can be used to estimate the number of acid-fast bacteria present (i.e., Bacterial Index), determine the type and severity of disease, as well as assess response to therapy.

Crush (Squash) Preparation

With the crush or squash preparation tissue is crushed between two glass slides. This technique is applied mostly for the intraoperative diagnosis of central nervous system (CNS) tumors (10,11). This topic is covered in great detail in Chapter 11. To make a "brain smear" one or more small (1–2 mm) representative pieces of tissue should be placed at one end of a clean, labeled glass slide (Figure 2.14). A second glass slide is then used to lightly press down and rapidly smear the tissue along the slide. The two slides should be pulled apart in opposite directions while pressure is continuously applied. Too much pressure causes crush artifact, whereas too little pressure can cause thick smears that are hard to interpret. The prepared smear must be immediately inserted into fixative. For firm pieces of tissue that do not smear well, a brief period of air-drying (e.g., 1 minute) may help with tissue adhesion to the

slide. The remaining tissue not used should be returned to the vial and/or fixed to prevent it drying out. When only limited tissue is received with a stereotactic biopsy, crush preparations alone should be made, because frozen sections consume more tissue. Most CNS lesions are soft and hence amenable to this technique. However, crush smears may not be suitable for all lesions. With tissue that is too tough and rubbery (e.g., nerve sheath tumor, desmoplastic carcinoma, craniopharyngioma) a frozen section may be superior, unless the material is heavily calcified.

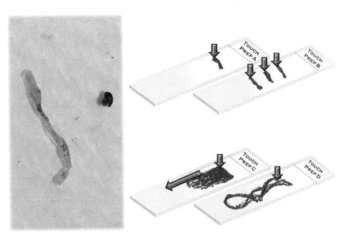

FIGURE 2.1 Optimal and suboptimal TP techniques. A TP of the tissue core shown on the left can be performed in several ways. The core can be touched on to the surface of a glass slide once (Touch Prep A), or it can be touched several times (Touch Prep B). It is best to touch the core along the short axis of the slide as shown in Touch Preps A and B. The core can also be touched and then dragged (smeared) along the slide (Touch Prep C). However, optimal TPs involve minimal core manipulation. Hence, dragging the tissue core all over the slide (Touch Prep D) is discouraged. TP, touch preparation.

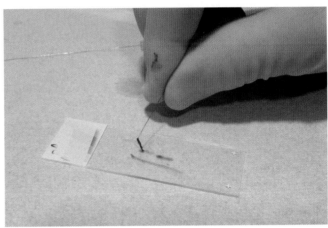

FIGURE 2.3 "Drag" preparation method. The core biopsy shown is being gently dragged along the surface of the slide.

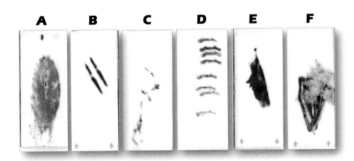

FIGURE 2.2 Different cytology slide preparations. FNA smear (A). TP of a CNB performed twice (B). TP of a CNB performed twice combined with dragging the core (C). TP of a CNB performed multiple times (D). TP combined with evenly smearing the core along the slide (E). Vigorous TP dragging and smearing the core all over the slide (F). All slides were DQ-stained. CNB, core needle biopsy; DQ, Diff-Quik; FNA, fine needle aspiration; TP, touch preparation.

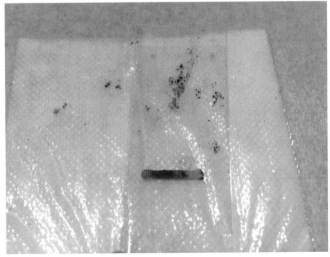

FIGURE 2.4 "Roll" preparation method. This firm core biopsy of bone is shown being lightly rolled on a glass slide.

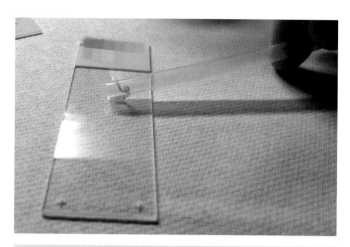

FIGURE 2.5 "Roll" preparation method. This soft tissue core is shown stuck to a plastic needle cover allowing it to be gently rolled on the slide.

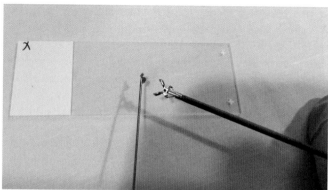

FIGURE 2.8 Tissue biopsy TP. This lung biopsy specimen was procured with a biopsy forceps, but transferred to a needle to gently touch it on to the surface of the slide and minimize crushing of delicate cells. TP, touch preparation.

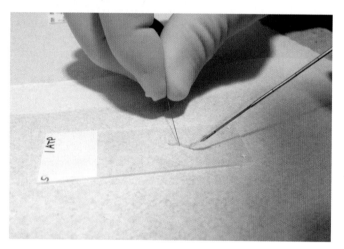

FIGURE 2.6 "Touch and Pick" preparation method. This tissue core is shown being gently touched on to the surface of a clean glass slide and then being picked up with a needle without dragging or smearing it.

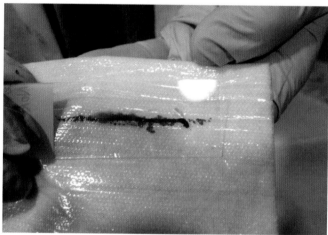

FIGURE 2.9 "Slide to Tissue" TP method. In the case shown a glass slide was gently pressed on to a bloody core biopsy that was received on a Telfa® pad. TP, touch preparation.

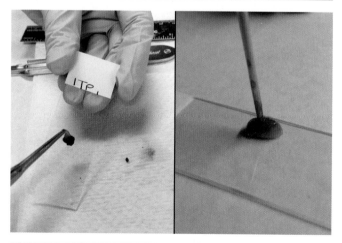

FIGURE 2.7 Tissue biopsy TP. In these examples tissue specimens that are larger than a core required a forceps to hold the sample in order to perform a TP. TP, touch preparation.

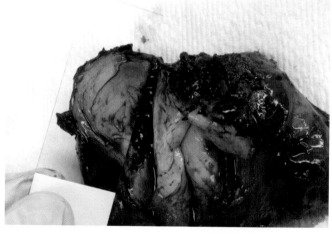

FIGURE 2.10 Imprint method. A clean glass slide is shown being gently pressed on to a freshly cut surface of this tan sarcoma to prepare an imprint of the tumor.

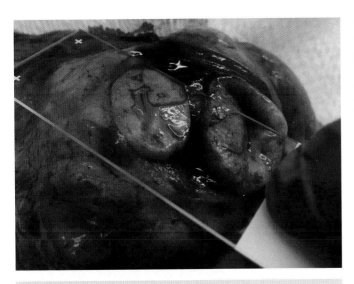

FIGURE 2.11 Imprint method. A clean glass slide is shown being gently pressed down on the cut surface of this metastatic sarcoma nodule in a lung resection.

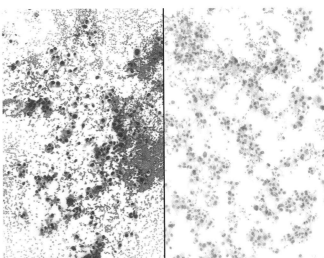

FIGURE 2.13 Comparison of TP and cytoscrape methods. The TP (left image) contains fewer tumor cells than the cytoscrape preparation (right image) performed on the same high-grade sarcoma. (Left: DQ-stained TP, low power; Right: Pap stained cytoscrape, low power.) DQ, Diff-Quik; TP, touch preparation.

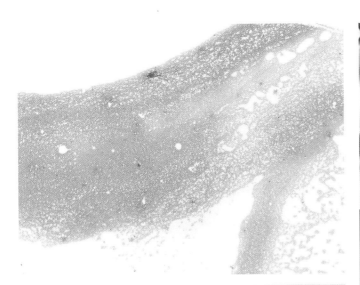

FIGURE 2.12 Blood dilution. The TP of lung tissue in this example is markedly hypocellular and consists predominantly of blood because excess blood was not soaked up before the tissue touched the slide's glass surface (DQ-stained TP, low power). DQ, Diff-Quik; TP, touch preparation.

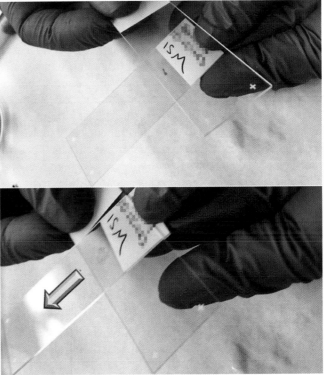

FIGURE 2.14 Crush technique. This intraoperative preparation shows (top) small pieces of brain tissue placed very close at one edge of a clean glass slide. A second glass slide (bottom) is then used to press down and firmly crush the tissue while very quickly and evenly smearing the material in the direction (arrow) depicted, away from the frosted labeled edge of the slide.

FIXATION AND STAINING

Prepared slides can be either air-dried or wet fixed. Wet fixation involves immediate immersion of the slide in 95% ethyl alcohol (ethanol). This is a dehydrating agent that causes cell shrinkage as it replaces water. Rapid fixation of slides is necessary in order to preserve cytologic details. Hence, the jar containing fixative solution should be placed near the area where slides are being made. Fixation determines what stains will be used. A Romanowsky stain such as Wright's stain, May-Grunwald-Giemsa stain (MGG), or DQ stain is based on air-drying fixation. The DQ stain is ideal for ROSE because it can be performed rapidly and only needs three solutions. Papanicolaou (Pap) and hematoxylin and eosin (H&E) stains are based on wet fixation. Unfixed, air-dried slides can be used for Pap staining but they require rehydration. Fixation and staining procedures for intraoperative use is covered in Chapter 3 Fixation and Staining Methods.

PROBLEMS AND PITFALLS

Loss of Material

Friable tissue cores, such as those taken from predominantly necrotic or inflammatory lesions, may fragment easily if overly manipulated. Small fragments can get lost with processing. Mucinous or necrotic tissue is sometimes very sticky, making it difficult to remove some or all of the tissue from the slide after a TP. This can result in lack of tissue available for permanent cell block processing. In such cases, the use of a concurrent FNA or omission of a TP may be helpful. It is also best to perform TPs with uncoated slides, because coated slides may further cause tissue to stick to the slide. Excess adherence of tissue to a slide may deplete the tissue of cells (Figures 2.15 and 2.16). If all the lesional cells get transferred onto the glass slide from a CNB, the specimen may be interpreted as being adequate onsite but result in a suboptimal histological specimen that is also inadequate for ancillary studies (12). In a study that evaluated 38 cases of lung adenocarcinoma that were subject to onsite evaluation of core biopsies, researchers revealed that 11% of these cases had an inadequate core while the TPs had adequate tumor cells (13). In another study of 1,100 CNBs associated with TPs, Tong et al found a marked difference in cellularity between the cores and TPs in 84 (8%) of their cases (4). Four (4.3%) of these cases

had diagnostic cells in either the CNB or touch prep, but not in both. In this particular study, lung was the site that was most affected by such loss of diagnostic cells. In an *ex vivo* experiment, Rekhtman et al showed that there can be a marked decrease in DNA content from CNBs that underwent vigorous TPs compared to those that were subject to a single less disruptive imprint (14). They documented a 25% decrease in DNA content with an even larger loss when cores were dragged along the length of the slide. Hence, when preparing slides it is important to avoid excessively forceful touch or imprint preparations. For this reason, CNB specimens should not be dragged for >1 cm along a slide. Procuring additional samples including concomitant FNA may be required in order to ensure there is sufficient lesional cellularity for ancillary studies. It remains to be tested whether touching cells on slides damages their cell surface such that it could impact certain biomarker (e.g., Her2/neu immunohistochemistry) testing.

Artifacts

TPs and imprints may result in artifacts that are slightly different to FNA and histological sections. Smearing or rubbing tissue on a slide can result in streaking artifacts of cells (Figures 2.17–2.19), in addition to crushing of cells or stripping them of their cytoplasm leaving behind only bare nuclei. For ultrasound-guided biopsies, excess ultrasound gel can contaminate samples and obscure material on slides (Figures 2.20 and 2.21). If tissue surfaces are not well exposed during intraoperative imprint preparations, ink used for margin evaluation may stick to the slide and thereby obscure cells (Figure 2.22). Aggressive TPs can cause too many cells and/or large fragments of tissue to stick to the slide. This not only results in loss of valuable tissue for ancillary studies, but frequently these fragments are too thick to properly evaluate (Figure 2.23). If fragments of bone break off and stick to the slide they may impede coverslipping of slides (Figure 2.24). TPs and imprint slides dry quickly when exposed to air. Such air-drying artifact may impact their interpretation (Figure 2.25). For example, air-drying artifact can sometimes cause cells to appear overly enlarged and atypical. Therefore, multiple imprints should not be made if the slides are intended for wet fixation. One approach to minimizing air-drying artifact that has been recommended is to hydrate the slide with a few drops of normal saline for a few minutes (15).

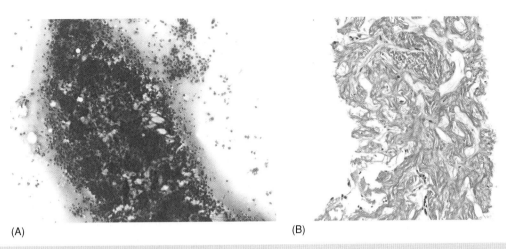

(A)   (B)

FIGURE 2.15   TP-related tissue depletion. The TP of the CNB from this intrahepatic cholangiocarcinoma shows abundant tumor cells (A). The corresponding histopathology section of this CNB is depleted of tumor cells and shows only residual fibrous stroma (B). ((A) DQ-stained TP, low power; (B) H&E-stained tissue core, medium power.) CNB, core needle biopsy; DQ, Diff-Quik; TP, touch preparation.

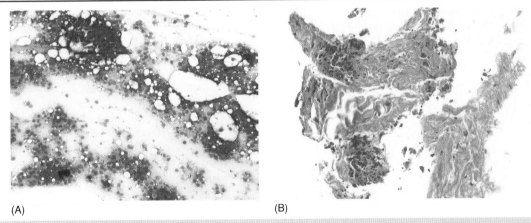

(A)   (B)

FIGURE 2.16   TP-related tissue depletion. The TP from a friable lymph node biopsy with metastatic melanoma shows abundant tumor cells (A). The corresponding histopathology section shows a fragmented biopsy associated with robust tissue manipulation and processing, and only residual fibrous stroma with melanosis that is lacking tumor cells to perform molecular testing (B). ((A) DQ-stained TP, medium power; (B) H&E-stained tissue core, medium power.) DQ, Diff-Quik; H&E, hematoxylin and eosin; TP, touch preparation.

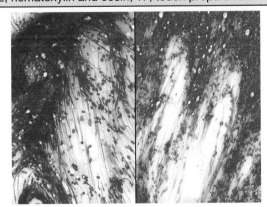

FIGURE 2.17   Streaking artifact. These TPs show marked streaking artifact of cells caused by forceful dragging of a core biopsy on the slide. The (left) specimen with non-Hodgkin lymphoma is difficult to differentiate from (right) the small cell carcinoma based on the cytomorphology of these TPs. (Right and Left: DQ-stained TPs, low power.) DQ, Diff-Quik; TP, touch preparation.

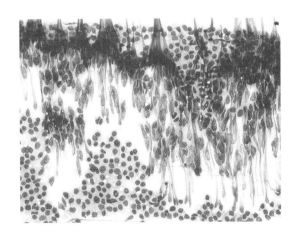

FIGURE 2.18   Streaking artifact. The TP of a diffuse large B-cell lymphoma shows several smudged cells caused by dragging of the CNB on the slide (DQ-stained TP, medium power). CNB, core needle biopsy; DQ, Diff-Quik; TP, touch preparation.

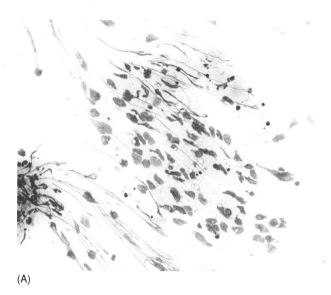

(A)

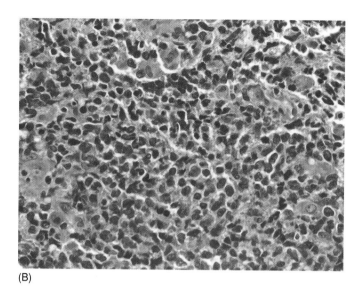

(B)

FIGURE 2.19 Streaking artifact. The TP of this non-Hodgkin lymphoma was incorrectly interpreted during immediate onsite evaluation as a spindle cell neoplasm (A). The stretched appearance of the lymphoma cells differ from the corresponding histopathology showing more round tumor cells (B). ((A) DQ-stained TP, medium power; (B) H&E-stained tissue core, medium power.) DQ, Diff-Quik; H&E, hematoxylin and eosin; TP, touch preparation.

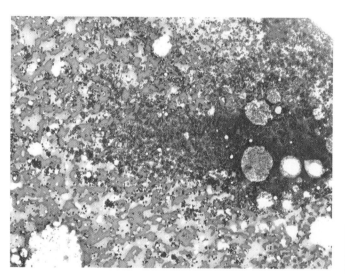

FIGURE 2.20 Ultrasound gel contamination. The presence of gel in this TP is shown as pink granular, amorphous material (DQ-stained TP, low power). DQ, Diff-Quik; TP, touch preparation.

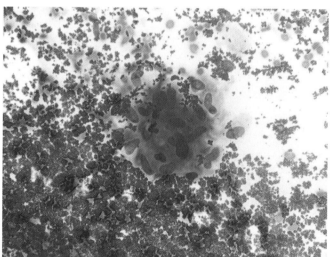

FIGURE 2.21 Ultrasound gel contamination. Excess gel in this case of granulomatous lymphadenitis can obscure diagnostic cellular material (DQ-stained TP, high power). DQ, Diff-Quik; TP, touch preparation.

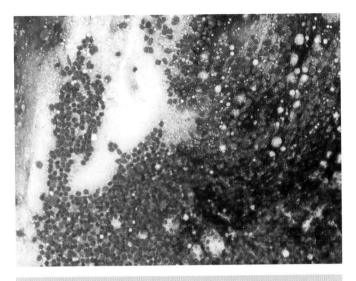

FIGURE 2.22 Specimen ink contamination. This intraoperative imprint preparation of a nodal lymphoma contains orange ink that was applied to the specimen surface (DQ-stained TP, low power). DQ, Diff-Quik; TP, touch preparation.

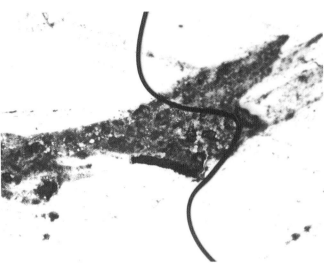

FIGURE 2.24 Bone TP. This TP of a bone biopsy resulted in several mineralized tissue fragments sticking to the slide. As a result, the coverslip was lifted up causing an air bubble to form (DQ-stained TP, low power). DQ, Diff-Quik; TP, touch preparation.

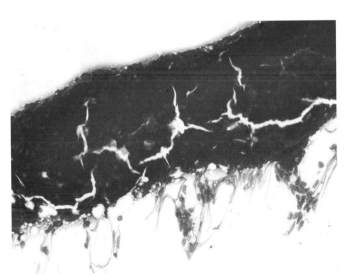

FIGURE 2.23 Thick TP. This TP of a lymphoma is too thick to reliably evaluate the cytomorphology (DQ-stained TP, low power). DQ, Diff-Quik; TP, touch preparation.

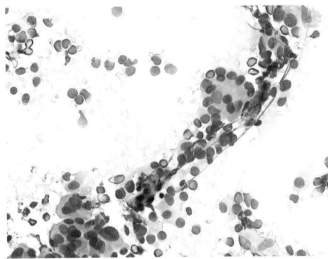

FIGURE 2.25 Air-drying artifact. Thyroid follicular cells showing faux nuclear inclusions due to air drying artifact (Pap-stained preparation, high power).

REFERENCES

1. Hahn PF, Eisenberg PJ, Pitman MB, Gazelle GS, Mueller PR. Cytopathologic touch preparations (imprints) from core needle biopsies: accuracy compared with that of fine-needle aspirates. *AJR Am J Roentgenol.* 1995;165:1277-1279.

2. Padmanabhan V, Barkan GA, Nayar R. Assessing needle core biopsy adequacy—survey of practices. *CAP Today.* 2016. http://www.captodayonline.com/assessing-needle-core-biopsy-adequacy-survey-practices-516/

3. Thrall MJ, Rivera AL, Takei H, Powell SZ. Validation of a novel robotic telepathology platform for neuropathology intraoperative touch preparations. *J Pathol Inform.* 2014;5:21.

4. Tong LC, Rudomina D, Rekhtman N, Lin O. Impact of touch preparations on core needle biopsies. *Cancer Cytopathol.* 2014;122:851-854.

5. Jacobson BC, Dubinchik IV, Swan N. A method of assessing the adequacy of trucut biopsy specimens obtained with a 19-gauge trucut core biopsy needle. *Acta Cytol.* 2006;50:141-146.

6. Chandan VS, Zimmerman K, Baker P, Scalzetti E, Khurana KK. Usefulness of core roll preparations in immediate assessment of neoplastic lung lesions: comparison to conventional CT scan-guided lung fine-needle aspiration cytology. *Chest.* 2004;126:739-743.

7. Abrahams C. The "Scrimp" technique—a method for the rapid diagnosis of surgical pathology specimens. *Histopathology.* 1978;2:255-266.

8. Ramakrishnaiah VP, Babu R, Pai D, Verma SK. Role of imprint/exfoliative cytology in ulcerated skin neoplasms. *Indian J Surg Oncol.* 2013;4:385-389.

9. Aryya NC, Khanna S, Shukla HS, Tripathi FM, Shukla VK. Role of rapid imprint cytology in the diagnosis of skin cancer and assessment of adequacy of excision. *Indian J Pathol Microbiol.* 1992;35:108-112.

10. Moss TH. Nicoll JAR, Ironside JW. *Intra-Operative Diagnosis of CNS Tumours.* London: Arnold; 1997:6-9.

11. Joseph JT. *Diagnostic Neuropathology Smears.* Philadelphia, PA: Lippincott Williams & Williams; 2007:7-11.

12. Tsou MH, Tsai SF, Chan KY, et al. CT-guided needle biopsy: value of onsite cytopathologic evaluation of core specimen touch preparations. *J Vasc Interv Radiol.* 2009;20:71-76.

13. Kurian EM, Ewing G. Frequency of discordance between touch preparations and corresponding lung core biopsies in patients with adenocarcinoma. *Modern Pathol.* 2014;27 (suppl 2):108A.

14. Rekhtman N, Kazi S, Yao J, et al. Depletion of core needle biopsy cellularity and DNA content as a result of vigorous touch preparations. *Arch Pathol Lab Med.* 2015;139:907-912.

15. Saqi A, Crapanzano JP. Optimization and triage of small specimens. In: Moreira AL, Saqi A, eds. *Diagnosing Non-Small Cell Carcinoma in Small Biopsy and Cytology.* New York, NY: Springer; 2015:61-76.

CHAPTER 3

Intraoperative Cytology

Liron Pantanowitz and Juan Xing

INTRODUCTION

Frozen sections are commonly used to render intraoperative pathology diagnoses. Touch imprints offer a more simple, cheaper, rapid, and reliable diagnostic alternative to frozen sections in order to accurately guide surgical management of the patient. The use of imprint cytology with fresh specimens was first reported by Dudgeon and Patrick in 1927 (1). It has since been shown that imprints may be equivalent to frozen section examination for several intraoperative situations, and increases the diagnostic accuracy when used as an adjunct with frozen section, without introducing much additional work (2–6). An intraoperative cytology touch preparation can often be rapidly performed and interpreted before a frozen section is even prepared. In a large comparative study of 2,250 intraoperative cytologies performed together with frozen sections, the diagnostic accuracy rate (99.2%) was significantly higher when both procedures were performed than when frozen sections were prepared alone (7).

Compared to frozen sections, imprint cytology has several advantages. These include (8):

- imprints can be performed rapidly
- slides can be prepared without special equipment
- they produce better nuclear details without frozen artifacts
- tissue is conserved for ancillary studies, especially when material is limited
- allows specimens to be easily sampled in multiple areas
- facilitates rapid triage of multiple specimens

Imprints can also provide valuable information when a frozen section cannot be easily performed (e.g., bone or fatty tissue), or when a frozen section interpretation is equivocal. Imprints may also limit contaminating the cryostat and lower the risk of staff exposure to infectious agents (9). Saving extra imprints allows interesting cases to be archived in cytology slide teaching sets.

Currently, intraoperative imprint cytology is underused, most probably due to the relative lack of experience with this technique among pathologists. The focus of this chapter is to highlight instances where intraoperative touch imprints are likely to be helpful.

IMPRINT TECHNIQUE

Prior to performing an imprint, careful gross examination of the specimen is required to help select the most appropriate areas for sampling. Solid tissue areas are suitable whereas necrotic, hemorrhagic, and cystic areas should ideally be avoided. If no gross lesion is identified, touch imprints can be obtained from different areas to increase the negative predictive value. Lymph nodes, for example, will need to be regularly sectioned and entirely sampled when looking for metastasis without an obviously visible lesion.

A touch imprint should be performed before the specimen is fixed. The freshly cut specimen surface must be well exposed. Blotting the surface gently will absorb excess blood that may dilute the cytology preparation and obscure cells. A clean, dry glass slide should then be gently and evenly pressed against the tissue surface (Figure 3.1) quickly (e.g., 2 seconds) to obtain an imprint. Tissue can either be touched to the slide or the slide can be brought into contact with the specimen. The aim is to get intact lesional cells to stick to the glass slide. Too much pressure or lateral movement may damage cells. Scraping the surface with a scapel blade (e.g., cytoscrape) of the same specimen can be performed to prepare a complementary direct smear for interpretation. As fibrotic tumors are unlikely to yield too many cells on an imprint, a scrape smear may be more helpful (10). Touch preps need to be performed in close proximity to a fixative jar, because air-drying artifact can occur quickly. For this reason it is best to prepare imprints one at time and immediately immerse them in fixative, rather than collecting multiple touch prep slides and later batch fixing all of them.

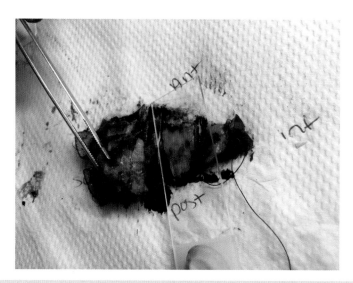

FIGURE 3.1 Imprint preparation technique. A dry glass slide is shown evenly pressed against the cut tissue surface of this subcutaneous dermatofibrosarcoma protuberans tumor to obtain a cytology imprint.

FIXATION AND STAINING METHODS

Fixation and staining techniques are critical in order to achieve the best cellular details using imprint cytology (11). Wet-fixation and air-drying are two fundamentally different methods for routine fixation. Romanowsky-type stains such as Wight's, May-Grunwald-Giemsa, and Diff-Quik (DQ) stains are based on air-dried specimens, while the Papanicolaou (Pap) and hematoxylin and eosin (H&E) stains are based on wet-fixed slides. DQ and rapid H&E stains are used more often than the rapid Pap stain during intraoperative consultations. Table 3.1 compares these three commonly used staining methods. Toluidine blue stain may also be used (Figure 3.2). This requires only one drop of stain, which can be subsequently destained and later restained with another method if needed.

Rapid H&E Stain

The protocol for a rapid H&E stain is shown in Table 3.2. H&E is common to surgical pathologists. The H&E stain is easiest to correlate cytomorphology with corresponding H&E-stained frozen tissue sections. After a direct imprint is immediately fixed in 95% ethyl alcohol for a few seconds, the slide can then be stained. The stain procedure is rapid to perform and should not delay an intraoperative evaluation. Stained slides need a coverslip prior to microscopic review.

DQ Stain

The DQ stain, a Romanowsky stain variant, can be used intraoperatively. The DQ stain is commonly used by cytopathologists. Commercial staining kits such as the PROTO-COL™ Hema 3™ Stain set (Fisher Diagnostics) are available (Figure 3.3). The DQ stain is quick and easy to perform. It often provides better cytoplasmic details than the H&E stain and highlights extracellular matrix. Table 3.3 provides the protocol of a DQ stain. Imprint slides should be air-dried and then stained. This stain procedure can be completed in 2 to 3 minutes. A DQ-stained slide can be interpreted unmounted. After the stained slide is completely dried, a coverslip can be added to preserve the slide. Alternatively, thick material could be scraped from a DQ-stained slide to enhance a cell block. This can be helpful in limited specimens, particularly since the scant material will retain the dark color of the stain and be easily visualized during processing of the specimen. The drawback is that the cells can be distorted when forcefully scraped from the slide, limiting the morphological evaluation.

Rapid Pap Stain

The rapid Pap stain is the least commonly used method for intraoperative diagnosis. Compared to the DQ stain, it takes longer. This stain provides better nuclear details, but may not produce a distinct background. Wet fixation of the slide is required. Refer to Table 3.4 for the stepwise procedure of performing a rapid Pap stain.

TABLE 3.1 Commonly Used Rapid Staining Methods

	Rapid H&E	DQ	Pap
Cell size	Smaller or similar to histologic specimens	Increased	Same as H&E
Nucleus	Crisp	Fair	Crisp
Nucleolus	Distinct	Visible	Distinct
Cytoplasm	Similar to histologic specimens	Excellent	Transparent, highlights keratin
Extracellular matrix	Poor	Excellent	Poor
Artifacts	Air-drying	Incomplete drying	Air-drying
Particular value	Most familiar to general pathologists	Hematolymphoid samples	Squamous cell carcinoma

DQ, Diff-Quik; H&E, hematoxylin and eosin; Pap, Papanicolaou.

TABLE 3.2 Rapid H&E Stain Procedure

Steps	Solution/Procedure	Time
1	95% alcohol	10 sec
2	Tap water	Rinse
3	Hematoxylin	1 min
4	Tap water	Rinse
5	Eosin Y	15 sec
6	95% alcohol	10 dips
7	100% alcohol	10 dips
8	Coverslip	

H&E, hematoxylin and eosin.

TABLE 3.3 DQ Stain Procedure

Steps	Solution/Procedure	Time
1	Dip slide in fixative solution	10 times
2	Allow excess to drain	
3	Dip slide into DQ Solution I	10 times
4	Allow excess to drain	
5	Dip slide into DQ Solution II	30 times
6	Allow excess to drain	
7	Rinse slide with water	

Note: Solution I contains xanthine dye. Solution II contains thiazine dye mixture.
DQ, Diff-Quik.

TABLE 3.4 Rapid Pap Stain Procedure

Steps	Solution/Procedure	Time
1	Tap water	Until clear
2	Hematoxylin	45 sec
3	Tap water	Rinse
4	Eosin 50	45 sec
5	95% alcohol	10 dips
6	100% alcohol	10 dips
7	Xylene	20 dips
8	Mount	

Pap, Papanicolaou.

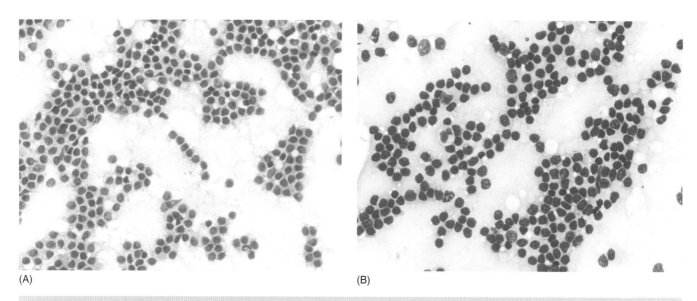

(A)   (B)

FIGURE 3.2 Nodal T-cell non-Hodgkin lymphoma. TPs show a monotonous population of abnormal lymphocytes. Lymphocyte nuclei are stained dark blue and their cytoplasm light blue with (A) Toluidine blue and (B) DQ stains. ((A) and (B) both medium power.) DQ, Diff-Quik; TP, touch preparation.

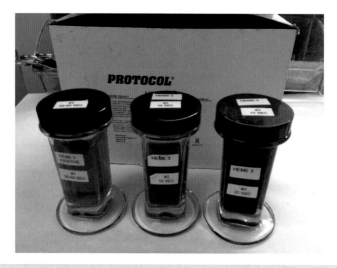

FIGURE 3.3 PROTOCOL™ Hema 3™ staining kit. Within 30 sec, this three-step staining procedure can be used to prepare an intraoperative cytology imprint.

SUITABLE SAMPLES

Hematolymphoid Specimens

Intraoperative imprint cytology is extremely helpful for the rapid examination of hematolymphoid specimens (e.g., lymph nodes, spleen), and other samples suspected of being involved by a lymphoproliferative lesion, leukemia, or plasma cell neoplasm (12,13). They permit accurate diagnoses and help triage samples for subsequent ancillary testing such as flow cytometry. DQ-stained imprints are preferred by hematopathologists. Preparing up to three unstained touch imprints is advisable for possible fluorescence in situ hybridization (FISH) studies.

Small Round Blue Cell Tumors

Small round blue cell tumors include small cell carcinoma, lymphoma, Ewing sarcoma/primitive neuroectodermal tumor (PNET), desmoplastic round cell tumor, embryonal rhabdomyosarcoma, small cell variant of various malignancies (e.g., osteosarcoma small cell variant), and blastomas of different organs (e.g., neuroblastoma (Figure 3.4), blastemal Wilms tumor, hepatoblastoma, medulloblastoma). Accurate intraoperative diagnosis of this group of tumors is critical because their management differs substantially. These tumors yield good touch preparations, which are reliable to rapidly render an intraoperative diagnosis and appropriately triage material for ancillary studies. On frozen section, these neoplastic cells can have significant crush and frozen tissue artifact, making them difficult to distinguish from lymphocytes. In addition, important morphological clues present in DQ-stained aspirates and touch imprints, such as lymphoglandular bodies, are lacking in frozen section slides of lymphoid lesions.

Bone Tissue

Intraoperative consultation of bone tumors is typically requested to provide a diagnosis and/or determine resection margin status. Cytology preparations can be helpful for these purposes (14–16). Well-mineralized fresh bone tissue, especially margins, may be too hard to perform a frozen section. In these cases, an imprint can either be made from the resection margin directly (Figure 3.5) or using bone fragments scraped from the surgical margin (Figure 3.6). In one study conducted on 52 patients with bone tumors/tumor-like conditions, although frozen section had better diagnostic sensitivity (88.2% for frozen section vs. 76.5% for imprint), it had less specificity than imprints (95% for frozen section vs. 100% for imprint) (17). Subtyping sarcomas may nevertheless be difficult on imprints, especially if key features such as osteoid or chondroid differentiation are not present. In general, metastases (e.g., metastatic carcinoma (Figure 3.7), melanoma

(Figure 3.8), plasmacytoma) easily yield adequate material to make a diagnosis using a touch preparation (18). Normal bone marrow elements (e.g., immature blood cells, megakaryocytes) are an expected finding (Figure 3.9), and should not be misdiagnosed as malignancy.

Small Biopsy Specimens

In the era of personalized medicine where ancillary studies such as molecular tests are important, preservation of adequate tissue is critical. Since intraoperative imprint cytology only requires a few lesional cells to make a diagnosis, when small specimens (e.g., core biopsy) are received, after performing a touch preparation, the entire tissue sample can be saved. Frozen section examination need only be performed in such cases if the imprint cannot reliably be used to render a definitive diagnosis. Touch preparations also work well for small specimens that are too small to easily scrape to produce a smear.

Sentinel Lymph Nodes

Performing touch imprints of lymph nodes to detect metastatic disease has been recommended by several authors due to the high accuracy rate of this cytologic technique (19,20). Touch imprint cytology appears to be particularly reliable for the intraoperative evaluation of sentinel lymph nodes in breast cancer patients (21–25). Imprints of sentinel nodes have similarly proven to be a reliable method for evaluation in skin melanoma patients (26,27). In one study involving breast cancer patients the sensitivity, specificity, and overall accuracy of imprint cytology for the diagnosis of sentinel node metastases were 84.6%, 96.6%, and 94.1%, respectively (28). In another related study, the positive predictive value was 100% and negative predictive value was 99% (29). Lobular breast carcinoma is often more difficult to identify in lymph nodes because these tumor cells tend to infiltrate in a single cell pattern, generally have lower grade nuclei, and morphologically may resemble sinus histiocytes or lymphoid cells. However, the sensitivity and specificity of intraoperative imprint cytology in evaluating lobular carcinoma has been shown to still be feasible and accurate (30).

Cytology imprints of sentinel nodes not only permit sampling without destroying tissue, but they are often easier to prepare when dealing with fatty lymph nodes. The major cause of false-negative imprints appears to be related to inadequate sampling (31). It is important to be aware that micrometastases (<2 mm) may not always be detected by imprints (32,33). Touch preparations should also not be used alone for the evaluation of sentinel nodes after neoadjuvant therapy (34). This may be related to the paucity of tumor cells, extensive fibrosis, lymphocyte depletion, and robust histiocytic infiltrate seen post-treatment. Combining touch imprint cytology with cytokeratin immunostaining of imprint slides has been shown by some investigators to improve the accuracy to diagnose nodal metastases (35–37). However, immunostained imprints can take up to 45 minutes to prepare. Performing immunohistochemistry on imprints has not been shown in all studies to significantly improve sensitivity (38) and would require a separate validation given that most laboratories validate immunostains on standard formalin-fixed paraffin-embedded tissue.

Touch preps of metastatic carcinoma are typically easy to recognize, even at low magnification, because carcinoma cells tend to cluster and thus stand out in a background of dyshesive lymphocytes (Figure 3.10). It is important not to over-interpret lymphohistiocytic aggregates as tumor clusters. Several carcinomas (e.g., lobular breast carcinoma) may present as isolated tumor cells. Other malignancies that may present with a dispersed pattern of plasmacytoid cells are neuroendocrine tumors, lymphoma, plasma cell neoplasia, and melanoma. Metastatic melanoma cells can vary from being polygonal to spindle shaped. Melanoma cells also usually have prominent nucleoli, can be binucleate, have intranuclear inclusions, and may be associated with melanin pigmentation. Melanin needs to be distinguished from hemosiderin (e.g., seen with dermatopathic lymphadenopathy) and exogenous pigments such as tattoo pigment, metallosis (e.g., seen with nearby metal joint prostheses), and graphite (e.g., seen with broken pencils on a slide).

Tumor Margins

Gross examination alone of surgical resection margins may not always be reliable. Utilizing frozen sections to examine extensive margins (e.g., an entire breast lumpectomy) is labor intensive, time consuming, and may destroy valuable tissue. A major advantage of imprint cytology is the ability to rapidly assess the entire surface of a tumor. If positive margins are detected with these touch imprints, a frozen section of this region can be undertaken for confirmation. Indeed, several studies have shown that intraoperative imprint cytology is accurate and reliable to evaluate surgical margins in breast lumpectomy specimens, squamous cell carcinoma of the oral cavity, partial nephrectomy specimens, biliary tract and pancreatic tumors, skin cancers, as well as bone tumors (39–47). Touch imprint cytology, however, is not recommended for the evaluation of all types of surgical margins such as with Mohs micrographic surgery (48), as well as lung bronchial resection margins (49). In bronchial resection margins, the presence of squamous metaplasia, radiation changes, submucosal glands, and peribronchial lymphocytes may all mimic carcinoma. Moreover, touch preparations appear to be of limited value when evaluating margins for invasive lobular carcinoma (50). The diagnostic accuracy of imprint cytology is unlikely to be

impacted by the mode of excision (i.e., by scalpel or electrocautery) (51). The limitation of performing imprints on surgical margins is that they cannot accurately estimate the distance of tumor from the surgical margin.

Neuropathology Samples

Intraoperative neuropathology consultation can be handled by frozen section and/or cytology techniques such as touch imprints, crush preparations, or scrapes (52–54). Neurosurgeons typically want to know if the brain lesion they biopsied is diagnostic of a neoplasm, infection, demyelination process, or some other condition. Central nervous system tissue has a high content of water and lipids causing marked freezing artifact, which hinders frozen section interpretation. Hence, employing cytology preparations for intraoperative diagnosis is often encouraged (55). Touch preps, however, are not helpful in all cases, particularly oligodendroglial lesions where the fried egg appearance that results with formalin fixation is missing and makes subclassification of these neoplasms difficult on touch imprint alone. They have also been shown to not be helpful in the diagnosis of hydatid cysts (56).

Breast Specimens

The role of imprint cytology for evaluating breast margins (section "Tumor Margins") and sentinel nodes (section "Sentinel Lymph Nodes") is discussed elsewhere in this chapter. Imprints have been recommended by several authors for the intraoperative evaluation of breast tumors (57–60). Excess fat may need to be trimmed away from breast lumps to avoid false-negative imprints. In these prior studies there were very few false-positive cases (<1%) and limited false-negative (around 5%) cases by the imprint method. However, it should be noted that it is often much easier to diagnose malignant tumors than benign breast tumors on imprint cytology. In addition, ductal carcinoma in situ (DCIS) is difficult to detect with touch preparation (61), as well as distinguish from invasive mammary carcinoma.

Thyroid Gland

Intraoperative consultation is most useful in cases previously diagnosed as suspicious for papillary carcinoma by fine needle aspiration (FNA) (62). Intraoperative imprint cytology can be of great value when evaluating such thyroid nodules (63–65). It is often easier to diagnose papillary thyroid carcinoma by cytomorphology than via frozen section (66). A correct intraoperative diagnosis of papillary thyroid carcinoma in this setting can allow a surgeon to perform a total thyroidectomy instead of just a lobectomy, eliminating the need for second surgery.

Imprint preparations of thyroid lesions resemble those seen on FNA. Colloid nodules show bland follicular cells and background colloid (Figure 3.11). Imprints of follicular neoplasms will have increased cellularity, predominantly microfollicles, bland to atypical follicular cells, and limited colloid. Hürthle cell change with nuclear enlargement and nucleoli may accompany lymphocytic thyroiditis. Imprint cytology cannot reliably diagnose follicular carcinoma or differentiate lymphocytic thyroiditis from low-grade lymphoma (67,68). Useful cytological features to establish a diagnosis of papillary thyroid carcinoma include papillae, overlapping enlarged and elongated nuclei, nuclear grooves, intranuclear cytoplasmic inclusions (Figure 3.12), powdery (open) chromatin, and peripherally located nucleoli. Nuclear grooves and pseudoinclusions are not usually evident on frozen sections. Nuclear grooves can occasionally be seen in other thyroid neoplasms such as hyalinizing trabecular tumor. Intranuclear inclusions can also be seen with melanoma, meningioma, well-differentiated lung adenocarcinoma, hepatocellular carcinoma, and renal cell carcinoma.

Parathyroid Glands

Intraoperative assessment is often required to confirm that parathyroid tissue was correctly removed during surgical exploration of the neck. The differential diagnosis for a parathyroid gland on gross examination is nodular thyroid tissue, lymph node, ectopic thymic tissue, and brown fat.

The diagnosis can be rapidly accomplished by touch preparation technique (69,70). Cytologic features diagnostic of parathyroid tissue include the presence of small uniform cells alone or in small groups, round to oval nuclei, salt-and-pepper chromatin, occasional naked nuclei, and small vacuoles both within the cytoplasm and background (71). With forceful imprints, delicate cytoplasm may be stripped away leaving behind only bare nuclei that may be nondiagnostic and difficult to distinguish from lymphocytes (72). Careful examination in such cases for even a few clusters of cells where cytoplasm remains is necessary. Similar to frozen section, imprints alone cannot reliably differentiate normal parathyroid tissue from an adenoma or hyperplasia.

Products of Conception

Frozen section is useful for rapidly identifying products of conception (POC) in endometrial specimens to rule out ectopic pregnancy. Villi usually contain abundant fluid and are thus subject to freezing artifact with frozen section. Hence, POC can instead be diagnosed by touch preparation (73,74). Touch imprints need to be carefully examined to find placental villi (Figure 3.13). Villi are surrounded by trophoblast and syncytiotrophoblast layers. Syncytiotrophoblasts are relatively easy to recognize (Figure 3.14). They are multinucleated giant cells with abundant vacuolated cytoplasm. Cytotrophoblasts, which are present in early gestation, may be harder to definitively diagnose. These are smaller, round mononuclear cells with minimal cytoplasm and contain only a single vesicular nucleus. Cytotrophoblasts can resemble other similar cells, such as large reactive squamous cells (74)

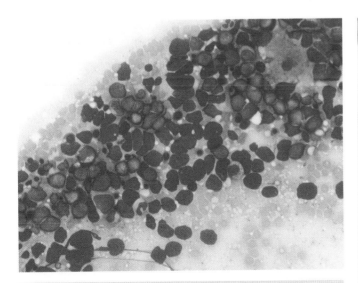

FIGURE 3.4 Bone marrow with metastatic neuroblastoma. TP showing medium sized tumor cells with indiscernible cytoplasm and nuclei with salt-and-pepper chromatin (Wright–Giemsa-stained TP, medium power). TP, touch preparation.

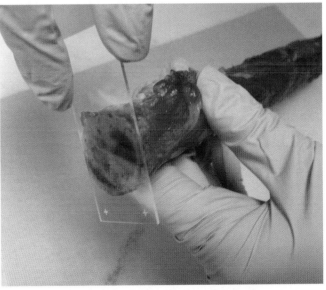

FIGURE 3.5 Bone margin imprint. A cytology imprint is performed by pressing a glass slide directly against the surgical resection margin.

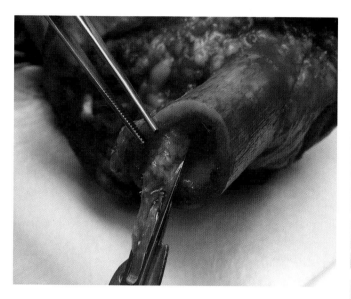

FIGURE 3.6 Bone margin TP technique. A cytology slide in this case is obtained by scraping out bone marrow with fragments from the surgical margin, which is then used to make a TP. TP, touch preparation.

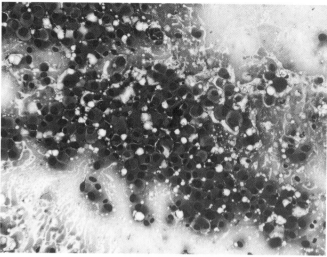

FIGURE 3.8 Melanoma metastatic to bone. Cellular imprint showing many discohesive epithelioid tumor cells. Note the presence of a rare binucleate cell, intranuclear inclusion, and macrophage with dark melanin pigment (DQ-stained TP, low power). DQ, Diff-Quik; TP, touch preparation.

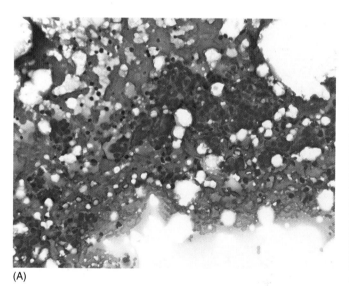

(A)

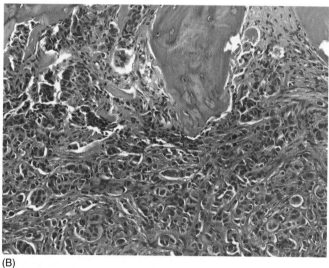

(B)

FIGURE 3.7 Breast ductal carcinoma metastatic to bone. Touch imprint demonstrating many clusters of carcinoma cells, which easily adhere to the glass slide during this touch preparation. The accompanying core biopsy shows extensive infiltration of the marrow cavity by nests of tumor cells. ((A) DQ-stained TP, low power; (B) H&E-stained bone biopsy, medium power.) DQ, Diff-Quik; H&E, hematoxylin and eosin; TP touch preparation.

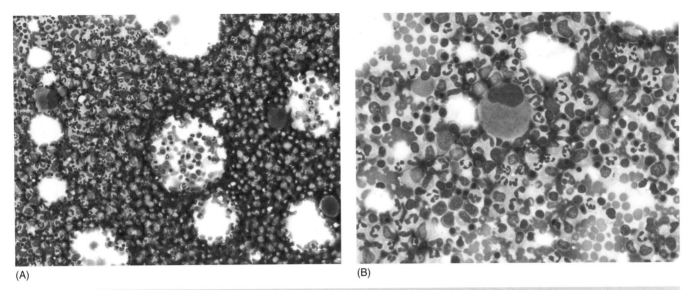

(A)

(B)

FIGURE 3.9   Normal bone marrow. TP showing trilineage hematopoiesis. The abundant myeloid cells may mimic acute inflammation. Erythroid precursors and large megakaryocytes may mimic malignant cells. ((A) DQ-stained TP, low power; (B) H&E-stained bone biopsy, medium power.) DQ, Diff-Quik; H&E, hematoxylin and eosin; TP, touch preparation.

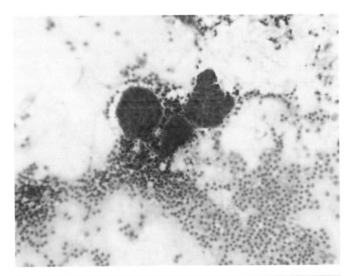

FIGURE 3.10   Axillary sentinel node with metastatic breast ductal carcinoma. TP showing cohesive clusters of carcinoma cells with a background of small lymphocytes (DQ-stained TP, low power). DQ, Diff-Quik; TP, touch preparation.

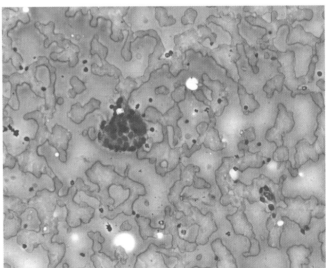

FIGURE 3.11   Benign colloid nodule. A bland macrofollicle is shown with abundant background colloid (DQ-stained TP, low power). DQ, Diff-Quik; TP, touch preparation.

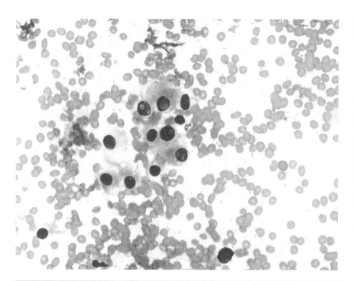

FIGURE 3.12 Papillary thyroid carcinoma. Scant atypical follicular cells are shown with intranuclear inclusions (DQ-stained TP, medium power). DQ, Diff-Quik; TP, touch preparation.

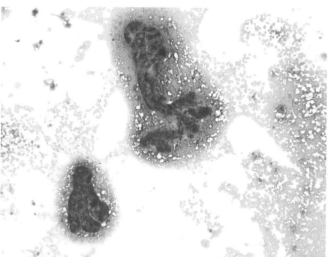

FIGURE 3.13 Placental villi. Touch imprint showing villi comprised of several trophoblastic cells (DQ-stained TP, low power). DQ, Diff-Quik; TP, touch preparation.

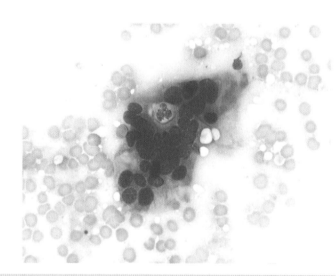

FIGURE 3.14 Syncytiotrophoblast. TP showing a single large multinucleated giant cell (DQ-stained TP, high power). DQ, Diff-Quik; TP, touch preparation.

UNSUITABLE SAMPLES

Imprint cytology will be of low yield for lesions that poorly exfoliate. This includes fibrous soft tissue tumors, tumors with marked desmoplasia, and neoplasms that were subject to chemoradiation therapy. Imprint cytology is also not suitable to evaluate the depth of tumor invasion (e.g., endometrial adenocarcinoma of the uterus). Intraoperative touch imprints cannot distinguish in situ carcinoma from invasive carcinoma, which may be critical for the surgical management of certain cancers. Frozen section is better suited for this purpose, and will also be superior to cytology preparations to distinguish infiltrating well-differentiated tumors (e.g., salivary gland adenoma vs. low-grade carcinoma). For evaluating ovarian tumors, frozen sections tend to be more beneficial because complex architecture and invasion are important features to be able to assess (75). However, intraoperative touch preparation can be helpful in certain ovarian cases such as granulosa cell tumors where "coffee bean" nuclear grooves (Figure 3.15) are easy to recognize (76). Imprint cytology is unsuitable to evaluate certain inflammatory processes, such as a lung biopsy for interstitial lung disease. During orthopedic surgery, joint tissue (synovium, capsule, or pseudocapsule) is frequently submitted to determine the neutrophil count for suspected infection in reimplantation arthroplasties. Performing touch preparations of these joint specimens is not advised, because the presence of neutrophils in these cytology preparations may be from peripheral blood, surface inflammatory exudate, or fibrin (Figure 3.16), and hence may not be indicative of neutrophils embedded within infected tissue.

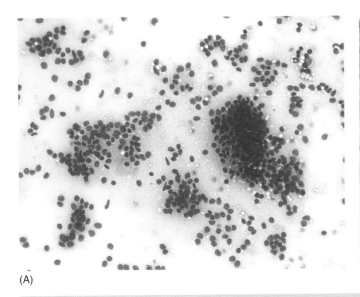

(A)

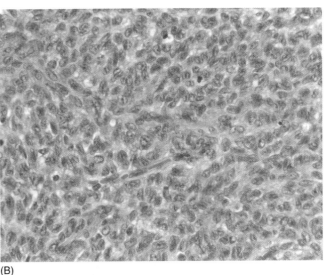

(B)

FIGURE 3.15 Ovarian granulosa cell tumor. Monotonous tumor cells have ovoid nuclei characterized by distinct nuclear grooves. ((A) DQ-stained TP, low power; (B) H&E-stained tissue, medium power.) DQ, Diff-Quik; H&E, hematoxylin and eosin; TP, touch preparation.

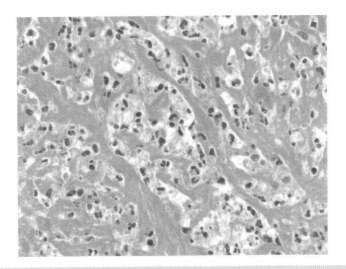

FIGURE 3.16 Joint tissue fibroinflammatory exudate. Neutrophils are shown admixed with fibrin, which is not representative of tissue involvement (H&E-stained tissue, high power). H&E, hematoxylin and eosin.

DIAGNOSTIC ERRORS

False-Positive Diagnoses

There are several reasons for false-positive intraoperative imprint cytology. Apart from misinterpretation errors, the presence of numerous reactive (nonlesional) cells or cauterized cells may be misleading. Rarely, granulomas may be misdiagnosed as neoplasms and vice versa. The cytomorphology of granulomas varies from loosely aggregated macrophages to compact epithelioid histiocytes with/without necrosis (Figure 3.17). Imprints with dysplasia or radiation atypia can also be over-interpreted as invasive malignancy. Moreover, imprints could be contaminated by tumor cells during tissue manipulation and slide preparation in the frozen section environment.

False-Negative Diagnoses

False-negative diagnoses may occur when imprints are hypocellular or nonrepresentative (i.e., sampling error). Hypocellularity may be attributed to tissue heterogeneity (e.g., fibrotic/sclerotic regions), failure of tumor cells to adhere to the glass slide, or if insufficient pressure is applied when preparing the imprint slide. There may be lack of adequate cellular pleomorphism, atypia, or mitoses in some cases, especially for well-differentiated neoplasms. Finally, when there is only focal extension of tumor to a margin, or when tumors closely approximate but do not actually reach a surgical margin, these cases may be missed on touch imprints.

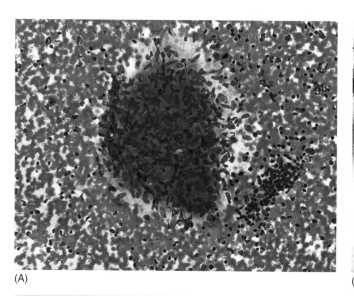

(A)

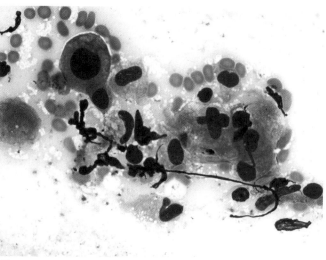

(B)

FIGURE 3.17 Non-necrotizing granulomas. (A) A cohesive group of spindled and epithelioid histiocytes are shown. (B) Occasional histiocytes may show reactive nuclear atypia that mimics malignancy. ((A) DQ-stained TP, low power; (B) DQ-stained TP, high power.) DQ, Diff-Quik; TP, touch preparation.

REFERENCES

1. Dudgeon LS, Patrick CV. A new method for the rapid microscopical diagnosis of tumours, with an account of 200 cases so examined. Br J Surgery. 1927;15:250-261.

2. Suen KC, Wood WS, Syed AA, et al. Role of imprint cytology in intraoperative diagnosis: value and limitations. J Clin Pathol. 1978;31:328-337.

3. Wilkerson JA, Bonnin JM. Intraoperative Cytology: An Adjunct to Frozen Sections. New York, NY: Igaku-Shoin; 1987.

4. Mair S, Lash RH, Suskin D, Mendelsohn G. Intraoperative surgical specimen evaluation: frozen section analysis, cytologic examination, or both? A comparative study of 206 cases. Am J Clin Pathol. 1991;96:8-14.

5. Suen KC, Wood WS, Syed AA, et al. Intraoperative surgical specimen evaluation: frozen section analysis, cytologic examination, or both? A comparative study of 206 cases. Am J Clin Pathol. 1991;96:8-14.

6. Sidaway MK, Silverberg SG. Intraoperative cytology: back to the future? Am J Clin Pathol. 1991;96:1-3.

7. Scucchi LF, Di Stefano D, Cosentino L, Vecchione A. Value of cytology as an adjunctive intraoperative diagnostic method. An audit of 2,250 consecutive cases. Acta Cytol. 1997;41:1489-1496.

8. Frishberg DP. Guide to the preparation of intraoperative touch preparations and other cytologic preparations. In: Marchevsky A, Balzer B, Abdul-Karim FW, eds. Intraoperative Consultation. Philadelphia, PA: Saunders; 2014: 6-15.

9. Eltoum IA, Tabbara S. Intraoperative cytologic diagnosis of granulomas: a retrospective study of 156 cases. Diagn Cytopathol. 1998;18:62-66.

10. Nochomovitz L, Sidaway M, Silverberg S, et al. Intraoperative Consultation. A Guide to Smears, Imprints, and Frozen Sections. Chicago, IL: ASCP Press; 1989.

11. Jörundsson E, Lumsden JH, Jacobs RM. Rapid staining techniques in cytopathology: a review and comparison of modified protocols for hematoxylin and eosin, Papanicolaou and Romanowsky stains. Vet Clin Pathol. 1999;28:100-108.

12. Feinberg MR, Bhaskar AG, Bourne P. Differential diagnosis of malignant lymphomas by imprint cytology. Acta Cytol. 1980;24:16-25.

13. Wilkerson JA. Intraoperative cytology of lymph nodes and lymphoid lesions. Diagn Cytopathol. 1985;1:46-52.

14. Wilkerson JA, Crowell WT. Intraoperative cytology of osseous lesions. Diagn Cytopathol. 1986;2:5-12.

15. Bui MM, Smith P, Agresta SV, et al. Practical issues of intraoperative frozen section diagnosis of bone and soft tissue lesions. Cancer Control. 2008;15:7-12.

16. Rahman K, Asif Siddiqui F, Zaheer S, et al. Intraoperative cytology-role in bone lesions. Diagn Cytopathol. 2010;38:639-644.

17. Bhaker P, Mohan H, Handa U, Kumar S. Role of intraoperative pathology consultation in skeletal tumors and tumor-like lesions. Sarcoma. 2014;2014:902104.

18. Kjurkchiev G, Valkov I. Role of touch imprint and core biopsy for detection of tumor metastases in bone marrow. Diagn Cytopathol. 1998;18:323-324.

19. Ghandur-Mnaymneh L, Paz J. The use of touch preparations (tissue imprints) in the rapid intraoperative diagnosis of metastatic lymph node disease in cancer staging procedures. Cancer. 1985;56:339-344.

20. Henry-Tillman RS, Korourian S, Rubio IT, et al. Intraoperative touch preparation for sentinel lymph node biopsy: a 4-year experience. Ann Surg Oncol. 2002;9:333-339.

21. Baitchev G, Gortchev G, Todorova A. Intraoperative sentinel lymph node examination by imprint cytology during breast surgery. Curr Med Res Opin. 2002;18:185-187.

22. Creager AJ, Geisinger KR, Shiver SA, et al. Intraoperative evaluation of sentinel lymph nodes for metastatic breast carcinoma by imprint cytology. Mod Pathol. 2002;15:1140-1147.

23. Limberis V, Romanidis C, Galazios G, et al. Intraoperative estimation of sentinel lymph nodes in breast cancer by imprint cytology. Eur J Gynaecol Oncol. 2009;30:85-87.

24. Guidroz JA, Johnson MT, Scott-Conner CE, et al. The use of touch preparation for the evaluation of sentinel lymph nodes in breast cancer. Am J Surg. 2010;199:792-796.

25. Calhoun BC, Chambers K, Flippo-Morton T, et al. Breast cancer detection in axillary sentinel lymph nodes: the impact of the method of pathologic examination. Hum Pathol. 2014;45: 2497-2501.

26. Creager AJ, Shiver SA, Shen P, et al. Intraoperative evaluation of sentinel lymph nodes for metastatic melanoma by imprint cytology. Cancer. 2002;94:3016-3022.

27. Nejc D, Pasz-Walczak G, Piekarski J, et al. 94% accuracy of intraoperative imprint touch cytology of sentinel nodes in skin melanoma patients. Anticancer Res. 2008;28:465-469.

28. Motomura K, Nagumo S, Komoike Y, et al. Accuracy of imprint cytology for intraoperative diagnosis of sentinel node metastases in breast cancer. Ann Surg. 2008;247:839-842.

29. Rubio IT, Korourian S, Cowan C, et al. Use of touch preps for intraoperative diagnosis of sentinel lymph node metastases in breast cancer. Ann Surg Oncol. 1998;5:689-894.

30. Howard-McNatt M, Geisinger KR, Stewart JH IV, et al. Is intraoperative imprint cytology evaluation still feasible for the evaluation of sentinel lymph nodes for lobular carcinoma of the breast? Ann Surg Oncol. 2012;19:929-934.

31. Sauer T, Engh V, Holck AM, et al. Imprint cytology of sentinel lymph nodes in breast cancer. Experience with rapid, intraoperative diagnosis and primary screening by cytotechnologists. Acta Cytol. 2003;47:768-773.

32. Shiver SA, Creager AJ, Geisinger K, et al. Intraoperative analysis of sentinel lymph nodes by imprint cytology for cancer of the breast. Am J Surg. 2002;184:424-427.

33. Barranger E, Antoine M, Grahek D, et al. Intraoperative imprint cytology of sentinel nodes in breast cancer. J Surg Oncol. 2004;86:128-133.

34. Elliott RM, Shenk RR, Thompson CL, Gilmore HL. Touch preparations for the intraoperative evaluation of sentinel lymph nodes after neoadjuvant therapy have high false-negative rates in patients with breast cancer. Arch Pathol Lab Med. 2014;138: 814-818.

35. Weinberg ES, Dickson D, White L, et al. Cytokeratin staining for intraoperative evaluation of sentinel lymph nodes in patients with invasive lobular carcinoma. Am J Surg. 2004;188:419-422.

36. Salem AA, Douglas-Jones AG, Sweetland HM, Mansel RE. Intraoperative evaluation of axillary sentinel lymph nodes using touch imprint cytology and immunohistochemistry. Part II. Results. Eur J Surg Oncol. 2006;32:484-487.

37. Fujishima M, Watatani M, Inui H, et al. Touch imprint cytology with cytokeratin immunostaining versus Papanicolaou staining for intraoperative evaluation of sentinel lymph node metastasis in clinically node-negative breast cancer. Eur J Surg Oncol. 2009;35: 398-402.

38. Lambah PA, McIntyre MA, Chetty U, Dixon JM. Imprint cytology of axillary lymph nodes as an intraoperative diagnostic tool. Eur J Surg Oncol. 2003;29:224-228.

39. Aryya NC, Khanna S, Shukla HS, et al. Role of rapid imprint cytology in the diagnosis of skin cancer and assessment of adequacy of excision. Indian J Pathol Microbiol. 1992;35:108-112.

40. Klimberg VS, Westbrook KC, Korourian S. Use of touch preps for diagnosis and evaluation of surgical margins in breast cancer. Ann Surg Oncol. 1998;5:220-226.

41. Bakhshandeh M, Tutuncuoglu SO, Fischer G, Masood S. Use of imprint cytology for assessment of surgical margins in lumpectomy specimens of breast cancer patients. Diagn Cytopathol. 2007;35: 656-659.

42. Valdes EK, Boolbol SK, Cohen JM, Feldman SM. Intra-operative touch preparation cytology; does it have a role in re-excision lumpectomy? *Ann Surg Oncol.* 2007;14:1045-1050.

43. D'Halluin F, Tas P, Rouquette S, et al. Intra-operative touch preparation cytology following lumpectomy for breast cancer: a series of 400 procedures. *Breast.* 2009;18:248-253.

44. Yadav GS, Donoghue M, Tauro DP, et al. Intraoperative imprint evaluation of surgical margins in oral squamous cell carcinoma. *Acta Cytol.* 2013;57:75-83.

45. Palermo SM, Dechet C, Trenti E, et al. Cytology as an alternative to frozen section at the time of nephron-sparing surgery to evaluate surgical margin status. *Urology.* 2013;82:1071-1075.

46. Ozsoy M, Klatte T, Wiener H, et al. Intraoperative imprint cytology for real-time assessment of surgical margins during partial nephrectomy: a comparison with frozen section. *Urol Oncol.* 2014;pii:S1078–1439(14)00273-7.

47. Tone K, Kojima K, Hoshiai K, et al. Utility of intraoperative cytology of resection margins in biliary tract and pancreas tumors. *Diagn Cytopathol.* 2015;43:366-373.

48. Florell SR, Layfield LJ, Gerwels JW. A comparison of touch imprint cytology and Mohs frozen-section histology in the evaluation of Mohs micrographic surgical margins. *J Am Acad Dermatol.* 2001;44:660-664.

49. Rakha EA, Haider A, Patil S, et al. Evaluation of touch preparation cytology during frozen-section diagnoses of pulmonary lesions. *J Clin Pathol.* 2010;63:675-677.

50. Valdes EK, Boolbol SK, Ali I, et al. Intraoperative touch preparation cytology for margin assessment in breast-conservation surgery: does it work for lobular carcinoma? *Ann Surg Oncol.* 2007;14:2940-2945.

51. Yadav GS, Donoghue M, Tauro DP, et al. Confounding factors and diagnostic accuracy of imprint cytology. *Acta Cytol.* 2014;58:53-59.

52. Burger PC. Use of cytological preparations in the frozen section diagnosis of central nervous system neoplasia. *Am J Surg Pathol.* 1985;9:344-354.

53. Hitchcock E, Morris CS, Sotelo MG, Salmon M. Comparison of smear and imprint techniques for rapid diagnosis in neuro-oncology. *Surg Neurol.* 1986;26:176-182.

54. Powell SZ. Intraoperative consultation, cytologic preparations, and frozen section in the central nervous system. *Arch Pathol Lab Med.* 2005;129:1635-1652.

55. Martinez AJ, Pollack I, Hall WA, Lunsford LD. Touch preparations in the rapid intraoperative diagnosis of central nervous system lesions. A comparison with frozen sections and paraffin-embedded sections. *Mod Pathol.* 1988;1:378-384.

56. Khamechian T, Alizargar J, Mazoochi T. The value of touch preparation for rapid diagnosis of brain tumors as an intraoperative consultation. *Iran J Med Sci.* 2012;37:105-111.

57. Tribe CR. A comparison of rapid methods including imprint cyto-diagnosis for the diagnosis of breast tumours. *J Clin Pathol.* 1973;26:273-277.

58. Helpap B, Tschubel K. The significance of the imprint cytology in breast biopsy diagnosis. *Acta Cytol.* 1978;22:133-137.

59. Esteban JM, Zaloudek C, Silverberg SG. Intraoperative diagnosis of breast lesions. Comparison of cytologic with frozen section techniques. *Am J Clin Pathol.* 1987;88:681-688.

60. De Rosa G, Boschi R, Boscaino A, et al. Intraoperative cytology in breast cancer diagnosis: comparison between cytologic and frozen section techniques. *Diagn Cytopathol.* 1993;9:623-631.

61. D'Halluin F, Tas P, Rouquette S, et al. Intra-operative touch preparation cytology following lumpectomy for breast cancer: a series of 400 procedures. *Breast.* 2009;18:248-253.

62. LiVolsi VA, Baloch ZW. Use and abuse of frozen section in the diagnosis of follicular thyroid lesions. *Endocr Pathol.* 2005;16:285-293.

63. Basolo F, Ugolini C, Proietti A, et al. Role of frozen section associated with intraoperative cytology in comparison to FNA and FS alone in the management of thyroid nodules. *Eur J Surg Oncol.* 2007;33:769-775.

64. Anila KR, Krishna G. Role of imprint cytology in intra operative diagnosis of thyroid lesions. *Gulf J Oncol.* 2014;1:73-78.

65. Ahmadinejad M, Aliepour A, Anbari K, et al.. Fine-needle aspiration, touch imprint, and crush preparation cytology for diagnosing thyroid malignancies in thyroid nodules. *Indian J Surg.* 2015;77(suppl 2):480-483.

66. Pyo JS, Sohn JH, Kang G. Diagnostic assessment of intraoperative cytology for papillary thyroid carcinoma: using a decision tree analysis. *J Endocrinol Invest.* 2017;40:305-311.

67. Balázs G, Fábián E, Lukács G, Juhász F. Rapid cytological diagnosis during thyroid surgery. *Eur J Surg Oncol.* 1992;18:1-6.

68. Tworek JA, Giordano TJ, Michael CW. Comparison of intraoperative cytology with frozen sections in the diagnosis of thyroid lesions. *Am J Clin Pathol.* 1998;110:456-461.

69. Geelhoed GW, Silverberg SG. Intraoperative imprints for the identification of parathyroid tissue. *Surgery.* 1984;96:1124-1131.

70. Shidham VB, Asma Z, Rao RN, et al. Intraoperative cytology increases the diagnostic accuracy of frozen sections for the confirmation of various tissues in the parathyroid region. *Am J Clin Pathol.* 2002;118:895-902.

71. Yao DX, Hoda SA, Yin DY, et al. Interpretative problems and preparative technique influence reliability of intraoperative parathyroid touch imprints. *Arch Pathol Lab Med.* 2003;127:64-67.

72. Ranchod M, Chan JKC, Kebew E. Parathyroid gland. In: Ranchod M, ed. *Intraoperative Consultation in Surgical Pathology.* New York, NY: Cambridge University Press; 2010:179-191.

73. Kinugasa M, Sato T, Tamura M. Cytological detection of trophoblasts for rapid diagnosis of pregnancy of unknown location. *Int J Gynaecol Obstet.* 2012;117:87-88.

74. Chen AL, Tambouret RH, Roberts DJ. Touch preps of products of conception for rule-out ectopic pregnancy: a viable alternative to frozen section. *Am J Clin Pathol.* 2016;145:752-756.

75. Stewart CJ, Brennan BA, Koay E, et al. Value of cytology in the intraoperative assessment of ovarian tumors: a review of 402 cases and comparison with frozen section diagnosis. *Cancer Cytopathol.* 2010;118:127-136.

76. Montag AG. Intraoperative consultation in gynecologic pathology. In: Taxy J, Husain A, Montag A, eds. *Biopsy Interpretation: The Frozen Section.* Philadelphia, PA: Wolters Kluwer; 2010:33-46.

CHAPTER 4

Gynecological System

Zaibo Li and Chengquan Zhao

INTRODUCTION

Touch imprint cytology can be used intraoperatively to evaluate ovarian, uterine, cervical, and other gynecological tumors, in addition to lymph nodes excised during staging of women with a presumed gynecological malignancy. Since aspiration cytology is not frequently used for preoperative evaluation of adnexal and uterine lesions, touch preparation cytology becomes important and may be the only cytological specimen for evaluation of these tumors prior to processing (1–3).

NORMAL

Ovary

The normal ovary is usually not evaluated with touch preparations, unless it is edematous, hemorrhagic, cystic, or concerning for a neoplasm at the time of oophorectomy. These tend to be hypocellular with some mesothelial cells, ciliated epithelial cells, stromal cells, and proteinaceous fluid.

Uterus and Cervix

Touch imprint cytology of the endometrium will depend on the age of the patient and stage of the menstrual cycle. Proliferative endometrium yields cohesive sheets of cells and short segments of tubular glands lined by pseudostratified cells with ovoid nuclei, mitoses, and dense cytoplasm. Nuclear overlap and mild to moderate nuclear size variation can be seen. The stroma usually contains homogeneous spindle-shaped cells with indistinct cytoplasm and bland nuclei. The background is usually clean with occasional thin-walled blood vessels. Touch imprints of secretory endometrium yield glandular cells arranged in a spread-out honeycomb architecture. The glandular cells have abundant cytoplasm with secretory vacuoles, well-defined cell borders, round nuclei, and more conspicuous nucleoli. Spindled stromal cells show more abundant cytoplasm. Mucoid material or predecidual changes can be seen. Touch imprints of menstrual endometrium is bloody with a few degenerated epithelial–stromal fragments mixed with neutrophils and nuclear debris. Touch imprints of atrophic endometrium can yield few loosely cohesive flat sheets or strips of glands lined by nonstratified uniform small columnar cells, which have monomorphic nuclei with smooth nuclear membranes and inconspicuous nucleoli. The stroma is usually fibrous and forms isolated tissue aggregates. The uterine cervix is lined by squamous mucosa and endocervical epithelium, but usually is not evaluated intraoperatively with touch preparations.

BENIGN ENTITIES

Ovary

Benign serous tumors are characterized by a ciliated epithelial cell lining resembling that seen in the fallopian tube. Such tumors include serous cystadenoma, adenofibroma, and cystadenofibroma depending on cyst formation and the stromal component. Benign serous tumors account for about 50% of all ovarian serous tumors and occur in women ranging in age from 40 to 60 years. Touch imprint of these tumors may show rare uniform bland columnar epithelial cells in a background of thin serous fluid with histiocytes. Tumor cells have a moderate amount of cytoplasm, well-defined cell borders, round/oval nuclei, and fine granular chromatin (4). Small nucleoli may be seen. If well-preserved, cilia may be seen. Detached ciliary tufts and psammoma bodies may be present. Spindle cells may be seen in serous adenofibroma and cystadenofibroma. The differential diagnosis includes epithelial inclusion cyst, hydrosalpinx, and borderline serous tumor.

Benign mucinous tumors (mucinous cystadenoma/cystadenofibroma) include tumors with a mucinous endocervical or gastrointestinal mucin-producing epithelial-lined cyst with (cystadenoma) or without prominent fibrous stroma (adenofibroma). Benign mucinous tumors occur in patients with a wide age range and account for 80% of all ovarian mucinous tumors. Touch imprints of benign mucinous tumors show few bland mucinous cells in a background of viscous mucin and macrophages. The mucinous cells are tall columnar with small, round, basally oriented bland nuclei, low nuclear:cytoplasmic (N:C) ratio, and mucinous cytoplasm. No cilia are seen. Fibroblasts may be seen in mucinous adenofibroma.

Benign Brenner tumors, with cells resembling those of the normal bladder can also be seen in the ovary. Touch imprints of a benign Brenner tumor may only yield few epithelial cells in clusters, sheets, or singly. The tumor cells resemble urothelial cells with bland appearing, small oval/coffee bean–shaped nuclei with nuclear grooves and conspicuous nucleoli. Extracellular metachromatic hyaline globules, squamous or glandular differentiation, and spindle-shaped fibrous cells may be seen (Figure 4.1).

In addition to epithelial-type tumors of the ovary, germ cell tumors can arise, particularly in younger women. Mature cystic teratoma (MCT) is a benign neoplasm derived from the ovum that differentiates into mature ectoderm, mesoderm, and/or endoderm. It is the most common germ cell tumor. Sebaceous material, hair, and teeth are commonly identified grossly. Touch imprint of the solid components may show squamous cells, keratinaceous material, amorphous clumps of cellular debris, and other differentiated cell types such as sebaceous cells, fat cells, and enteric or respiratory epithelium. Immature teratomas contain immature cellular elements, including commonly encountered neuroblastic tissue, in addition to mature differentiated components. The immature neuronal cells are small cells with scant cytoplasm and immature chromatin, imparting a "small round blue cell" morphology on touch prep. Dysgerminoma is a primitive germ cell tumor composed of primitive germ cells with no specific differentiation pattern. It accounts for 1% to 2% of ovarian malignancies, but is the most common malignant germ cell tumor of the ovary. Touch imprint cytology findings in dysgerminoma are identical to that of seminoma in males, showing a dual population of malignant germinoma cells and lymphocytes. Tumor cells are round, large, and discohesive with large anisokaryotic nuclei, prominent nucleoli, and foamy cytoplasm. Sharply punched-out vacuoles may be seen at the cell periphery. Multinucleated giant cells may also be seen. A "tigroid" background with interwoven lacy material is characteristic, although it can also be seen in other glycogen-rich tumors such as some squamous cell carcinomas, renal cell carcinomas, clear cell tumors, or synovial sarcomas. The differential diagnosis includes large cell lymphoma, melanoma, and poorly differentiated/undifferentiated carcinoma.

Thecoma is a benign ovarian stromal tumor mostly composed of thecoma cells. Pure thecomas are rare and are approximately one third as common as granulosa cell tumors. Thecoma occurs at an older age with a mean of 59 years and is uncommon before the age of 30 years. The cellularity of these imprint samples is variable with plump oval or spindle cells. Their nuclei are irregular and the cytoplasm of these tumor cells is abundant and fragile with vacuoles. Rare bizarre cells can be present. Thecoma cells are usually positive for inhibin and calretinin, but negative for cytokeratin and epithelial membrane antigen (EMA). The differential diagnosis includes massive edema, ovarian fibromatosis, stromal hyperplasia, stromal hyperthecosis, granulosa cell tumor, Sertoli–Leydig cell tumor, and stromal tumor.

Fibroma is a benign ovarian stromal tumor composed of fibroblasts. Fibroma accounts for 4% of all ovarian tumors and occurs at all ages, but more frequently manifests at middle age. Fibroma may be accompanied by two unusual clinical syndromes: Meigs' syndrome and Gorlin's syndrome (basal cell nevus syndrome). The cellularity of touch preps is usually low with scant thin spindle-shaped cells. However, cellular fibromas may show high cellularity. Rare bizarre cells can occur. Cells are usually positive for calretinin, but negative for inhibin, EMA, and cytokeratin. The differential diagnosis of spindle cell lesions of the ovary includes massive edema, ovarian fibromatosis, stromal hyperplasia, stromal hyperthecosis, granulosa cell tumor, Sertoli–Leydig cell tumor, stromal tumor, smooth muscle neoplasm, and metastatic spindle cell neoplasms.

Fibrothecoma is more common than pure thecoma or fibroma with a combination of fibroblasts and thecal cells. Their cellularity is variable with both thin spindle-shaped fibroma cells and more plump oval thecoma cells. Thecoma cells have irregular nuclei and abundant vacuolated cytoplasm (Figure 4.2).

Uterus

Endometrial hyperplasia includes simple and complex hyperplasia without or with atypia. Architecture is rarely appreciated on touch imprints; therefore, it is almost impossible to differentiate simple hyperplasia from complex hyperplasia on touch imprint cytology. Cytologically, touch imprint cytology of endometrial hyperplasia without cytologic atypia overlaps considerably with that of proliferative endometrium and regenerative endometrium, making it impossible to tell them apart. Similar to proliferative endometrium, the epithelial cells are columnar in shape with uniformly ovoid nuclei, finely granular chromatin, and small micronucleoli. Touch imprint cytology of endometrial hyperplasia with atypia overlaps significantly with that of low-grade endometrioid adenocarcinoma. The cytology is cellular with glandular epithelial cells that are stratified, crowded, and demonstrates loss of normal polarity. The nuclei are mildly pleomorphic with mild coarse chromatin and medium-sized nucleoli. Necrosis is absent.

Leiomyoma of the uterus is a benign smooth muscle tumor. It is the most common tumor in the uterus. These neoplasms occur most commonly in women aged 40 to 50 years. Touch imprints of leiomyoma usually show variable cellularity with spindle-shaped bland-appearing cells with indistinct cell borders, eosinophilic fibrillary cytoplasm, and cigar-shaped nuclei. Hyalinized material may be seen in the background. Cellular leiomyoma may show more hypercellularity. Epithelioid leiomyoma may show epithelioid cells. Tumor cells with bizarre nuclei may be seen in leiomyomas with bizarre nuclei (atypical leiomyoma) (Figure 4.3).

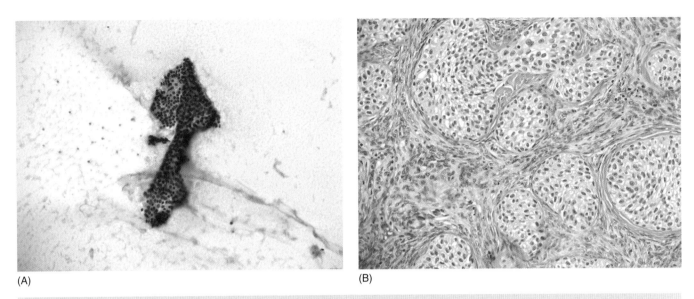

(A)

(B)

FIGURE 4.1   Brenner tumor. (A) Touch imprint of a benign Brenner tumor is shown yielding a cluster of epithelial cells. Tumor cells resemble urothelial cells with bland appearing, small oval/coffee bean–shaped nuclei with nuclear grooves and conspicuous nucleoli (H&E-stained, medium power). (B) Histologic section showing a typical Brenner tumor with nested urothelial cells in ovarian stroma (H&E-stained, medium power). H&E, hematoxylin and eosin.

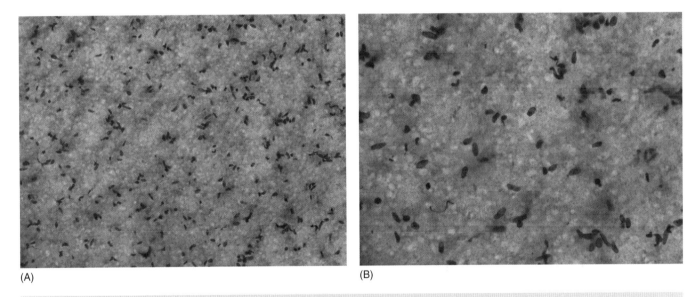

(A)

(B)

FIGURE 4.2   Fibrothecoma. (A and B) The touch imprint shown is hypocellular with thin spindle-shaped fibroma cells. Thecoma cells are not shown here (H&E-stained, medium and high power). (*C continued*)

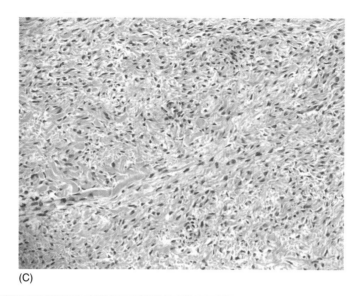

(C)

FIGURE 4.2 (*continued*) (C) Corresponding histologic section of this fibrothecoma (H&E-stained, medium power). H&E, hematoxylin and eosin.

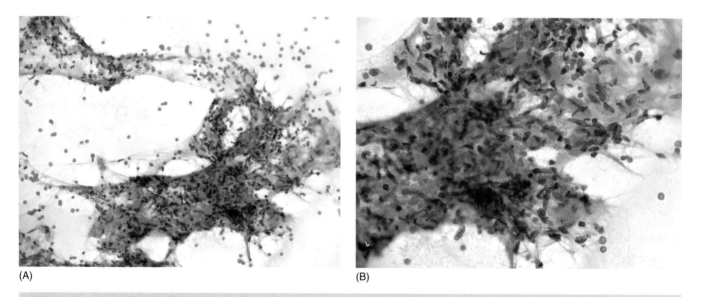

(A)   (B)

FIGURE 4.3   Leiomyoma. (A and B) Touch imprints show variable cellularity with spindle-shaped, bland-appearing cells with indistinct cell borders, eosinophilic fibrillary cytoplasm, and cigar-shaped nuclei (H&E-stained, medium and high power). H&E, hematoxylin and eosin.

MALIGNANT ENTITIES

Ovary

Serous tumors with increased proliferation or atypia may represent a serous borderline tumor (SBT) or serous carcinoma. SBT is a noninvasive serous tumor with greater epithelial proliferation and cytological atypia than benign serous tumors, but less than that of low-grade serous carcinoma. It accounts for about 15% of all ovarian serous tumors. Touch imprint of a SBT is more cellular than benign serous tumors. SBT cells are arranged in large sheets, crowded clusters, or branched papillae. SBT cells are more atypical than benign serous tumor cells with modest amount of cytoplasm, high N:C ratio, modest nuclear pleomorphism, irregular nuclear membrane, fine chromatin, and conspicuous nucleoli. Psammoma bodies may be seen. However, distinguishing SBT from low-grade serous carcinoma may not be possible by cytology alone. Touch imprints of serous carcinoma (low-grade and high-grade) are very cellular with small crowded clusters. There may also be large branching papillae, together with abundant individual cells. Cytological atypia depends on the tumor grade. Low-grade serous carcinoma cells usually show less atypia, smaller nuclei, less hyperchromasia, and more cytoplasm. High-grade serous carcinoma cells are hyperchromatic with large nuclei, high N:C ratio, irregular chromatin, and prominent nucleoli. Psammoma bodies may be seen (Figure 4.4). The differential diagnosis includes poorly differentiated endometrioid carcinoma or metastatic carcinoma.

Mucinous tumors are classified similar to serous tumors, with those having increased proliferation or atypia being classified as mucinous borderline tumor or mucinous carcinoma. Mucinous borderline tumor is a low-malignant potential mucinous tumor and is the second most common type of borderline ovarian tumor. It occurs in patients with a wide age range. Touch imprints of mucinous borderline tumor usually yield more cells than benign tumors. Small papillae may be seen in a background of mucin. Tumor cells have more atypia than benign cells, but less atypia than mucinous carcinoma cells. The nuclei are modestly atypical with conspicuous nucleoli. However, distinguishing borderline tumor from well-differentiated carcinoma may not be possible by cytology alone. Mucinous carcinoma is a malignant mucinous epithelial tumor with endocervical or gastrointestinal-type cells containing mucin (Figure 4.5). It accounts for 3% to 4% of primary ovarian carcinomas. Touch imprints of mucinous carcinoma usually yield hypercellular material with mucin in the background. Tumor cells are arranged in irregular clusters, syncytial fragments, or singly with obviously malignant atypia including prominent nuclear pleomorphism, coarse chromatin, multinucleation, and vacuolated cytoplasm. The main differential diagnosis is metastatic colorectal carcinoma or pancreatobiliary carcinoma. This distinction is very difficult based on cytology alone; immunohistochemical studies and clinical information are usually necessary.

Endometrioid carcinoma of the ovary is a malignant epithelial tumor resembling endometrioid carcinoma of the uterus. It accounts for 10% to 15% of all ovarian carcinomas. Touch imprint cytology of this tumor is identical to those from endometrioid carcinoma of the uterus. These specimens are hypercellular with sheets, three-dimensional clusters, microacini or complex papillae of tumor cells, and show modest eosinophilic cytoplasm, high N:C ratio, crowded enlarged hyperchromatic nuclei, coarse dark chromatin, and small conspicuous nucleoli. Mucoid material and hemosiderin-laden macrophages may be seen in the background. Cilia are absent (Figure 4.6).

Clear cell carcinoma is a malignant epithelial tumor with clear or eosinophilic, hobnail cells. It usually arises in endometriosis and occurs in women with an average age of 55 years. Touch imprints of this tumor can yield cellular material with a background of blood and necrosis, if they are not cystic. Tumor cells have irregular pleomorphic nuclei, fine chromatin, macronucleoli and abundant pale/eosinophilic cytoplasm (5,6). Metachromatic hyaline cytoplasmic inclusions or extracellular hyaline matrix may be seen.

Brenner tumors are a group of tumors with transitional-type cells (urothelial cells). They include benign, borderline, and malignant Brenner tumor (urothelial carcinoma arising in a benign Brenner tumor) (Figure 4.1). Touch imprints of borderline tumors differ from benign Brenner tumors due to the increased number of cercariform tumor cells with more atypia. Touch imprints of malignant tumors show obviously malignant urothelial cells in a background of benign-appearing urothelial cells (7).

Undifferentiated ovarian carcinoma is usually a high-stage tumor with a poor prognosis. Touch imprints yield anaplastic malignant epithelial cells without any differentiation. Tumor cells are usually single with fragile cytoplasm, naked nuclei, and apoptotic debris. This diagnosis usually requires the exclusion of other tumor types with immunohistochemical stains.

Two types of small cell carcinoma occur in the ovary, including small cell carcinoma of the ovary with hypercalcemia and small cell carcinoma of pulmonary type. Small cell carcinoma of pulmonary type shows similar touch imprint cytology to that of small cell carcinoma of the lung. Small cell carcinoma of the ovary with hypercalcemia shows two types of cells, small cells and large cells. The small cells have hyperchromatic nuclei and scant cytoplasm, whereas the large cells have abundant cytoplasm, vesicular nuclei, and prominent nucleoli (Figure 4.7).

Adult granulosa cell tumor (AGCT) is a low-grade malignant sex cord-stromal tumor composed of granulosa cells with limited fibroblasts and theca cells. AGCT accounts for about 1% of all ovarian tumors and the majority of granulosa cell tumors. It occurs more often in postmenopausal women. Their tumor cells can secrete estrogen that stimulates endometrium hyperplasia or carcinoma. AGCTs can be solid or cystic, and when cystic their cellularity may be low. A touch imprint of the solid AGCT is more hypercellular with cords, rosettes, trabeculae, papillary fronds, or individual granulosa cells (8,9). Granulosa cells are uniformly small with scant wispy cytoplasm, high N:C ratio, and indistinct cell border. Their nuclei are round/oval with fine chromatin and small distinct nucleoli. Irregular nuclear membranes, coffee bean–shaped nuclei, and nuclear grooves are characteristic. The Call–Exner body, a small cavitary space with matrix material surrounded by granulosa cells, may be seen in some cases. AGCT cells are usually positive for inhibin, CD99, smooth muscle action, and calretinin, but negative for EMA. Cytokeratin reactivity is variable. The differential diagnosis includes Brenner tumor, sex cord tumor with annular tubules, Sertoli cell tumor, and reactive mesothelial cells. Both Brenner tumor and sex cord tumor with annular tubules may show prominent nuclear grooves.

Juvenile granulosa cell tumor (JGCT) is a distinct type of GCT composed of a mixture of granulosa and theca cells and occurs mainly in children and young adults. Touch imprints may show follicles of granulosa cells and thecal cells (10). Compared to AGCT cells, JGCT granulosa cells are more atypical with dark round nuclei and more abundant cytoplasm. Nuclear grooves are rare, and nuclear pleomorphism and mitotic activity are more common. Thecal cells have elongated blunt-ended, more hyperchromatic nuclei with less distinct nucleoli.

Sertoli–Leydig cell tumor (SLCT) is a mixed sex cord-stromal tumor composed of variable Sertoli cells and Leydig cells. SLCTs are rare ovarian tumors and range from well-differentiated to poorly differentiated types. SLCTs occur at all ages, but are more common in young women. Clinically, virilization only develops in one third of the cases. The prognosis is related to the degree of differentiation. SLCT is composed of Sertoli cells, Leydig cells, and possible heterologous elements such as mucinous cells, hepatocytes, neuroendocrine cells, skeletal muscle, and cartilage. Sertoli cells may form cords, tubules, and trabeculae, and there may also be individual cells seen on imprints that are columnar in shape with uniform oval nuclei, irregular chromatin, and abundant finely granular cytoplasm. Leydig cells are large and monomorphic with uniform round nuclei, smooth nuclear membranes, fine chromatin, variable nucleoli, and pseudoinclusions. Reinke crystals, which are elongated rectangular eosinophilic structures, may rarely be seen. Metachromatic hyaline material may also be seen. Sertoli cells are usually positive for inhibin and calretinin, variably positive for cytokeratin, but negative for EMA. Leydig cells are positive for inhibin, calretinin, and Melan A.

Malignant mixed Müllerian tumor (MMMT/carcinosarcoma) is rare in the ovary and is a bimorphic neoplasm with malignant epithelial and mesenchymal components. Endometrial stromal sarcoma (ESS) is also rare in the ovary, but when it occurs, has the same morphology as ESS of the uterus (Figure 4.8). Metastatic colorectal, pancreatobiliary, and breast carcinoma are the most common metastatic tumors seen in the ovary. Their touch imprints show similar morphology to the primary tumors (Figure 4.9).

Uterus

Endometrioid carcinoma is the most common malignant tumor in the uterus and accounts for 70% to 80% of all endometrial cancers. It includes well-differentiated (Federation of Gynecology and Obstetrics (FIGO) grade 1), moderately differentiated (FIGO grade 2), and poorly differentiated (FIGO grade 3) carcinoma depending on architecture and cytological features. The touch imprint appearance of endometrioid carcinoma of the uterus significantly varies among tumors with different grades. Touch imprint cytology of grade 1 endometrioid carcinoma resembles that of endometrial hyperplasia with atypia. The specimens are cellular with glandular epithelial cells that are stratified, crowded, and demonstrate loss of normal polarity. The tumor cell nuclei are mildly pleomorphic with mild coarse chromatin and medium-sized nucleoli. Necrosis is absent. Touch imprint cytology of grade 2 endometrioid carcinoma is more cellular with sheets, three-dimensional clusters, and microacini or complex papillae of tumor cells, comprised of cells which show modest eosinophilic cytoplasm, high N:C ratio, crowded enlarged hyperchromatic nuclei, coarse dark chromatin, and conspicuous nucleoli (Figure 4.10). Necrosis and hemosiderin-laden macrophages may be seen in the background. Touch imprint cytology of grade 3 endometrioid carcinoma is variably cellular with a background of necrosis. Tumor cells are mostly single cells with prominent nuclear pleomorphism, hyperchromasia, prominent coarse chromatin, and less glandular differentiation (Figure 4.11). It may be impossible to differentiate grade 3 endometrioid carcinoma from undifferentiated carcinoma.

Serous carcinoma is uncommon in the uterus. When present, it is a high-grade carcinoma with worse prognosis than endometrioid carcinoma. It is considered to represent the prototypical type II endometrial carcinoma.

Touch imprints of this tumor are identical to those seen from serous carcinoma of the ovary. The imprints are cellular with small crowded clusters that may also have large branching papillae, together with abundant individual cells. Cytological atypia depends on the tumor grade. Low-grade serous carcinoma cells usually show less atypia, smaller nuclei, less hyperchromasia, and more cytoplasm. High-grade serous carcinoma cells are hyperchromatic with large nuclei, high N:C ratio, irregular chromatin, and prominent nucleoli (Figure 4.12).

Clear cell carcinoma is rare in the uterus and accounts for only 2% of endometrial carcinomas. It is considered to be a type II endometrial carcinoma. Touch imprints of this tumor resemble those of ovarian clear cell carcinoma. Tumor cells have irregular pleomorphic nuclei, fine chromatin, macronucleoli, and abundant pale/eosinophilic cytoplasm. Metachromatic hyaline cytoplasmic inclusions or extracellular hyaline matrix may be seen (Figure 4.13).

Undifferentiated ovarian carcinoma usually presents with a high stage with a poor prognosis. It can be monomorphic or mixed with a well-differentiated endometrioid carcinoma (dedifferentiated endometrioid carcinoma). Touch imprints yield anaplastic malignant epithelial cells without any differentiation. Tumor cells are usually single with fragile cytoplasm, naked nuclei, and apoptotic debris. Low-grade malignant glandular cells may be seen in dedifferentiated endometrioid carcinoma.

MMMT/carcinosarcoma is a high-grade malignancy of the uterus and is composed of both a malignant mesenchymal component and malignant epithelium, with adenocarcinoma being the most common epithelial component. MMMT is considered to represent a carcinoma that has undergone spindle cell or sarcomatous differentiation. Although MMMT is a biphasic neoplasm with high-grade malignant epithelial and mesenchymal components, a dual malignant cell population is often not appreciated on touch imprint cytology. The cytology usually shows carcinoma (11), and a definitive diagnosis is best made on histologic examination.

Leiomyosarcoma is the most common sarcoma in the uterus and accounts for 1% to 2% of uterine malignancies. Most leiomyosarcomas exhibit spindle- or irregularly shaped cells with marked nuclear pleomorphism, hyperchromasia, and coarse chromatin. Tumor cells with atypical mitoses, multinucleated tumor giant cells, and necrosis may be seen. Epithelioid tumor cells may be seen in epithelioid leiomyosarcoma and myxoid background may be seen in myxoid leiomyosarcoma (Figure 4.14).

ESS is a malignant tumor composed of cells resembling endometrial stromal cells. There are two types; low-grade ESS and high-grade ESS. It is the second most common uterine sarcoma, but only accounts for less than 1% of uterine malignancies. Low-grade ESS cells are small with scant cytoplasm and oval nuclei resembling stromal cells seen in proliferative endometrium. They have minimal cytologic atypia and are usually indistinguishable from normal stromal fragments and cells. High-grade ESS cells exhibit more marked cytologic atypia with hyperchromasia, nuclear pleomorphism, irregular nuclear membrane contours, and increased mitotic figures.

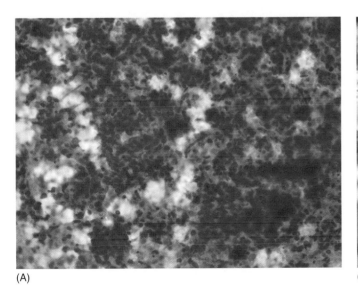
(A)

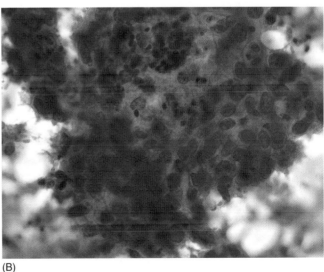
(B)

FIGURE 4.4 High-grade serous carcinoma of the ovary. (A) The touch imprint from this serous carcinoma is hypercellular with crowded clusters (H&E-stained, medium power). (B) Carcinoma cells are hyperchromatic with large nuclei, high N:C ratios, irregular chromatin, and prominent nucleoli (H&E-stained, high power). H&E, hematoxylin and eosin; N:C, nuclear:cytoplasmic.

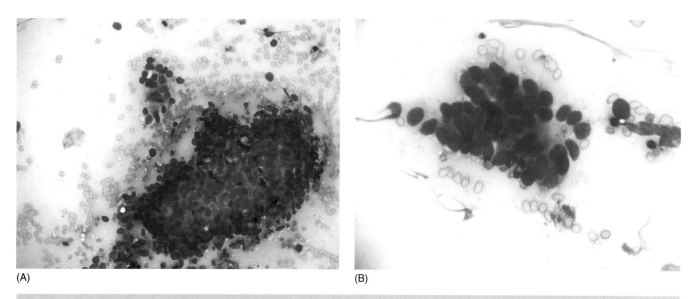

(A)   (B)

FIGURE 4.5 Mucinous carcinoma of the ovary. (A) Touch imprint showing tumor cells arranged in an irregular cluster (DQ, medium power). (B) Tumor cells are shown with a glandular structure. These tumor cells have prominent nuclear pleomorphism (DQ, high power). DQ, Diff-Quik.

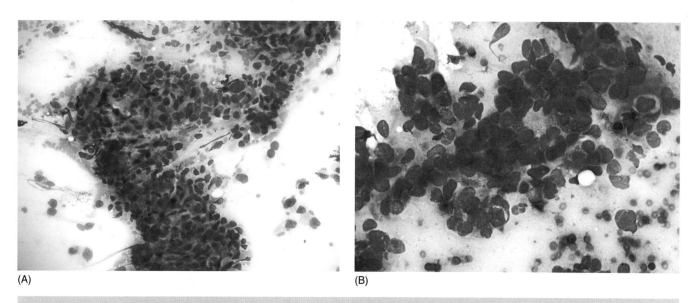

(A)   (B)

FIGURE 4.6 Endometrioid carcinoma of the ovary. (A) This touch imprint is hypercellular with sheets of tumor cells (DQ, medium power). (B) Tumor cells show modest eosinophilic cytoplasm, high N:C ratios, crowded enlarged hyperchromatic nuclei, coarse dark chromatin, and small conspicuous nucleoli. Cilia are absent (DQ, high power). DQ, Diff-Quik; N:C, nuclear:cytoplasmic.

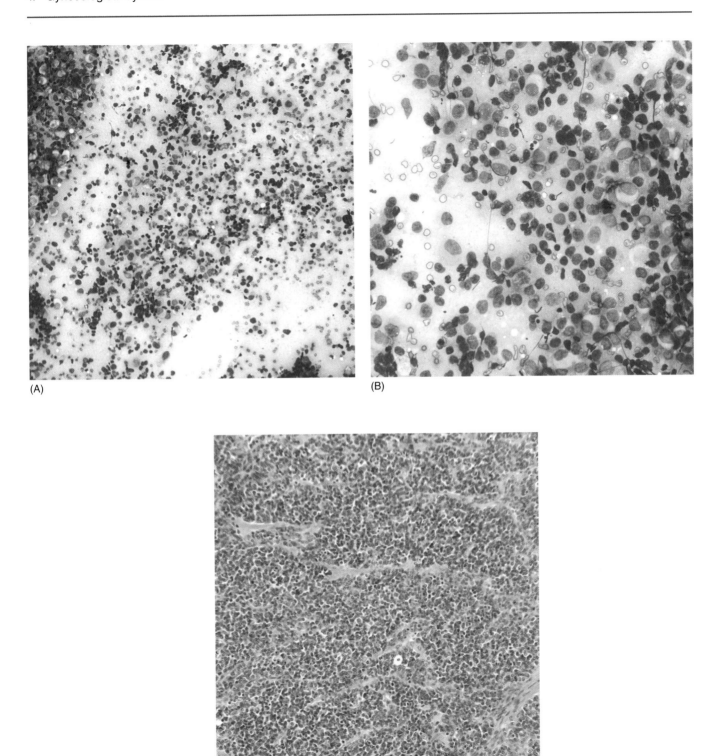

(A)

(B)

(C)

FIGURE 4.7 Small cell carcinoma of the ovary. (A) Touch imprint showing individual small cells (DQ, medium power). (B) Tumor cells have scant cytoplasm, smudged chromatin, and apoptotic bodies (DQ, high power). (C) Histologic section of small cell carcinoma of the ovary (H&E-stained, medium power). DQ, Diff-Quik; H&E, hematoxylin and eosin.

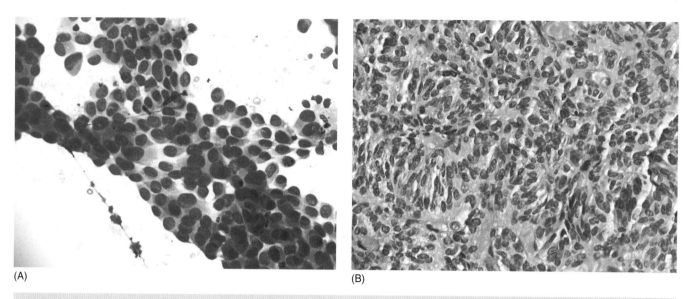

(A)   (B)

FIGURE 4.8 Metastatic high-grade ESS. (A) Touch imprint showing stromal sarcoma cells with marked cytologic atypia, hyperchromasia, nuclear pleomorphism, and irregular nuclear membrane contours (DQ, high power). (B) Histologic section of metastatic high-grade ESS (H&E-stained, high power). DQ, Diff-Quik; ESS, endometrial stromal sarcoma; H&E, hematoxylin and eosin.

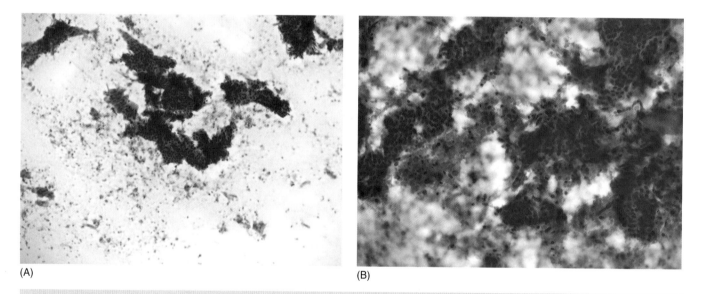

(A)   (B)

FIGURE 4.9 Metastatic colonic adenocarcinoma to the ovary. (A) Touch imprint showing clusters of glandular tumor cells in a necrotic background (H&E-stained, low power). (B) Tumor cells are demonstrated with a glandular architecture and show hyperchromatic nuclei, irregular nuclear membranes, and coarse chromatin in a background of necrosis (H&E-stained, medium power). H&E, hematoxylin and eosin.

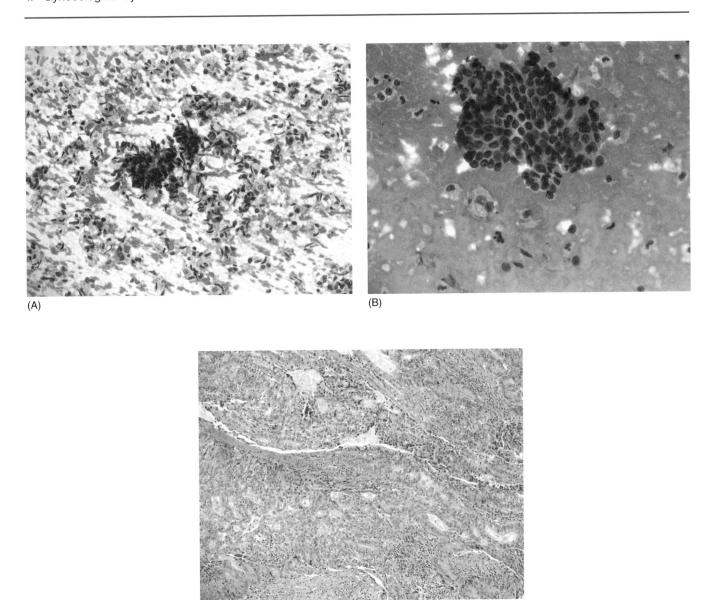

(A)

(B)

(C)

FIGURE 4.10 Endometrial endometrioid carcinoma, FIGO grade 2. (A and B) Touch imprints showing single cells and clusters of tumor cells, which show modest eosinophilic cytoplasm, high N:C ratio, crowded enlarged hyperchromatic nuclei, coarse dark chromatin, and conspicuous nucleoli (H&E-stained, medium and high power). (C) Histologic section of this FIGO grade 2 endometrioid carcinoma (H&E-stained, low power). FIGO, Federation of Gynecology and Obstetrics; H&E, hematoxylin and eosin; N:C, nuclear:cytoplasmic.

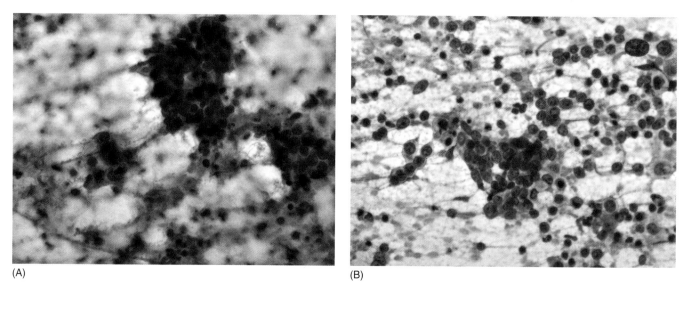

(A)   (B)

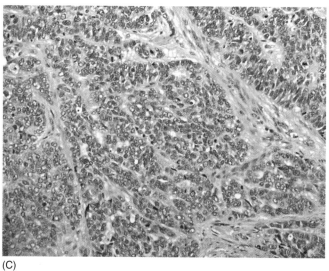

(C)

FIGURE 4.11 Endometrial endometrioid carcinoma, FIGO grade 3. (A and B) Touch imprints showing tumor cells in a background of necrosis. The tumor cells show prominent nuclear pleomorphism, hyperchromasia, prominent coarse chromatin, and no obvious glandular differentiation (H&E-stained, medium and high power). (C) Histologic section of the corresponding FIGO grade 3 endometrioid carcinoma of the uterus (H&E-stained, medium power). FIGO, Federation of Gynecology and Obstetrics; H&E, hematoxylin and eosin.

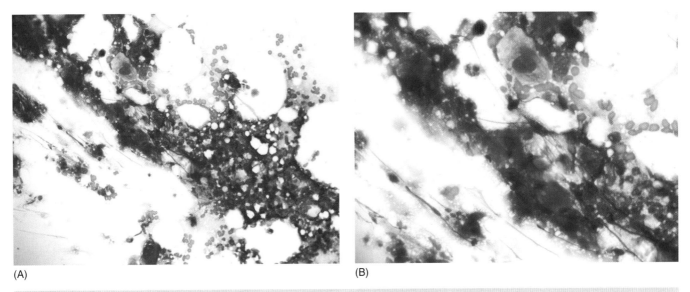

FIGURE 4.12 Serous carcinoma of the uterus. (A and B) Touch imprints showing mostly sparse individual cells with large nuclei, high N:C ratio, irregular chromatin, and prominent nucleoli (DQ, medium & high power). DQ, Diff-Quik; N:C, nuclear:cytoplasmic.

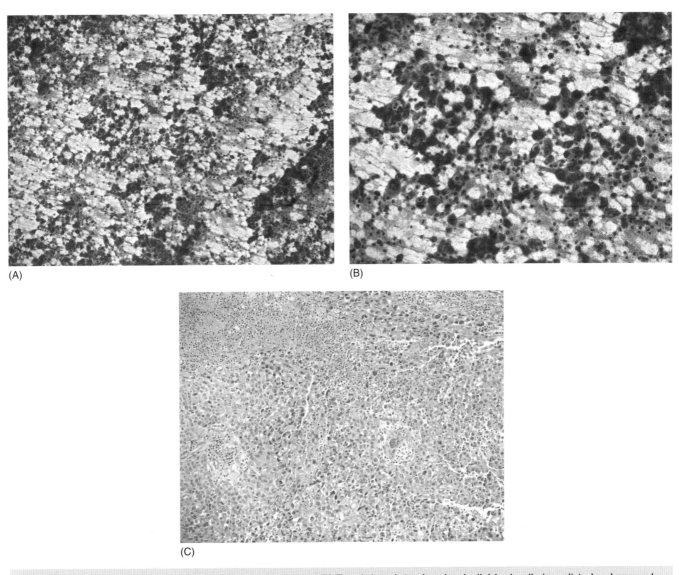

FIGURE 4.13 Clear cell carcinoma of the uterus. (A and B) Touch imprints showing individual cells in a dirty background. Tumor cells have irregular pleomorphic nuclei, fine chromatin, macronucleoli, and abundant pale/eosinophilic cytoplasm (H&E-stained, medium and high power). (C) Histologic section of this clear cell carcinoma (H&E-stained, low power). H&E, hematoxylin and eosin.

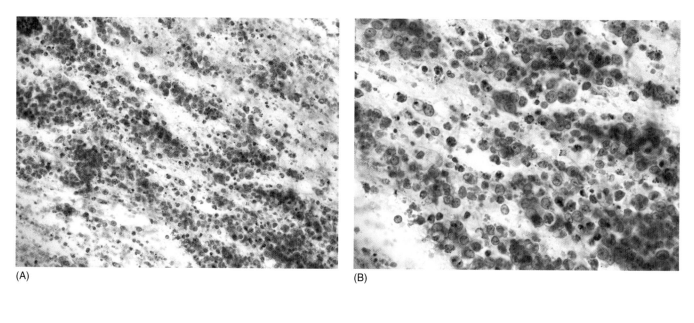

(A)   (B)

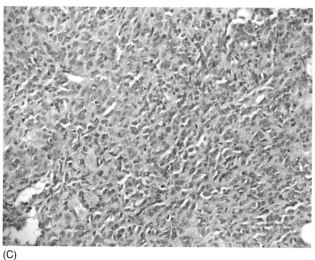

(C)

FIGURE 4.14   High-grade sarcoma of the uterus. (A and B) Touch imprints are cellular with many single sarcoma cells that exhibit marked cytologic atypia with hyperchromasia, nuclear pleomorphism, and irregular nuclear membrane contours (H&E-stained, medium and high power). (C) Histologic section of high-grade sarcoma without apparent differentiation (H&E-stained, medium power). H&E, hematoxylin and eosin.

REFERENCES

1. DeMay RM. *The* Art and Science of Cytopathology. Chicago, IL: ASCP Press; 2012.

2. Shahid M, Zaheer S, Mubeen A, et al. The role of intraoperative cytology in the diagnostic evaluation of ovarian neoplasms. Acta Cytol. 2012;56:467-473.

3. Alvarez Santín C, Sica A, Melesi S, et al. Contribution of intraoperative cytology to the diagnosis of ovarian lesions. Acta Cytol. 2011;55:85-91.

4. Volmar KE, Herman CM, Creager AJ. Fine-needle aspiration cytology of endometrioid adenofibroma of the ovary. Diagn Cytopathol. 2004;31:38-42.

5. Vrdoljak-Mozetic D, Stanković T, Krasević M, et al. Intraoperative cytology of clear cell carcinoma of the ovary. Cytopathology. 2006;17:390-395.

6. Kuwashima Y, Uehara T, Kurosumi M, et al.. Cytological distinction between clear cell carcinoma and yolk sac tumor of the ovary. Eur J Gynaecol Oncol. 1996;17:345-350.

7. Singh RI, Rosen L, Reddy VB, et al. Intraoperative imprint cytology of ovarian transitional cell (Brenner) tumors: a retrospective study. Diagn Cytopathol. 2014;42:660-663.

8. Deb P, Malik A, Sinha KK. Intraoperative scrape cytology: adult granulosa cell tumor of ovary. J Cytol. October 2011;28:207-209.

9. Ali S, Gattuso P, Howard A, et al. Adult granulosa cell tumor of the ovary: fine-needle-aspiration cytology of 10 cases and review of literature. *Diagn Cytopathol*. 2008;36:297-302.

10. Shintaku M, Sangawa A, Matsumoto T, Ohtsuka K. Juvenile granulosa cell tumor of the ovary: imprint cytology findings. *Acta Cytol*. 2002;46:1173-1175.

11. Ventura KC, Filipowicz EA, Molina CP, et al. Diagnosis of recurrent uterine carcinosarcoma by fine-needle aspiration cytology: report of a case. *Diagn Cytopathol*. 2000;23:108-113.

CHAPTER 5

Respiratory System

Sara E. Monaco

INTRODUCTION

The respiratory system has become a common source of biopsy specimens given the high incidence of lung carcinomas, and the need to perform multiple ancillary studies on these specimens for theranostic purposes (Table 5.1) (1). In addition, there is a wide spectrum of infectious and nonneoplastic entities that can give rise to lesions or masses in the respiratory system, and pathological sampling is critical in order to exclude malignancy (Table 5.2). There

TABLE 5.1 Types of Biopsy Specimens Seen in the Respiratory System

- Endobronchial biopsy
- CT-guided or US-guided core needle biopsy
- Electromagnetic navigational (superdimensional) bronchoscopy (ENB)-guided biopsy
- Endobronchial ultrasound (EBUS)-guided procore biopsy
- Mediastinoscopy lymph node biopsies

TABLE 5.2 Differential Diagnosis for Lesions in the Respiratory System

Benign
- Reactive bronchial epithelial cells
- Histiocytic lesions (e.g., foamy macrophages, granulomatous inflammation)
- Inflammatory lesions (e.g., abscess)

Neoplasm (Benign and Malignant)
- Pulmonary hamartoma
- Sclerosing hemangioma
- Papillomas
- Salivary gland type tumor (SGTT)
- Clear cell tumors
- Langerhans cell histiocytosis
- Lymphoma and other lymphoproliferative lesions
- Neuroendocrine tumors (e.g., carcinoid, small cell carcinoma)
- Metastatic tumor (e.g., carcinoma, melanoma, sarcoma)
- Primary lung carcinoma
- Mesenchymal tumors (e.g., sarcoma)
- Malignant melanoma

are also a variety of different approaches to sample these masses, from exfoliative cytology to aspiration cytology and small needle biopsies (2). This chapter gives an overview of the normal and neoplastic entities that can be seen in touch imprints and core needle biopsies from respiratory specimens.

NORMAL

The main normal elements to consider in specimens are benign bronchial epithelium, reactive pneumocytes, alveolar macrophages, epithelioid histiocytes, and inflammatory cells. These benign specimens may show a spectrum of atypia, without a discrete second or foreign population present with marked pleomorphism.

Bronchial Epithelial Cells

Bronchial epithelial cells tend to show columnar morphology with an apical terminal bar and cilia, in addition to a basally located, round nucleus (Figures 5.1 and 5.2). The overall nuclear-to-cytoplasmic ratio is low. These cells are typically seen in small strips or as single cells and the presence of cilia or terminal bars usually make them easy to identify and exclude malignancy. However, in touch preparations that are thick, there can be overlap of the cell clusters and a lack of readily identifiable cilia. Cilia can usually be seen on one edge of such cell groups when using fine focus and the nuclei will be similar to the bronchial cells in the background (Figure 5.2). Occasionally the bronchial cells will appear as multinucleated or syncytial cells, which may be due to manipulation of the cells during touch preparation or in the acquisition of the biopsy (3). Bronchial cells can undergo reactive changes with more prominent nucleoli, which may make them difficult to differentiate from a well-differentiated adenocarcinoma (ADC); however, these reactive cells will show a spectrum of changes and will not have a large or irregular nucleolus. These cells can also show metaplastic changes, like goblet cell metaplasia (Figure 5.1C). In goblet cell metaplasia, the cells will have large apical vacuoles, occasionally cilia will be seen, and the nuclei will not show atypia. These cells are also seen in cohesive groups intermixed with ciliated bronchial epithelial cells. The pitfall is to not misinterpret these cells as evidence of a signet ring type ADC, which should have more atypia, targetoid mucin droplets within the vacuoles, more discohesion, and a lack of cilia. A lack of bronchial cells, granulomas, or tumor cells on a touch imprint may indicate that the biopsy is not from the lesion of interest, and additional sampling should be performed. When sampling lung lesions via CT or ultrasound-guidance, radiologists may sample surrounding soft tissue elements, as opposed to the lesion itself, and this would be a nondiagnostic biopsy (Figure 5.3).

Alveolar Macrophages

Alveolar macrophages appear as discohesive cells with low nuclear-to-cytoplasmic ratios, moderate-to-abundant vacuolated cytoplasm, and oval-to-reniform nuclei. Foamy histiocytes with multiple small cytoplasmic vacuoles can be seen with lipoid pneumonia, postobstructive changes, exogenous material (e.g., mineral oil ingestion), or infection (e.g., atypical mycobacteria) (Figure 5.4). Foamy macrophages can also be seen in association with mucinous neoplasms, so called muciphages, but in this context should also be seen with vacuolated neoplastic cells and a thick mucinous background. Histiocytes can also have black finely granular anthracotic pigment, hemosiderin, or other debris in them. On touch imprints, there can be more clustering of histiocytes than appreciated on smears, and thus, the nuclear features are extremely important to exclude malignancy. When histiocytes get activated, they can also cluster and have more prominent nucleoli, imparting an "epithelioid appearance," which can be seen in granulomas (Figures 5.5–5.7). These epithelioid histiocytes should not be confused with ADC, and in some cases, immunostains on the corresponding biopsy can help to make this distinction given that histiocytes are positive for CD68, while negative for cytokeratin. Necrotizing granulomas can be particularly challenging given that the necrotic background and epithelioid histiocytes can be overcalled as malignant (Figure 5.5). Rheumatoid nodules can mimic necrotizing granulomas given the presence of multinucleated giant cells and debris (Figure 5.7),

but should have degenerated, elongated, carrot-type cells as well (4). When granulomatous inflammation is identified on a touch imprint, this is a good opportunity to collect material for microbial cultures in order to exclude mycobacterial or fungal infection.

Inflammatory Cells and Infection

Inflammatory cells, other than histiocytes (e.g., neutrophils, lymphocytes), can also be seen, and should be mentioned when present in a touch preparation. If an abundance of neutrophils are present, often with inflammatory debris, this likely represents an abscess (Figure 5.8). These types of core biopsies can fall apart easily and be difficult to remove from the slide after touch preparation. Thus, a gentle touch is suggested, as the majority of material should be preserved for microbial cultures and special stains. In this scenario, dedicated cores that are untouched should strongly be recommended to increase the utility of ancillary studies. Touch preparations on lymphocyte-rich lesions are particularly helpful to recognize the need for flow cytometry if a lymphoproliferative disorder is in the differential diagnosis. Furthermore, plasma cells can be readily identifiable on Diff-Quik stained material by their perinuclear halo, eccentrically located nucleus, and deep basophilic cytoplasm, which are often more difficult to identify on H&E-stained material. Thus, touch preparations for lung lesions with inflammatory cells are very helpful.

A variety of infections could be seen in the respiratory system, including mycobacterial and fungal infections. *Mycobacterium tuberculosis* will appear as necrotizing granulomatous inflammation and rare organisms may be identified with acid fast bacillus (AFB) staining or later from microbial cultures (Figure 5.5). Fungal infections show yeast or hyphal elements, which can be highlighted with a Grocott-Gomori's methenamine silver (GMS) stain (Figures 5.9 and 5.10). Touch imprint is valuable in cases suspicious for infection because the specimen can be triaged appropriately upfront for cultures and special stains. Some microorganisms may be identifiable at the time of onsite evaluation (e.g., negative staining of mycobacteria with a Diff-Quik stain). This is especially important, as some organisms are not readily identifiable on H&E-stained sections of the core biopsy, and the growth of these organisms can be slow if microbial cultures are relied upon alone.

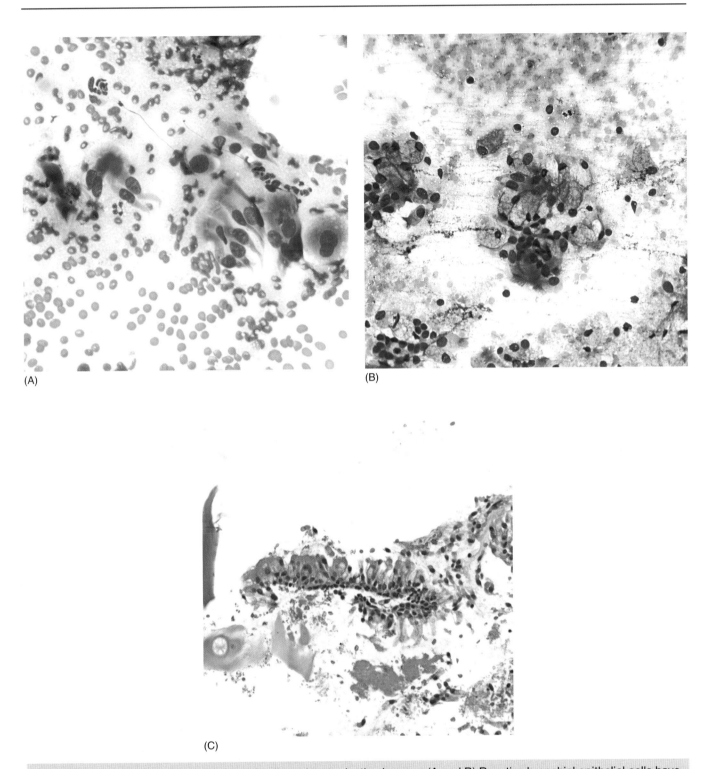

(A)

(B)

(C)

FIGURE 5.1 Reactive bronchial epithelial cells and metaplastic changes. (A and B) Reactive bronchial epithelial cells have a characteristic columnar shape, cilia, and terminal bars. (C) Occasionally, there will be evidence of goblet cell metaplasia, intermixed with reactive bronchial epithelial cells, which should not be over-interpreted as signet ring type ADC. ((A) and (B) DQ-stained TP, high power; (C) H&E-stained core, high power.) DQ, Diff-Quik; H&E, hematoxylin and eosin; TP, touch preparation.

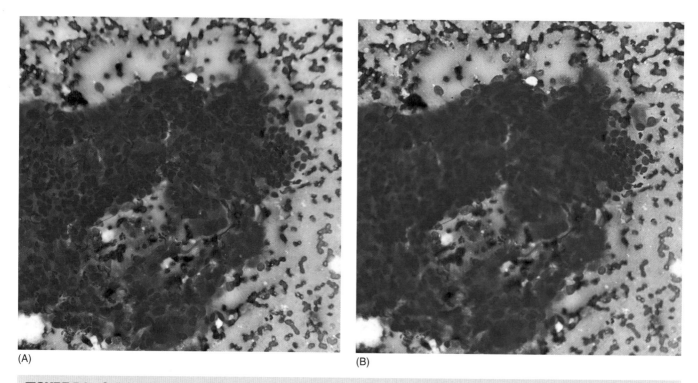

(A)   (B)

FIGURE 5.2 Cellular clusters of reactive bronchial epithelial cells. Using the fine focus to focus up and down in cellular, thick areas can highlight important features, such as cilia, as seen in this case of reactive bronchial epithelial cells. ((A) and (B) DQ-stained TP, high power.) DQ, Diff-Quik; TP, touch preparation.

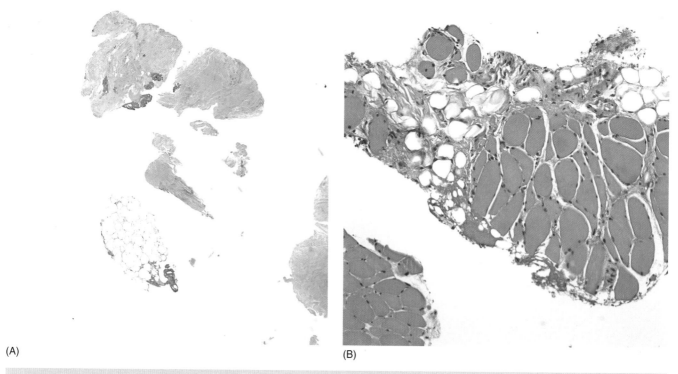

(A)   (B)

FIGURE 5.3 Normal soft tissue elements in nondiagnostic biopsies. More tissue does not always mean better tissue. In these two cases, the core biopsies reveal benign soft tissue elements, including fibrous tissue, adipose tissue, and skeletal muscle. ((A) and (B) H&E-stained core, low & medium power.) H&E, hematoxylin and eosin.

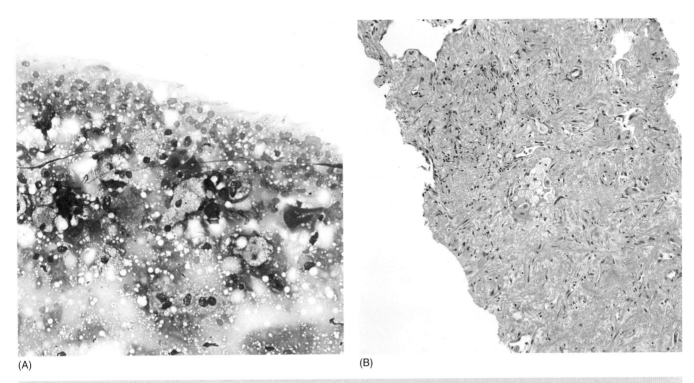

(A)

(B)

FIGURE 5.4 Foamy macrophages. Macrophages with multiple small, clear vacuoles can be seen with lipoid pneumonia, changes from obstruction, and exogenous factors (e.g., Mineral oil). ((A) DQ-stained TP, high power; (B) H&E-stained core, medium power.) DQ, Diff-Quik; H&E, hematoxylin and eosin; TP, touch preparation.

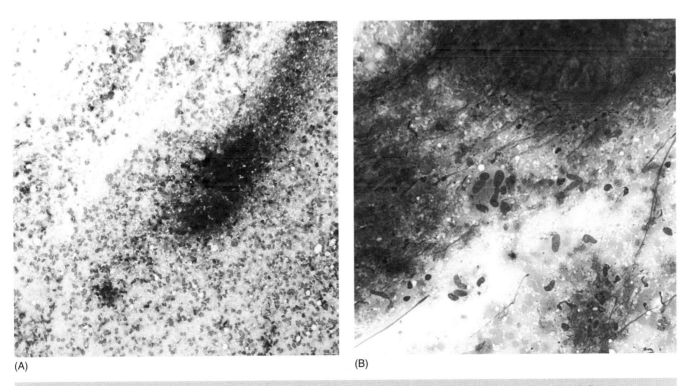

(A)

(B)

FIGURE 5.5 Necrotic granulomas. (A) Necrotizing granulomas will typically show acute inflammatory or noninflammatory granular debris on TP, which can mimic necrosis. It is important to ask the physician to target more peripheral areas in these scenarios. (B) If you look closely, most cases will have multinucleated giant cells. (*continued*)

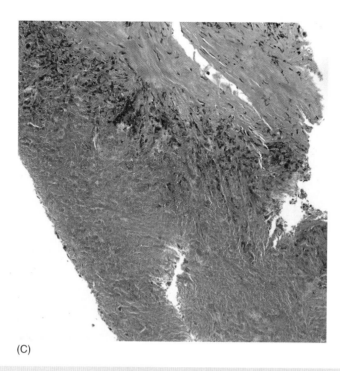

(C)

FIGURE 5.5 (*continued*) (C) On core biopsy, zonation is more apparent with viable epithelioid and multinucleated histiocytes on the periphery with central necrosis. ((A) and (B) DQ-stained TP, high power; (C) H&E-stained core, medium power.) DQ, Diff-Quik; H&E, hematoxylin and eosin; TP, touch preparation.

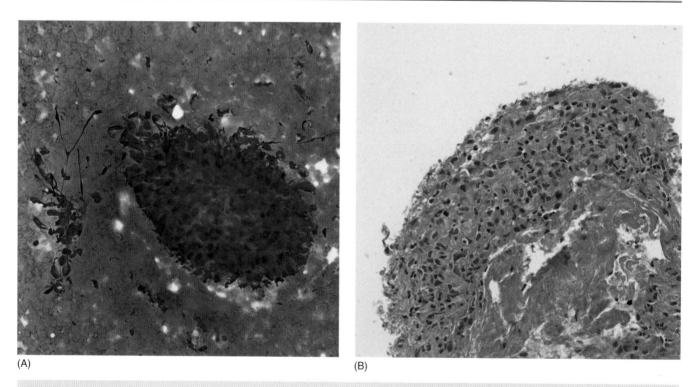

(A)   (B)

FIGURE 5.6 Cellular granulomas. (A) Cellular granulomas can appear similar to non-small cell carcinomas, but careful examination will usually reveal associated small lymphocytes and oval-to-reniform nuclei with occasional prominent nucleoli. (B) In the core biopsy these tend to look very pink because of the abundant cytoplasm; however, this feature can be difficult to recognize on thick touch preparations where nuclear and cytoplasmic detail are not as easily discerned. ((A) DQ-stained TP, high power; (B) H&E-stained core, high power.) DQ, Diff-Quik; H&E, hematoxylin and eosin; TP, touch preparation.

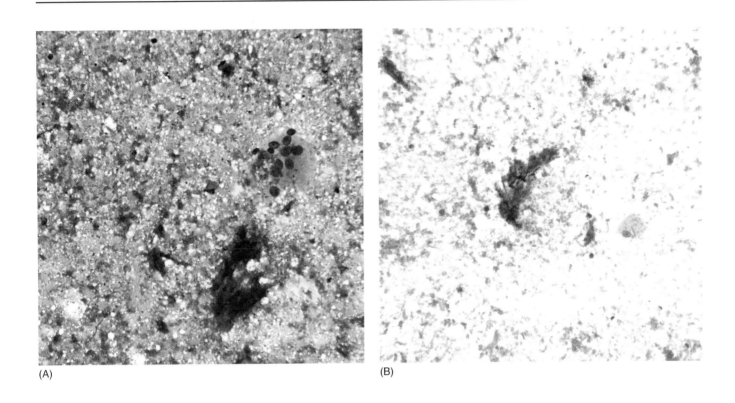

(A)

(B)

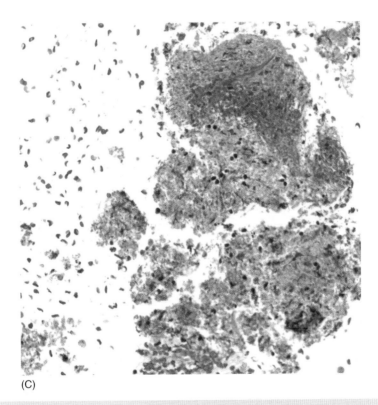

(C)

FIGURE 5.7 Rheumatoid nodule. The cytology shows granular debris with scattered macrophages, multinucleated giant cells, and degenerating cells, in a patient with long standing rheumatoid arthritis. ((A) DQ-stained TP, high power; (B) Pap-stained smear, high power; (C) H&E-stained core, high power.) DQ, Diff-Quik; H&E, hematoxylin and eosin; TP, touch preparation.

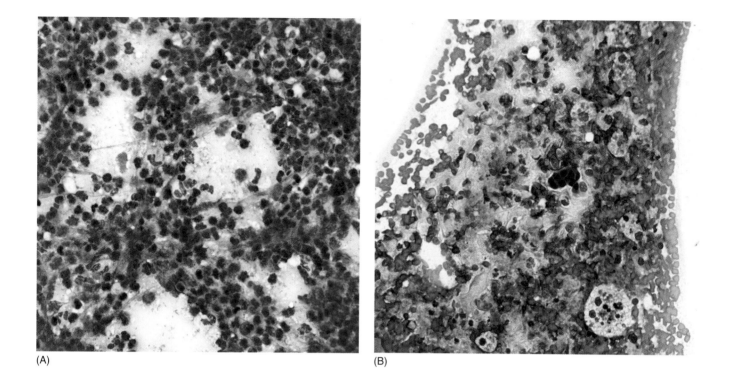

(A)   (B)

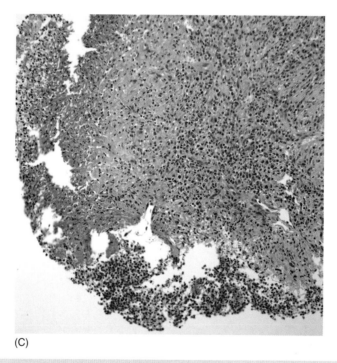

(C)

FIGURE 5.8 Lung abscess. (A) The TP shows purulent material with numerous neutrophils and inflammatory debris. (B) In addition, some TPs may highlight more of the chronic and histiocytic inflammatory component. (C) The core biopsy highlights the wall of an abscess showing fibrinopurulent material and fibrous tissue with dense chronic inflammation. ((A) and (B) DQ-stained TP, high power; (C) H&E-stained core, medium power.) DQ, Diff-Quik; H&E, hematoxylin and eosin; TP, touch preparation.

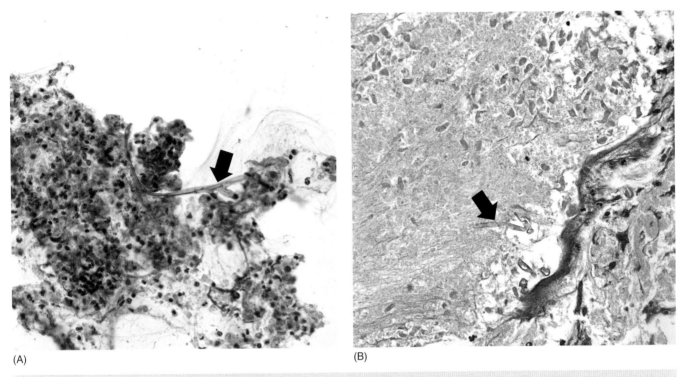

(A)

(B)

FIGURE 5.9 Mucormycosis infection in the lung. Fungal hyphal elements are identified, which appear as wide nonseptate hyphae (arrow) within an inflammatory background mixed with debris. ((A) Pap-stained smear, high power; (B) H&E-stained core, high power.) H&E, hematoxylin and eosin.

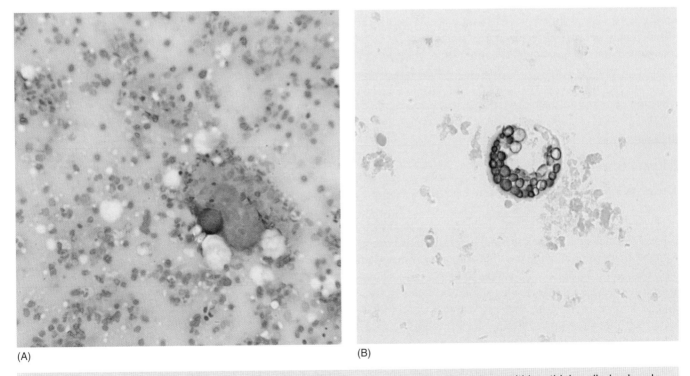

(A)

(B)

FIGURE 5.10 Coccidiomycosis infection in the lung. (A) Small cystic endospores are seen within a thick walled spherule. (B) These small cysts are highlighted on the Grocott-Gomori's methanamine silver (GMS) stain. ((A) H&E-stained TP, high power; (B) Grocott stain, high power.) H&E, hematoxylin and eosin; TP, touch preparation.

BENIGN ENTITIES

Reactive Changes

Reactive changes can be seen in the lung due to inflammation, infection, treatment (e.g., chemotherapy and radiation), and other conditions (Figures 5.11 and 5.12). The key finding is a lack of an obvious second or "foreign" population, in addition to the presence of cilia, cytoplasmic vacuolization, and an abundance of cytoplasm (so that the nuclear-to-cytoplasmic ratio is not increased). These findings favor a reactive process. On Romanowsky-stained touch imprints, the increase in nuclear size with air-drying can make reactive processes look more concerning, and thus, a conservative approach is suggested if the findings do not clearly look malignant, in order to avoid overcalling malignancy onsite. Furthermore, benign and reactive processes tend to have quantitatively less cells with atypia. In general, if there is pronounced inflammation, then one should also increase the threshold for committing to malignancy and rule out the possibility of an infectious or reactive process first.

Radiation Type Changes

Changes seen in the lung after radiation include hyalinized interstitial fibrosis, epithelial atypia, and histiocytic infiltration (Figures 5.11 and 5.12). The histiocytes can appear foamy. Given the hyalinized fibrosis, these lesions may be difficult to aspirate with fine needle aspiration (FNA), and are hence best sampled with a core biopsy. Touch imprints may not be very cellular, which is one clue favoring the absence of a neoplasm. Slight atypia should not be over-interpreted as malignancy. Radiation type changes are known to cause nuclear enlargement, but there is also a simultaneous increase in two-tone or vacuolated cytoplasm, resulting in an overall low nuclear-to-cytoplasmic ratio.

Neoplasms

Salivary Gland Type Tumors

There are a variety of salivary gland type tumors (SGTT) that can arise from the bronchial glands to form a primary lung mass, or manifest in the lungs as a metastatic tumor from a head and neck salivary gland primary tumor. Most of these tumors will have a biphasic appearance with metachromatic background stromal material and bland-appearing epithelioid cells, which should be a clue to their diagnosis given that most lung carcinomas are not associated with metachromatic stromal material (Figure 5.13). The epithelioid cells frequently have scant cytoplasm, which imparts a basaloid appearance and may mimic small cell carcinoma on a touch imprint. However, these SGTTs lack the pleomorphism, paranuclear blue bodies, and apoptotic debris that are seen with small cell carcinoma. The biphasic-appearing SGTTs in the lung include adenoid cystic carcinoma, pleomorphic adenoma, basal cell neoplasms,

and epithelial-myoepithelial carcinomas. Core biopsies can be very helpful in these cases to determine architecture and for performing immunostains to confirm the presence of myoepithelial cells (p63, S100) and/or epithelial cells (cytokeratin, epithelial membrane antigen). A mucoepidermoid carcinoma of the lung can mimic a primary squamous cell carcinoma (SqCC), ADC, or adenosquamous cell carcinoma. In these tumors, there are typically clusters of squamoid type cells with interspersed mucin vacuoles. The pitfall would be to misinterpret these SGTTs as SqCCs given the positivity for p63 and/or p40. Thus, careful review of the morphology and use of additional stains (mucicarmine and myoepithelial markers) is critical.

Solitary Fibrous Tumor

Solitary fibrous tumors (SFTs) are spindle cell tumors that may be difficult to aspirate, and thus, core biopsy may be a useful way to obtain diagnostic material for confirmatory ancillary studies. On touch preparations, these tumors appear as discohesive and cohesive bland spindle cells (Figure 5.14). They can appear cohesive on imprints given the collagenous stroma. A careful search for malignant features is also important such as necrosis, mitoses, and marked pleomorphism. Confirmatory immunostains include CD34, CD99, and bcl2. In addition, nuclear STAT6 expression has been shown to be a specific marker for SFT (5). The spindled tumor cells are negative for cytokeratin, S100, and desmin.

Pulmonary Hamartoma

Hamartomas in the lung appear as stable, slow growing peripheral lung masses that are rounded (ie, peripheral coin lesions). These have been shown to be true neoplasms given the presence of clonal rearrangements of chromosome 6p, involving the HMGI(Y) gene. These tumors have a variable appearance that includes a mixture of cartilaginous islands, immature chondromyxoid material, fat, and benign epithelial cells. These features can mimic a SGTT; however, there are key radiological differences that should be considered, including the fact that hamartomas will typically be peripheral in location, show slow or no growth over an extended time period, and lack significant atypia or basaloid cells. A core biopsy or touch imprint showing cartilaginous fragments with true chondrocytes is helpful, in conjunction with the appropriate clinical-radiological findings.

Neuroendocrine Neoplasms

Neuroendocrine tumors of well to moderate differentiation (e.g., typical and atypical carcinoid tumors) will show bland-appearing plasmacytoid cells with inconspicuous nucleoli (Figure 5.15). In contrast to small cell or large cell neuroendocrine carcinomas (LCNECs), these lower-grade tumors tend to have transgressing vessels, more plasmacytoid features, less pleomorphism, and less necrosis or apoptosis. Usually, these tumors are easy to aspirate, resulting in less of a need for a core biopsy. However, when seen in core biopsies compared to FNA smears, they may exhibit more of a nested appearance with fine

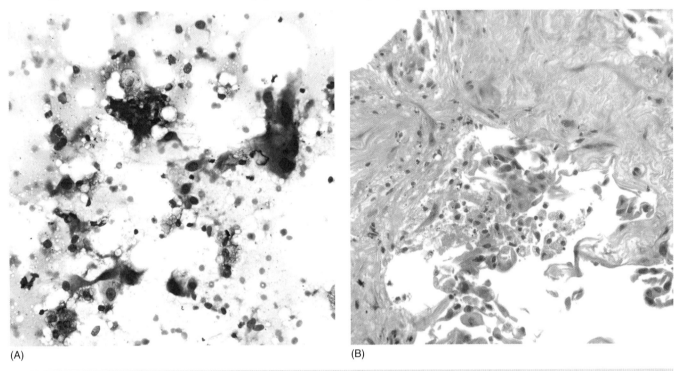

(A)

(B)

FIGURE 5.11 Radiation change. Radiation change should not be misinterpreted as malignancy. The key features are a lack of a definitive foreign tumor cell population, presence of nuclear and cytoplasmic enlargement (low nuclear-to-cytoplasmic ratio), and cytoplasmic vacuolization and stretching. ((A) DQ-stained TP, high power; (B) H&E-stained core, high power.) DQ, Diff-Quik; H&E, hematoxylin and eosin; TP, touch preparation.

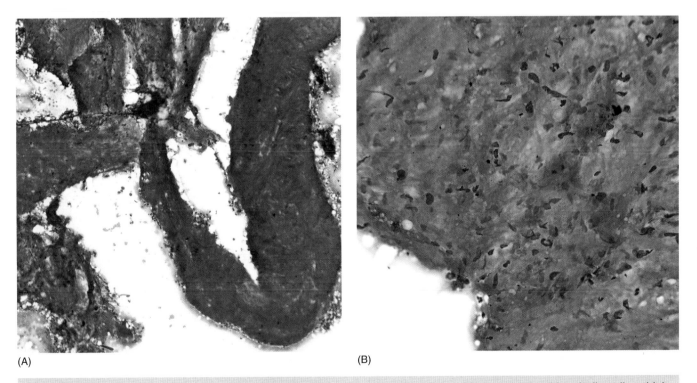

(A)

(B)

FIGURE 5.12 Radiation fibrosis. This case of radiation fibrosis shows fragments of fibrous tissue with spindle cells, which on subsequent core biopsy looks relatively hypocellular and hyalinized, with particular accentuation of hyalinized fibrosis around blood vessels. ((A) and (B) DQ-stained TP, low & high power; (continued)

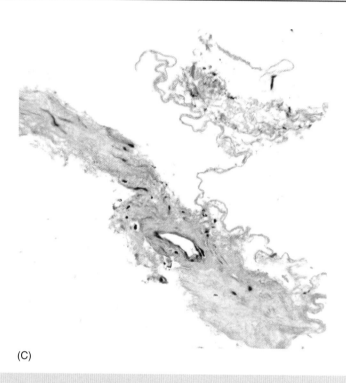

(C)

FIGURE 5.13   *(continued)* (C) H&E-stained core, high power.) DQ, Diff-Quik; H&E, hematoxylin and eosin; TP, touch preparation.

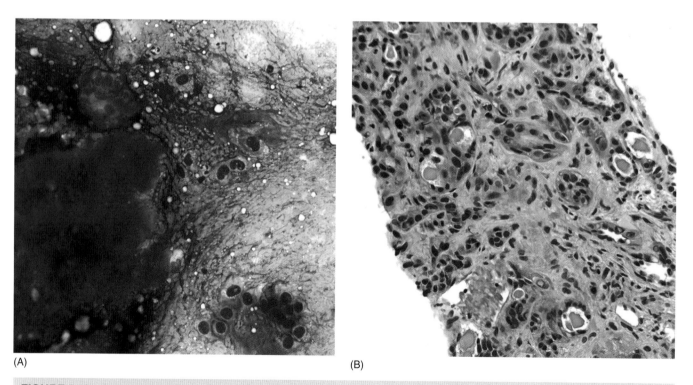

(A)   (B)

FIGURE 5.13   Salivary gland type tumor. (A) Cellular myxoid material with discohesive cells and clusters of cells are seen on the touch preparation. (B) On the core biopsy, there are gland-like cell clusters with eosinophilic material in the lumens within a cellular myxoid background containing myoepithelial cells. *(continued)*

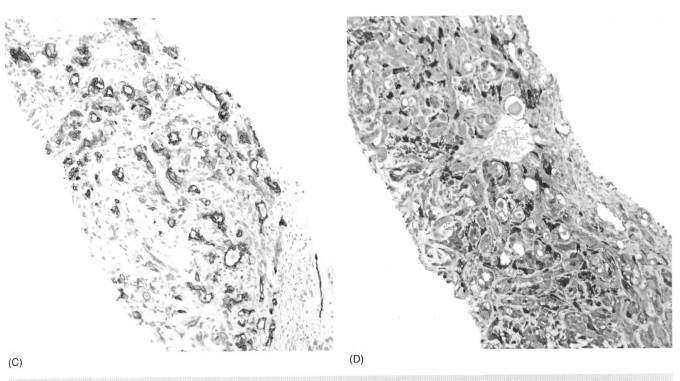

(C)

(D)

FIGURE 5.13 (*continued*) (C) The cytokeratin and (D) S100 stains highlight the epithelial and myoepithelial components. ((A) DQ-stained TP, high power; (B) H&E-stained core, high power; (C) Cytokeratin AE1/AE3 immunostain; (D) S100 immunostain.) DQ, Diff-Quik; H&E, hematoxylin and eosin; TP, touch preparation.

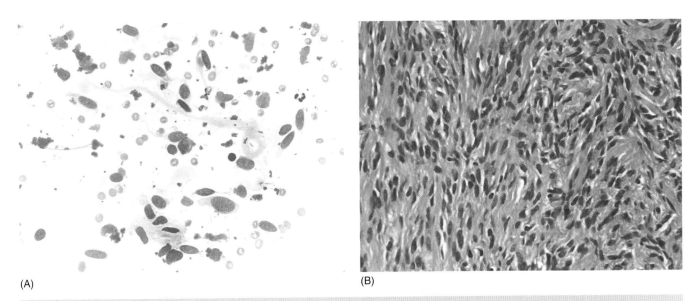

(A)

(B)

FIGURE 5.14 Solitary fibrous tumor. (A) The TPs show bland-appearing, plump spindle cells with scant cytoplasm and stripped oval nuclei. Contaminating ultrasound gel can be seen as scattered particulate matter in this TP. (B) The core biopsy shows a cellular spindle cell neoplasm with short fascicles. (*continued*)

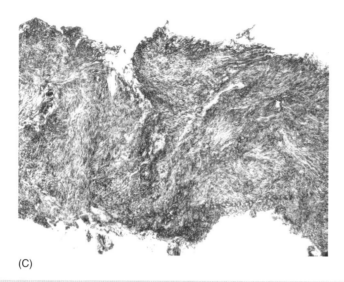

(C)

FIGURE 5.14 *(continued)* (C) The tumor cells are positive for CD34. ((A) DQ-stained TP, high power; (B) H&E-stained core, high power; (C) CD34 immunostain.) DQ, Diff-Quik; H&E, hematoxylin and eosin; TP, touch preparation.

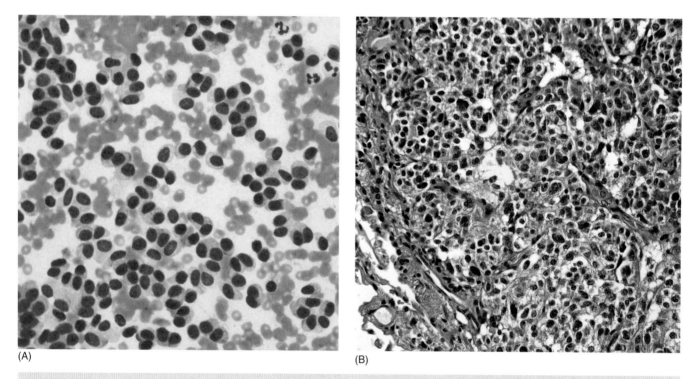

(A)   (B)

FIGURE 5.15 Carcinoid tumor (well-differentiated neuroendocrine tumor). (A) On touch imprints, well-differentiated neuroendocrine tumors show plasmacytoid features, granular cytoplasm, and nuclear monotony in vague, loosely cohesive groups. (B) On the core biopsy, there is a nested appearance to the tumor with fine blood vessels in between. ((A) DQ-stained TP, high power; (B) H&E-stained core, high power.) DQ, Diff-Quik; H&E, hematoxylin and eosin; TP, touch preparation.

interspersed blood vessels. Carcinoid tumors, especially those in the periphery of the lung, can also show spindle cell features, and be in the differential diagnosis of a SFT. Confirmatory immunostains to support neuroendocrine differentiation (e.g., synaptophysin, chromogranin) and low-moderate Ki67 (typically below 20%) are important.

MALIGNANT ENTITIES

Malignant lung tumors are predominantly primary lung carcinomas; however, mesenchymal tumors, lymphoproliferative disorders, and metastatic tumors can also occur. Given that lung carcinoma is the most common cause of cancer-related deaths, there has been a great deal of research on subtyping and classifying these tumors for optimal treatment. The classification now goes beyond simply stating what histological type of carcinoma is present, but further defining the exact subtype and molecular profile of these tumors. Table 5.3 illustrates the lung classification system for malignancies proposed by the International Association for the Study of Lung Cancer (IASLC)/American Thoracic Society (ATS)/European Respiratory Society (ERS), which was specifically proposed for small biopsies and cytology specimens (Table 5.3) (6–9). This highlights the significance of

TABLE 5.3 Terminology for Small Biopsy Diagnoses of Lung Cancer based on the IASLC/ATS/ERS Classification

IASLC/ATS/ERS Classification of Lung Carcinoma

Adenocarcinoma (ADC)
  ADC, describe all morphological patterns identified
  ADC with lepidic pattern (only if pure)
  Mucinous ADC with lepidic pattern (only if pure)
  Invasive Mucinous ADC
  ADC with fetal features
  ADC with colloid features
  ADC with enteric features
  NSCLC, favor ADC
Squamous cell carcinoma (SqCC)
  SqCC (can mention if keratinizing, non-keratinizing or basaloid
    features are identified)
  NSCLC, favor SqCC
Non-small cell carcinoma, not otherwise specified
**Non-small cell carcinoma with neuroendocrine morphology and
  positive neuroendocrine immunostains, possible large cell
  neuroendocrine carcinoma**
**Non-small cell carcinoma with neuroendocrine morphology
  (neuroendocrine immunohistochemical markers fail to
  demonstrate neuroendocrine differentiation)**
**Non-small cell carcinoma with spindle and/or giant cell
  carcinoma (mention if component of adenocarcinoma or
  squamous cell carcinoma are identified)**
Small cell neuroendocrine carcinoma

Source: From Ref. (2).

histological subtyping of non-small cell carcinoma and provides standardized terminology for diagnoses in small specimens (6).

Adenocarcinoma

ADC is part of the non-small cell lung carcinomas, and a great deal of research has been done on these tumors resulting in numerous molecular genetic abnormalities that have therapeutic or prognostic significance (10). The most recent guidelines released by the College of American Pathologists (CAP), IASLC, and Association for Molecular Pathology (AMP) in 2013, recommend testing for at least *EGFR* and *ALK* in pulmonary ADCs (1). However, most academic medical centers are also testing for additional mutations, such as *KRAS*, *PI3K*, and *BRAF* (Table 5.4).

Touch imprints of well-to-moderately differentiated ADCs of the lung usually show cellular two-dimensional clusters with acinar (glandular) arrangement, prominent nucleoli, and glassy-to-vacuolated cytoplasm (Figure 5.16). Tumors with a papillary pattern may show three-dimensional papillae with fibrovascular cores (Figure 5.17). Tumors with signet-ring morphology tend to have more discohesive cells with low nuclear-to-cytoplasmic ratios and a plasmacytoid appearance that may be difficult to identify as tumor on imprint cytology. However, targetoid mucin vacuoles, large vacuoles, and nuclear pleomorphism should provide clues that a signet-ring ADC is in the differential diagnosis. Tumors with mucinous features can have a mucinous background and may be difficult to remove from the slide after a touch imprint, as the mucin is sticky and may adhere to the slide leaving little remaining material for permanent processing in formalin. In these cases, additional untouched core biopsies are helpful to maximize the material available for processing. In the cytology laboratory, filtering these specimens or wrapping the core biopsies in filter paper at the time of collection can be helpful to avoid loss of small mucinous fragments. In addition, lung FNAs can be used with core biopsies to maximize tissue for ancillary studies (Figure 5.18). Poorly differentiated ADCs may show a more discohesive appearance with single pleomorphic cells or cohesive three-dimensional clusters within a background of desmoplasia or necrosis. Desmoplastic stroma will appear as metachromatic tissue fragments on the touch imprint, and can be challenging to distinguish from metachromatic stroma seen in biphasic SGTTs and chondromyxoid material from hamartomas at the time of onsite evaluation (Figure 5.19). Poorly differentiated ADC can also be difficult or impossible to distinguish from a poorly differentiated SqCC or LCNEC, which is why a core biopsy can be helpful to ensure that there is material for ancillary studies.

The differential diagnosis for ADC is shown in Table 5.5. Immunostains that are typically positive in pulmonary ADC include thyroid transcription factor 1 (TTF1) (nuclear staining) and NapsinA (cytoplasmic staining), and these stains may be used together in a double stain to conserve material in small biopsies for molecular testing (Figure 5.18D). Other markers that can be positive are surfactant protein A (SPA) and cytokeratin 7. Mucin can be highlighted by a mucicarmine special stain or PAS and PASD stains. Squamous markers such as p40, p63, and CK5/6 should be negative (11). Of note, ADC of the lung with mucinous features can be negative for TTF1, and may show positivity for intestinal markers like CK20 and CDX2; thus, correlation with the patient's history and number of lesions is essential. Furthermore, TTF1 is not only positive in lung ADC, but can be seen in LCNEC of the lung, extrapulmonary and pulmonary small cell carcinoma, carcinomas arising from the thyroid, and carcinomas arising in other locations (e.g.,

endometrial ADC). Lung ADC is also often tested with molecular studies looking for *EGFR*, and *KRAS* mutations, in addition to *EML4-ALK* rearrangements, as tumors with these molecular abnormalities may benefit from certain targeted therapies. Core biopsies can be very helpful in acquiring material for these ancillary studies, and have been shown to provide sufficient material for ancillary studies in over 90% of cases, similar to the yield with FNAs (12). *BRAF* and *PI3K* are also being tested for ADC at many academic medical centers (Table 5.4). There has also been an increased interest in testing for immunotherapy biomarkers, like PD-L1 (programmed death-ligand 1), to identify patients who may respond better to immunotherapy agents targeting the interaction between PD-L1 and PD-1. This includes the recent classification of ADC proposed by the IASLC/ATS/ERS recognizes five major patterns of lung ADC: lepidic, acinar, papillary, solid, and micropapillary, as well as subtype variants such as mucinous, colloid, fetal, and enteric (7). The solid and micropapillary patterns are important to identify given their poorer prognosis; however, subclassification

TABLE 5.4 Lung Cancer and Ancillary Testing

Subtype of Lung Cancer	Immunostaining Pattern	Molecular Testing
ADC	TTF1+, CK7+, p40 or p63 -, CK5/6-	Mutation testing for *EGFR* (*others commonly tested for include: KRAS, BRAF*, and *PI3K*) FISH testing for *ALK, ROS,* others
SqCC	p40 or p63+, CK5/6+, CK7-, TTF1-	No routine molecular studies
LCNEC	Synaptophysin+, CD56+, TTF1+/-	No routine molecular studies
Small cell carcinoma	Synaptophysin+, CD56+, TTF1+	No routine molecular studies

ADC, adenocarcinoma; *ALK*, anaplastic lymphoma kinase; CK, cytokeratin; *EGFR*, epidermal growth factor receptor; *FGFR*, fibroblast growth factor receptor; *KRAS*, Kirsten rat sarcoma viral oncogene; LCNEC, large cell neuroendocrine carcinoma; PI3, phosphatidylinositol 3; SqCC, squamous cell carcinoma; TTF, thyroid transcription factor.

TABLE 5.5 Differential Diagnoses for Non-Small Cell and Small Cell Lung Carcinoma

Adenocarcinoma	Squamous Cell Carcinoma	Small Cell Carcinoma
Poorly differentiated SqCC	Poorly differentiated ADC	Basaloid SqCC
Adenosquamous cell carcinoma	Adenosquamous cell carcinoma	LCNEC
LCNEC	Salivary gland-type tumors of the bronchial glands, especially mucoepidermoid carcinoma	Salivary gland-type tumors with basaloid features (primary or metastatic)
Metastatic extra-pulmonary ADC	Nonepithelial tumors (e.g., sarcoma, melanoma)	Well-to-moderately differentiated neuroendocrine neoplasms (e.g., carcinoid or atypical carcinoid)
Benign/reactive epithelial cells (e.g., goblet cell metaplasia)	Metastatic extra-pulmonary SqCCs (e.g., head and neck, uterine cervix, esophageal)	Metastatic small round blue cell tumors
Treatment-related atypia (e.g., chemotherapy, radiation)	Benign/reactive epithelial cells (e.g., squamous metaplasia)	Lymphoma/leukemia
Granulomatous inflammation	Treatment-related atypia (e.g., chemotherapy, radiation)	Benign lymphoid cells

ADC, adenocarcinoma; LCNEC, large cell neuroendocrine carcinoma; SqCC, squamous cell carcinoma.

of ADC into these patterns can be challenging on imprint cytology, as well as in cytology aspirates (9). Currently, subclassification of ADC is not performed on cytology specimens, but there are morphological clues that can sometimes help to separate the poor prognostic solid-type ADC from other subtypes (13).

Squamous Cell Carcinoma

SqCCs differ from ADC in that they tend to show large clusters of tumor cells, which have dense cytoplasm, coarser chromatin, pleomorphism, and a syncytial arrangement within a necroinflammatory background. In keratinizing SqCC, there can be single cells with cytoplasmic extensions (e.g., tadpole cells) or anucleate squames. In order to see the cytoplasmic orangeophilia, an alcohol-fixed touch imprint stained with the Papanicolaou stain or rapid-Papanicolaou stain (for onsite evaluation) can be helpful (Figure 5.20). Some of these cases can be cystic and have a predominance of inflammatory cells, so a careful search for pleomorphic cells is essential before dismissing a case as an inflammatory lesion. Some SqCC cases may also have a tigroid appearance in the background on imprint cytology, which can indicate the glycogenated nature of their tumor cells and be a helpful diagnostic clue (Figure 5.21). On a cellular basis, there tends to be more pleomorphism and coarse chromatin without distinct nucleoli, when compared to ADC. The nuclear-to-cytoplasmic ratio varies depending on the degree of differentiation, with lower nuclear-to-cytoplasmic ratios in well-to-moderately differentiated SqCC due to the presence of moderate-to-abundant dense cytoplasm. On permanent H&E sections from a core biopsy, intercellular bridges and keratin pearls can be helpful clues for SqCC. The difficulty arises with nonkeratinizing SqCC, which can have nucleoli mimicking ADC, particularly those with a solid pattern.

The differential diagnosis for SqCC is shown in Table 5.5. Basaloid SqCC can mimic neuroendocrine tumors, but has been shown to have adenoid-cystic like areas with palisading of the nuclei along the edges of clusters and metachromatic material (14). Immunostains are helpful to show that the tumor cells are positive for p40/p63 or CK5/6, while negative for TTF1 and synaptophysin (Figure 5.20–5.21). Some medical centers are now testing SqCCs for *FGFR1* amplification, which may have theranostic importance (15). The mutations seen in ADC such as *EGFR*, *KRAS*, and *ALK* mutations are not seen in SqCC. However, if an *EGFR* mutation was seen in a tumor suspected to be a SqCC, it would more likely be an adenosquamous cell carcinoma, which should be a consideration if there is a dual population of tumor cells by morphology and immunohistochemical analysis (e.g., some tumor cells are positive for TTF1, while other tumor cells stain positive for p40). In addition to adenosquamous cell carcinoma and poorly differentiated ADCs, other diagnoses to include in the differential for SqCC would include mucoepidermoid carcinoma (metastatic or primary from bronchial glands) and squamous metaplasia or papilloma.

Non-Small Cell Carcinoma, Not Otherwise Specified (NOS)

In some non-small cell carcinomas the tumor cells do not show definitive morphological features of ADC or SqCC. In these cases, immunohistochemical stains should be performed to at least favor an ADC or SqCC, and to exclude a neuroendocrine tumor or metastasis, depending on the clinical scenario (Figure 5.22). In tumors that cannot be definitively subclassified due to insufficient material for stains or negativity for key immunostains, the IASLC/ATS/ERS classification recommends the term, NSCLC NOS. If the stains do help to classify the tumor into an ADC or SqCC, the guidelines recommend using NSCLC, favor ADC, or NSCLC, favor SqCC (7). In pleural based tumors, it is reasonable to also consider the possibility of mesothelioma, which can mimic an ADC, and should thus be excluded (Figure 5.23).

Small Cell Carcinoma

Small cell carcinoma (SCC) is a poorly differentiated neuroendocrine tumor that has traditionally been separated from NSCLC given its poor prognosis, propensity to present with metastatic or advanced disease, and the fact that it is typically treated with chemotherapy and radiation. For these reasons, an accurate diagnosis is critical. On touch imprints, these tumors have small-to-intermediate sized cells measuring 2-3 times the size of a mature lymphocyte, in addition to smaller apoptotic dark nuclei and paranuclear blue bodies. Although the cells can appear to be discohesive, there is often at least some clustering, particularly on touch imprints (Figure 5.24). The areas of cohesion are helpful since they highlight the nuclear molding and scant cytoplasm of the cells with hyperchromatic, round nuclei that have a stippled chromatin pattern ("salt and pepper" appearance) and mitoses. Although nuclear crush artifact can be seen in aspirates, this is usually minimized in light touch preparations. There should also be an absence of lymphoglandular bodies as may be seen with lymphoma. A panel of immunostains can be helpful, to prove that the tumor cells are positive for TTF1 and neuroendocrine markers (e.g., synaptophysin, chromogranin, or CD56), in addition to showing a high proliferation index with Ki67, and negativity for p40 and LCA (CD45). The differential diagnosis of SCLC includes benign lymphocytes, lymphoma, well-to-moderately differentiated neuroendocrine tumors, benign/reactive changes like reserve cell hyperplasia, and poorly differentiated or basaloid appearing tumors (Table 5.5). A core biopsy for SCLC would really only be performed if there was insufficient aspirate material for immunohistochemical work-up, given that these tumors do not currently undergo routine molecular testing.

Large Cell Neuroendocrine Carcinoma

LCNEC is another high-grade neuroendocrine carcinoma that is grouped as a NSCLC, despite its worse prognosis and response to SCLC regimens (16). There are several overlapping features between LCNEC and SCLC, which can make definitive classification difficult. In general, the LCNECs have neuroendocrine features with some molding and cytoplasmic granularity, but in contrast to SCLC there is often a more prominent nucleolus and more cytoplasm imparting a "pink" appearance on the permanent H&E-stained sections of the core biopsy (Figure 5.25). This is in contrast to the very dark "blue" appearance seen with SCLC where tumor cells have only scant cytoplasm (19). Both tumors can show nuclear molding, mitoses, necrosis, and intermediate-sized nuclei. Other entities to consider in the differential diagnosis include ADC, atypical carcinoid, combined tumors, and other pleomorphic tumors such as melanoma. Immunophenotypically and morphologically, LCNEC can overlap with ADC given that they are both TTF1 positive and have prominent nucleoli. However, LCNEC will show positive staining with neuroendocrine markers, and currently do not undergo routine molecular testing.

Large Cell Carcinomas

Large cell carcinoma (LCC) represents an undifferentiated NSCLC with no definitive squamous, glandular, or neuroendocrine differentiation. Based on the recommendations from the IASLC/ATS/ERS classification, LCCs should not be a diagnosis made in small biopsies or cytology specimens (7). In general, the imprints of these tumors will look like poorly differentiated NSCLC and immunostains will confirm the absence of glandular, squamous, or neuroendocrine differentiation. An appropriate immunostain panel should include TTF1, p40, and neuroendocrine markers (e.g., synaptophysin, chromogranin). The differential diagnosis of LCC includes poorly differentiated ADC, poorly

differentiated SqCC, sarcomatoid carcinoma, epithelioid sarcoma, anaplastic lymphoma, metastatic non-pulmonary poorly differentiated carcinomas, germ cell tumors, and melanoma.

Lymphoma

Lymphomas are rare as primary lung tumors, but can occur. Proper triage of these specimens is crucial. Thus, in a patient with a history of lymphoma or suspicion for lymphoma, a touch imprint from the core biopsy can help to indicate if flow cytometry or additional lymphoma work-up is necessary. These touch preparations show discohesive cells with lymphoglandular bodies, and are rather monotonous-appearing for lymphoproliferative disorders. Triage of these specimens should include material for flow cytometry, immunohistochemical stains, and fluorescence in situ hybridization (FISH) studies. Core biopsies are somewhat problematic for flow cytometry, and thus aspirates may be a more ideal specimen to send for flow cytometry given that minimal manipulation is required and lymphoid cells tend to be fragile (17). Flow cytometry or FISH studies can help to confirm light-chain restriction or clonality, respectively. Immunostains can help with subclassification, especially for markers that are not evaluable by flow cytometry such as cyclin D1, Ki67, and others.

Malignant Melanoma

Melanoma presenting in the lung is usually metastatic, and may arise in the absence of a known primary tumor (e.g., tumor of unknown origin). Imprints of these tumors usually reveal discohesive large cells with prominent nucleoli, plasmacytoid features, and binucleation (Figure 5.26). Pigment may be seen, and will appear as dusty cytoplasmic material within tumor cells or histiocytes (melanophages). Intranuclear inclusions can also be seen. Immunostains are crucial for this diagnosis to confirm that the tumor cells are negative for cytokeratins, but are positive for melanoma markers (e.g., S100, MelanA, HMB45, MiTF, tyrosinase, SOX10). A limited immunopanel is important given that melanoma samples are likely to require molecular testing to look for *BRAF* mutations to guide treatment with *BRAF* inhibitors like vemurafenib.

Metastatic Tumors

A large variety of carcinomas and other neoplasms can metastasize or involve the lungs. The clinical history in these cases is important, in addition to knowing the number of lung lesions present. Patients with a prior malignancy and multiple lung lesions are more likely to have a metastasis. The most common metastatic tumors seen in the lung are from the breast, colon, head and neck, gastrointestinal tract, and bladder. Many of these tumors mimic non-small cell carcinoma, and should be negative for TTF1. Thus, in a patient with a lung mass that is TTF1 negative, and that also has a history of another neoplasm, additional immunostains should be used to exclude a metastasis. The distinction between primary lung ADC versus a metastatic ADC is crucial; molecular testing requirements may differ as well as treatment (e.g., surgery vs. no surgery). Metastatic urothelial carcinoma can be particularly problematic because it may mimic SqCC and stain with squamous cell markers (e.g., p63) (Figure 5.27). Newer immunomarkers like GATA3 can be helpful, which should be positive in bladder and breast carcinomas, but negative in SqCC; however, some studies have reported weak GATA3 expression in some

SqCC cases, so its specificity may not be as good as originally thought (18). A plethora of other rare tumors can metastasize or involve the lung, such as germ cell tumors in young patients (Figure 5.28).

Sarcoma

Sarcomas and other mesenchymal neoplasms can arise as primary lung tumors, or present as metastases. The key features on a touch imprint to look for in these tumors are a predominance of spindle cells, dyscohesion, background metachromatic material (e.g., chondromyxoid or osteoid material), and marked pleomorphism, in addition to a clinical history of sarcoma. The most common sarcomas to involve the lung include synovial sarcoma, myxofibrosarcoma, leiomyosarcoma, osteosarcoma, and angiosarcoma (Figures 5.29 and 5.30). A core biopsy is often essential to examine architecture and perform important ancillary (e.g., FISH) studies in mesenchymal tumors.

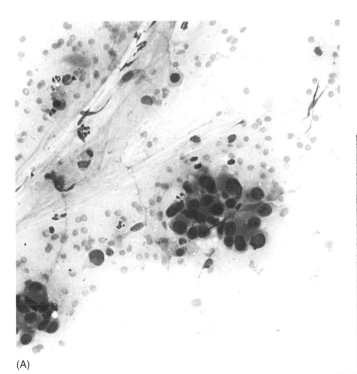

(A)

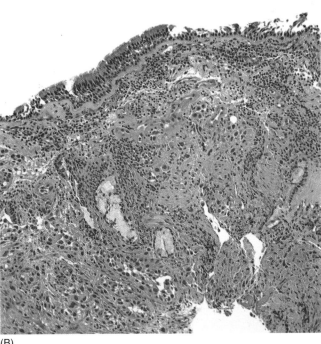

(B)

FIGURE 5.16 Lung ADC. (A) This ADC seen on touch preparation shows glassy cytoplasm and nucleoli, with vague glandular arrangement. (B) The core biopsy shows tumor cells with cytoplasmic vacuolization forming glands beneath the bronchial epithelium. ((A) DQ-stained TP, high power; (B) H&E-stained core, high power.) ADC, adenocarcinoma; DQ, Diff-Quik; H&E, hematoxylin and eosin; TP, touch preparation.

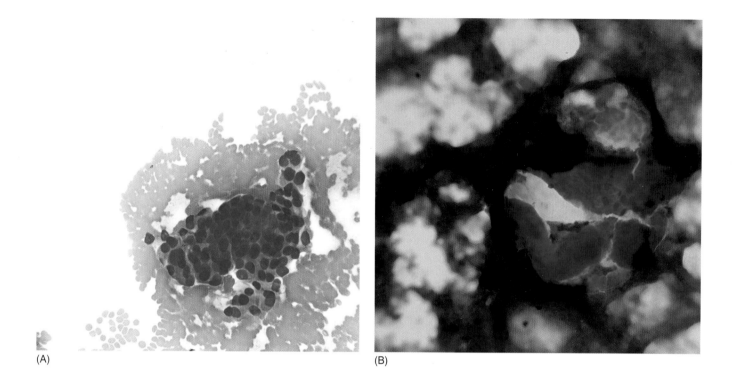

(A)   (B)

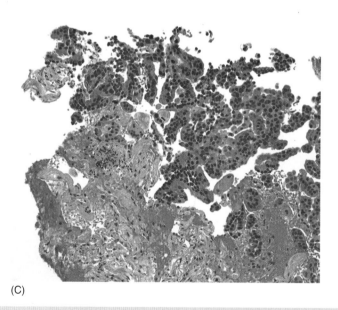

(C)

FIGURE 5.17 Lung ADC with papillary features and *EGFR* mutation. (A) The TPs show clusters of tumor cells with depth of focus and a suggestion of papillary features, (B) even on the dense TP from a bloody core biopsy. (C) The core biopsy shows an ADC of the lung with a papillary pattern, which was originally positive for an exon 18 *EGFR* mutation (conferring sensitivity to TKI), then acquired an Exon 20 resistance mutation. ((A) and (B) DQ-stained TP, high power; (C) H&E-stained core, high power.) ADC, adenocarcinoma; DQ, Diff-Quik; H&E, hematoxylin and eosin; TP, touch preparation.

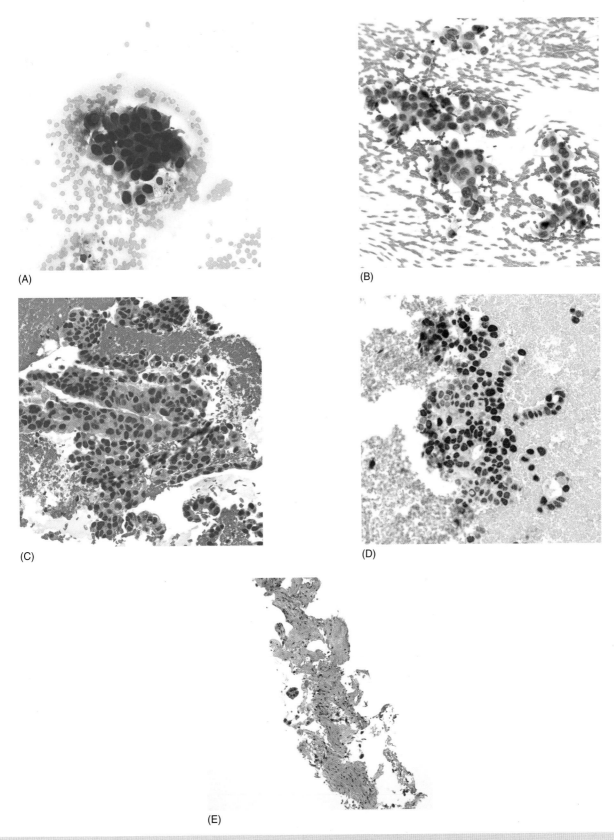

FIGURE 5.18 Lung ADC with cell block and core. This case illustrates an ADC with (A–B) cellular smears and (C) cell block, where an additional core biopsy was performed for ancillary studies (E), but was insufficient. The presence of a cellular cell block fortunately allowed (D) immunostains and molecular testing to be performed. Thus, the combination of and core biopsy can be helpful in the event that one of them is insufficient. ((A) DQ-stained smear, high power; (B) Pap-stained smear, high power; (C) H&E-stained cell block, high power; (D) TTF1 and Napsin A double immunostains on cell block; (E) H&E core, high power.) ADC, adenocarcinoma; DQ, Diff-Quik; H&E, hematoxylin and eosin.

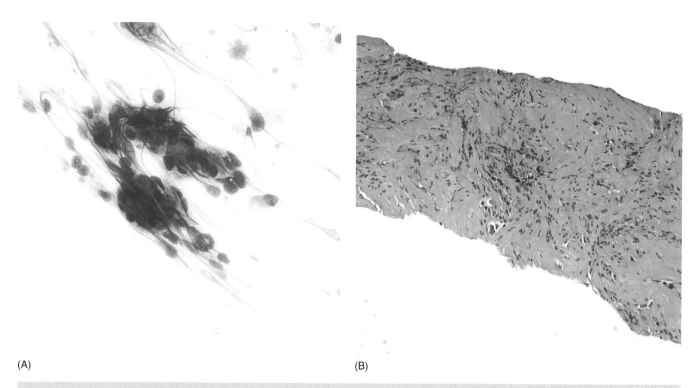

(A)   (B)

FIGURE 5.19 Lung ADC arising in scar. (A) This TP shows streaking artifact in tumor cell groups and scant cellularity overall, (B) which correlates with the findings in the core biopsy where there is extensive fibrous background given that the tumor is arising in an apical scar. ((A) DQ-stained TP, high power; (B) H&E-stained core, low power.) ADC, adenocarcinoma; DQ, Diff-Quik; H&E, hematoxylin and eosin; TP, touch preparation.

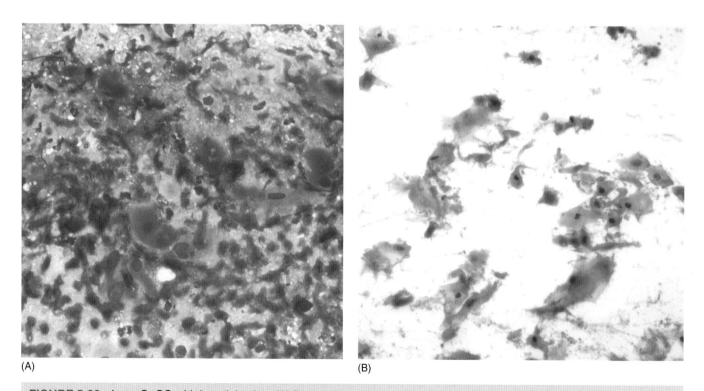

(A)   (B)

FIGURE 5.20 Lung SqCC with keratinization. (A) Discohesive single cells with dense cytoplasmic tails and anucleate ghost cells are seen in this TP. (B) A Pap-stained TP can be helpful in these scenarios, to highlight the cytoplasmic orangeophilia from keratinization that may not be as easily appreciated on routine H&E-stains of the core biopsy, and can help in subclassification. (*continued*)

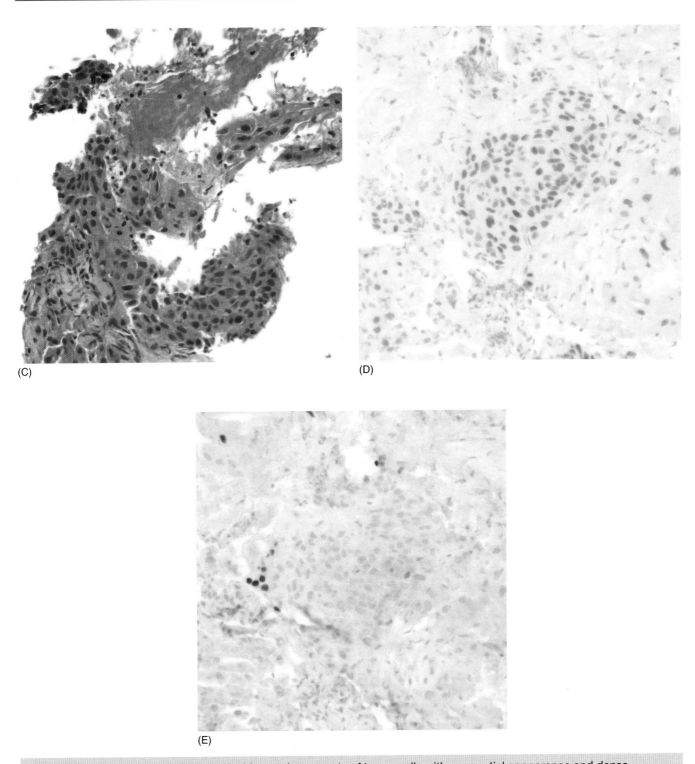

(C)

(D)

(E)

FIGURE 5.20 (*continued*) (C) The core biopsy shows nests of tumor cells with a syncytial appearance and dense eosinophilic cytoplasm, which are (D) positive for p40 and (E) negative for TTF1. ((A) DQ-stained TP, high power; (B) Pap-stained TP, high power; (C) H&E-stained core, high power; (D) p40 immunostain; (E) TTF1 immunostain.) DQ, Diff-Quik; H&E, hematoxylin and eosin; SqCC, squamous cell carcinoma; TP, touch preparation.

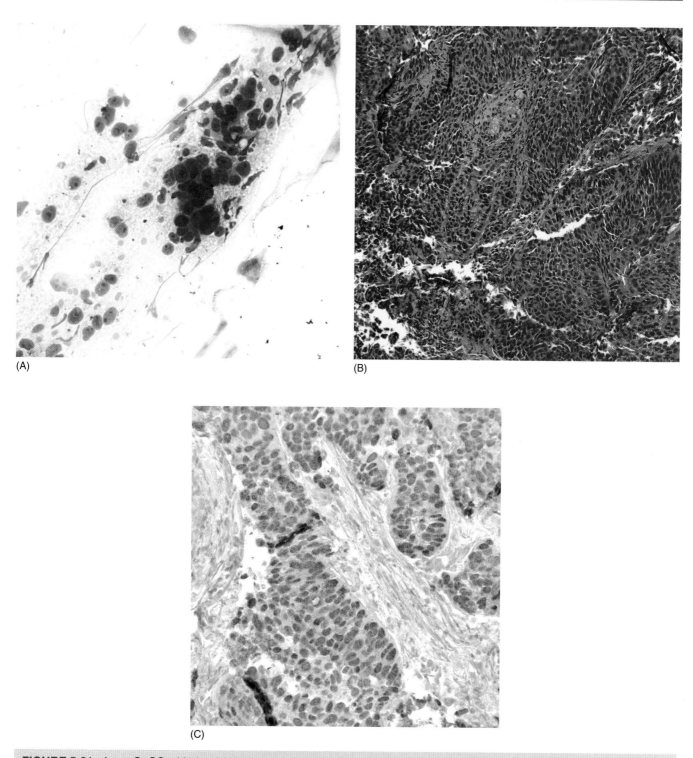

(A)

(B)

(C)

FIGURE 5.21 Lung SqCC with tigroid background. (A) The TP on this SqCC shows poorly differentiated tumor cells with a tigroid or lace-like background. (B) The tumor cells have a nested pattern without discernable glandular formation and (C) are positive for p40, confirming their squamous differentiation. ((A) DQ-stained TP, high power; (B) H&E-stained core, medium power; (C) p40 immunostain.) DQ, Diff-Quik; H&E, hematoxylin and eosin; SqCC, squamous cell carcinoma; TP, touch preparation.

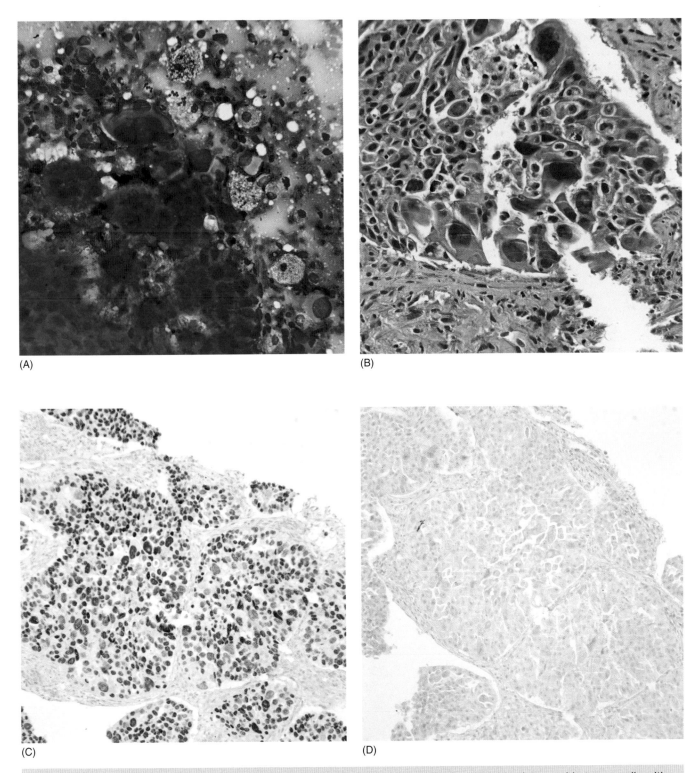

FIGURE 5.22 Poorly differentiated lung non-small cell carcinoma. (A) The TP shows highly pleomorphic tumor cells with multinucleation suggestive of a pleomorphic or giant cell carcinoma. (B) Similar morphology is seen on the corresponding core biopsy. Immunostains performed on the core biopsy show (C) positivity for TTF1 and (D) a negative p40 immunostain. ((A) DQ-stained TP, high power; (B) H&E-stained core, high power; (C) TTF1 immunostain; (D) p40 immunostain.) DQ, Diff-Quik; H&E, hematoxylin and eosin; TP, touch preparation.

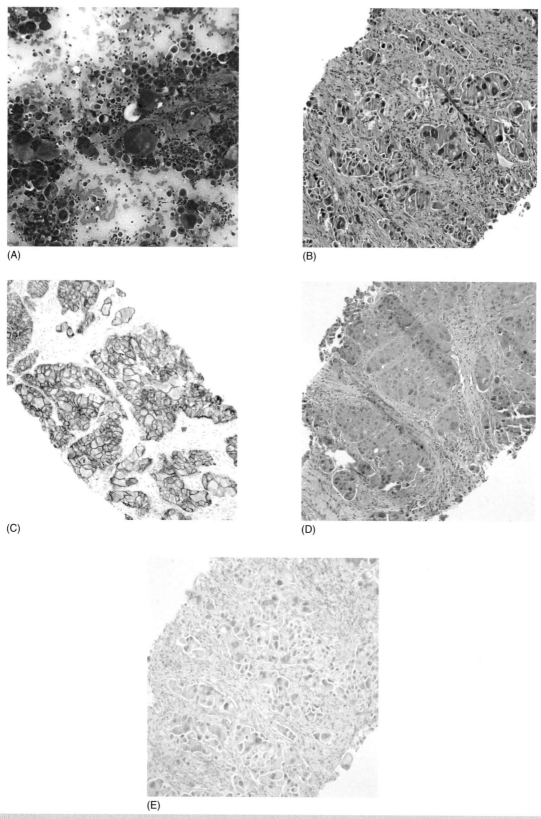

FIGURE 5.23 Poorly differentiated lung ADC mimicking mesothelioma in a pleural based lung mass. (A) This TP shows pleomorphic, large tumor cells that are loosely cohesive and have a few signet-ring type cells, within a background of inflammatory cells. (B) The core biopsy shows similar tumor cells and highlights some of the cytoplasmic vacuolization favoring an ADC over mesothelioma. Stains confirm that the tumor cells are positive for (C) MOC31 and (D) mucicarmine (D), but are (E) negative for calretinin. ((A) DQ-stained TP, high power; (B) H&E-stained core, high power; (C) MOC31 immunostain; (D) mucicarmine special stain; (E) calretinin immunostain.) ADC, adenocarcinoma; DQ, Diff-Quik; H&E, hematoxylin and eosin; TP, touch preparation.

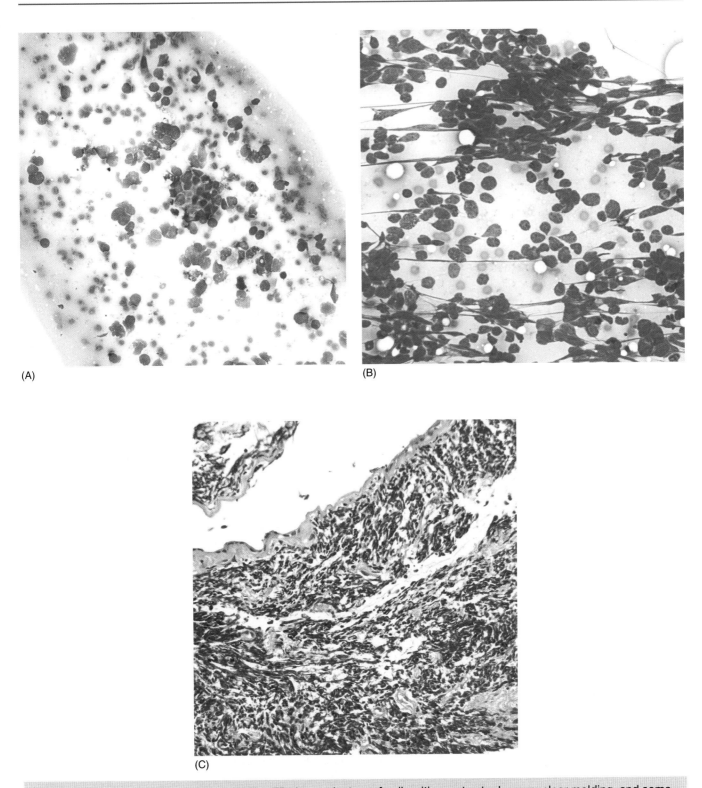

FIGURE 5.24 Small cell carcinoma. (A) The TP shows clusters of cells with scant cytoplasm, nuclear molding, and some discohesive cells. (B) In comparison to the FNA smear seen in B, the TP has less smearing and crush artifact, which can help in making a diagnosis and excluding lymphoma. (C) Even the core biopsies typically have crush artifact, making the morphology difficult to evaluate in comparison to the TP. However, the value of a cell block or core biopsy in such cases is to obtain material for immunostains to exclude a lymphoma or basaloid neoplasm (e.g., basaloid SqCC). ((A) DQ-stained TP, high power; (B) DQ-stained smear, high power; (C) H&E-stained core, high power.) DQ, Diff-Quik; FNA, fine needle aspiration; H&E, hematoxylin and eosin; SqCC, squamous cell carcinoma; TP, touch preparation.

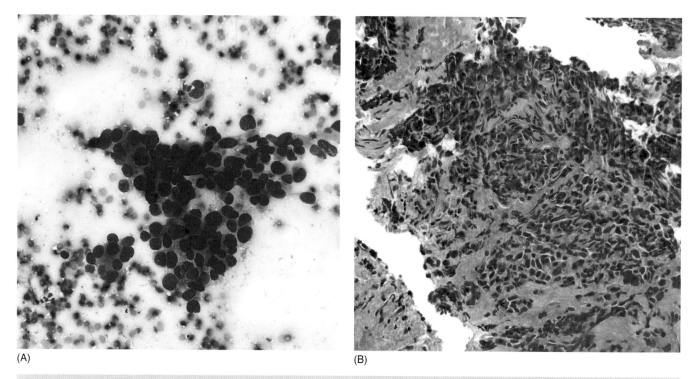

(A)   (B)

FIGURE 5.25 Large cell neuroendocrine carcinoma. (A) The TP is cellular and shows single and clusters of intermediate to large cells with rosette-like configuration. (B) The cell block highlights the "pink" appearance of the tumor cells due to their moderate amounts of eosinophilic, granular cytoplasm. ((A) DQ-stained TP, high power; (B) H&E-stained core, high power.) DQ, Diff-Quik; H&E, hematoxylin and eosin; TP, touch preparation.

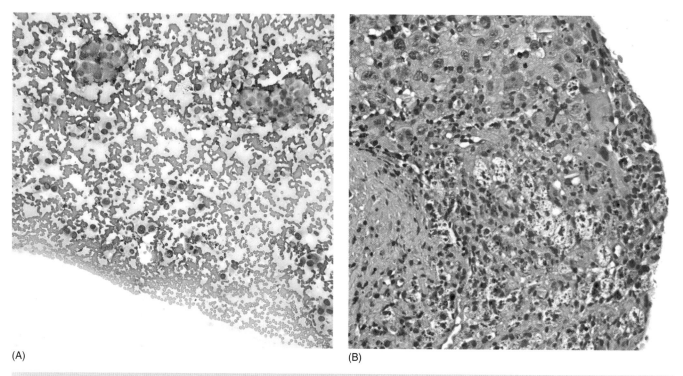

(A)   (B)

FIGURE 5.26 Metastatic malignant melanoma with pigment. (A) Tumor cells appear in clusters and as single cells and have prominent dusty cytoplasmic pigment, seen together with histiocytes containing melanin pigment in the background. (B) The core biopsy shows the pleomorphic tumor cells with melanin pigment, (*continued*)

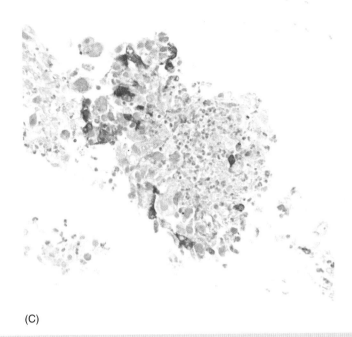

(C)

FIGURE 5.26 (*continued*) (C) which stain positive for S100. ((A) DQ-stained TP, high power; (B) H&E-stained core, medium power; (C) S100 immunostain.) DQ, Diff-Quik; H&E, hematoxylin and eosin; TP, touch preparation.

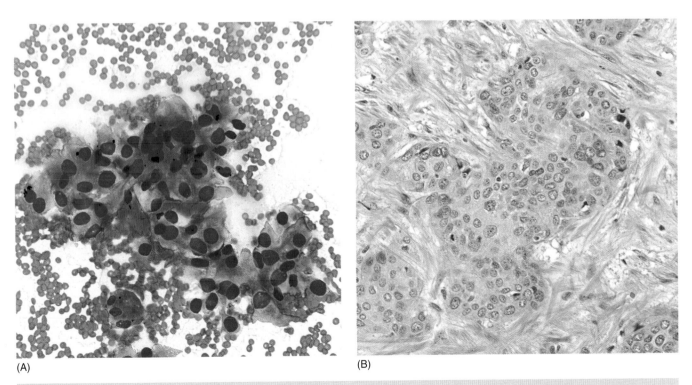

(A)

(B)

FIGURE 5.27 Metastatic urothelial carcinoma. (A) The TP shows loosely cohesive tumor cells with abundant cytoplasm. (B) The tumor cells form nests that have a vague squamoid appearance on the core biopsy, (*continued*)

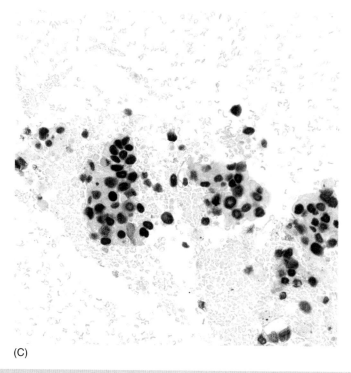

(C)

FIGURE 5.27 (*continued*) (C) that stain positive for GATA3, confirming their urothelial origin. ((A) DQ-stained TP, high power; (B) H&E-stained core, high power; (C) GATA3 immunostain.) DQ, Diff-Quik; H&E, hematoxylin and eosin; TP, touch preparation.

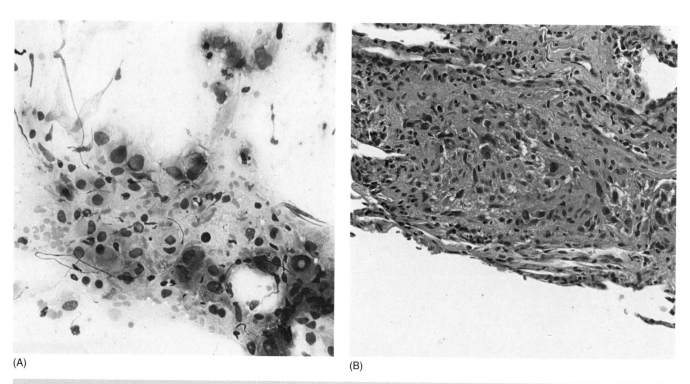

(A)   (B)

FIGURE 5.28 Metastatic germ cell tumor in the lung. (A) The TP and (B) core biopsy show loosely cohesive clusters of tumor cells with large nuclei and prominent macronucleoli, in addition to moderately abundant cytoplasm and a lymphohistiocytic background. (*continued*)

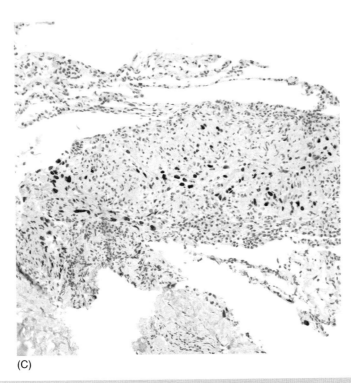

(C)

FIGURE 5.28 (*continued*) (C) The tumor cells show nuclear staining for SALL4. ((A) DQ-stained TP, high power; (B) H&E-stained core, high power; (C) SALL4 immunostain.) DQ, Diff-Quik; H&E, hematoxylin and eosin; TP, touch preparation.

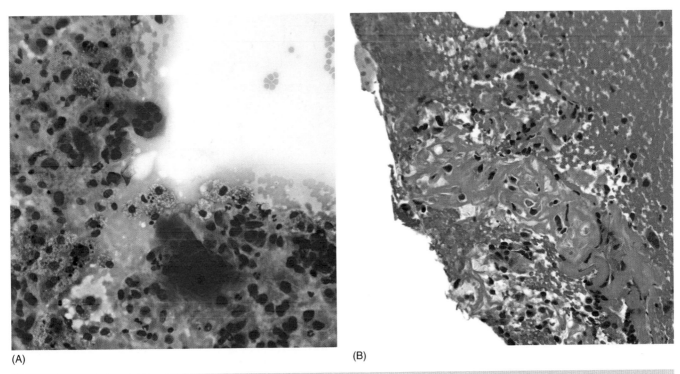

(A)   (B)

FIGURE 5.29 Metastatic osteosarcoma in the lung. (A) The TP shows a population of epithelioid cells and osteoclastic giant cells within a bloody background. (B) The core biopsy reveals osteoid with embedded neoplastic cells. ((A) DQ-stained TP, high power; (B) H&E-stained core, high power.) DQ, Diff-Quik; H&E, hematoxylin and eosin; TP, touch preparation.

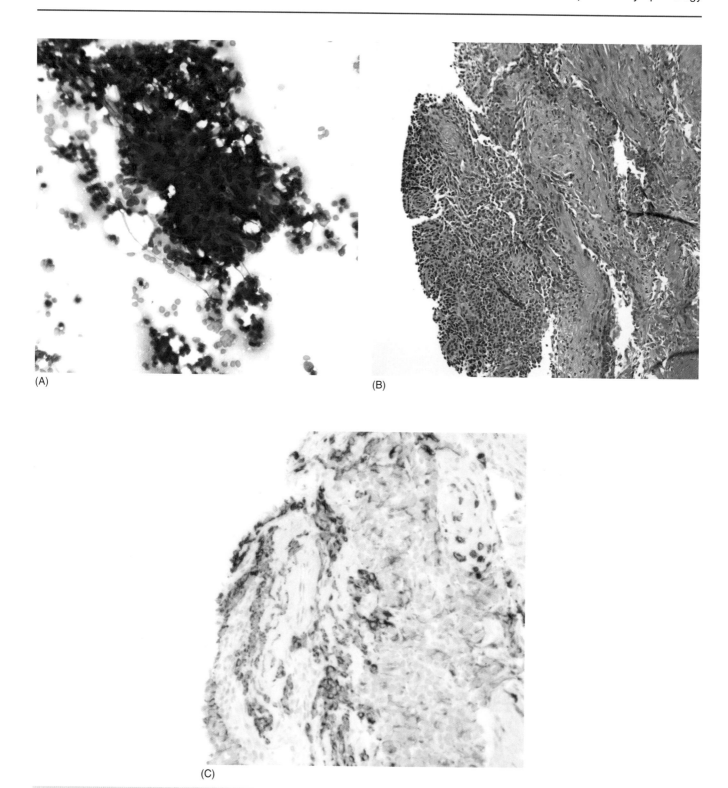

FIGURE 5.30 Synovial sarcoma. (A) The TP demonstrates cellular fragments of tissue with monotonous epithelioid cells and a necrotic background. (B) The core biopsy shows similar tumor cells that (C) stain positive cytokeratin. The findings in this case were morphologically similar to the patient's prior synovial sarcoma of the lung, compatible with recurrence. ((A) DQ-stained TP, high power; (B) H&E-stained core, medium power; (C) Cytokeratin immunostain.) DQ, Diff-Quik; H&E, hematoxylin and eosin; TP, touch preparation.

REFERENCES

1. Lindeman NI, Cagle PT, Beasley MB, et al. Molecular testing guideline for selection of lung cancer patients for EGFR and ALK tyrosine kinase inhibitors: guideline from the College of American Pathologists, International Association for the Study of Lung Cancer, and Association for Molecular Pathology. *J Thorac Oncol.* 2013;8:823-859.

2. Khalbuss WE, Monaco SE, Pantanowitz L. Lung and respiratory cytopathology. In: *ASCP Quick Compendium of Cytopathology.* ASCP Press, Chicago, IL; 2013:chap 12, 212-257.

3. Monaco SE, Schuchert MJ, Khalbuss WE. Diagnostic difficulties and pitfalls in rapid onsite evaluation of endobronchial ultrasound guided fine needle aspiration. *Cytojournal.* 2010;7:9.

4. Kalugina Y, Petruzzelli GJ, Wojcik EM. Fine-needle aspiration of rheumatoid nodule: a case report with review of diagnostic features and difficulties. *Diagn Cytopathol.* 2003;28:322-324.

5. Demicco EG, Harms PW, Patel RM, et al. Extensive survey of STAT6 expression in a large series of mesenchymal tumors. *Am J Clin Pathol.* 2015;143:672-682.

6. Travis WD, Brambilla C, Muller-Hermilink H, Curtis CH. *Pathology and Genetics Tumours of the Lung, Pleura, Thymus and Heart.* Lyon, France: IARC, 2004.

7. Travis WD, Brambilla E, Noguchi M, et al. International association for the study of lung cancer/American Thoracic Society/European Respiratory Society international multidisciplinary classification of lung ADC. *J Thorac Oncol.* 2011;6: 244-285.

8. Rossi G, Pelosi G, Graziano P, Barbareschi M, Papotti M. A reevaluation of the clinical significance of histological subtyping of non-small cell lung carcinoma: diagnostic algorithms in the era of personalized treatments. *Int J Surg Pathol.* 2009;17:206-218.

9. Rodriguez EF, Monaco SE, Dacic S. Cytologic subtyping of lung ADC by using the proposed International Association for the Study of Lung Cancer/American Thoracic Society/European Respiratory Society (IASLC/ATS/ERS) ADC classification. *Cancer Cytopathol.* 2013;121:629-637.

10. Dacic S, Shuai Y, Yousem S, Ohori P, Nikiforova M. Clinicopathological predictors of EGFR/KRAS mutational status in primary lung ADCs. *Mod Pathol.* 2010;23:159-168.

11. Ocque R, Tochigi N, Ohori NP, Dacic S. Usefulness of immunohistochemical and histochemical studies in the classification of lung ADC and squamous cell carcinoma in cytologic specimens. *Am J Clin Pathol.* 2011;136:81-87.

12. Coley SM, Crapanzano JP, Saqi A. FNA, core biopsy, or both for the diagnosis of lung carcinoma: obtaining sufficient tissue for a specific diagnosis and molecular testing. *Cancer Cytopathol.* 2015;123:318-326.

13. Rodriguez EF, Dacic S, Pantanowitz L, Khalbuss WE, Monaco SE. Cytopathology of pulmonary adenocarcinoma with a single histological pattern using the proposed International Association for the Study of Lung Cancer/American Thoracic Society/European Respiratory Society (IASLC/ATS/ERS) classification. *Cancer Cytopathol.* 2015;123:306-317.

14. Joshi D, Shivkumar VB, Sharma SM, Gangane N. Cytomorphologic diagnosis of basaloid squamous cell carcinoma: a case report. *Acta Cytol.* 2009;53:89-92.

15. Jiang T, Gao G, Fan G, Li M, Zhou C. FGFR1 amplification in lung squamous cell carcinoma: a systematic review with meta-analysis. *Lung Cancer.* 2015;87:1-7.

16. Rossi G, Cavazza A, Marchioni A, et al. Role of chemotherapy and the receptor tyrosine kinases KIT, PDGFRalpha, PDGFRbeta, and Met in large-cell neuroendocrine carcinoma of the lung. *J Clin Oncol.* 2005;23:8774-8785.

17. Boyd JD, Smith GD, Hong H, Mageau R, Juskevicius R. Fine-needle aspiration is superior to needle core biopsy as a sample acquisition method for flow cytometric analysis in suspected hematologic neoplasms. *Cytometry B Clin Cytom.* 2015;88: 64-68.

18. Clark BZ, Beriwal S, Dabbs DJ, Bhargava R. Semiquantitative GATA-3 immunoreactivity in breast, bladder, gynecologic tract, and other cytokeratin 7-positive carcinomas. *Am J Clin Pathol.* 2014;142:64-71.

19. Rekhtman N. Neuroendocrine tumors of the lung. *Arch Pathol Lab Med.* 2010;134:1628-1638.

CHAPTER 6

Hematopathology

Liron Pantanowitz

INTRODUCTION

Touch preparations and imprints have proven utility in the evaluation of hematolymphoid tissues to determine adequacy, render diagnoses, and to triage specimens for ancillary studies (1–3). Imprint cytology can be readily and rapidly applied to hematology specimens or tissues suspected of being involved by leukemia/lymphoma that are received during intraoperative consultations, at the surgical bench when grossing pathology specimens, as well as during rapid onsite evaluation (ROSE) of a core needle biopsy (CNB). However, hematopathology is challenging because of the broad diversity of lesions that may be encountered, morphological overlap of several entities, and the difficulty differentiating these diseases based on cytomorphology alone (4,5). Therefore, the practice of cytopathology involving hematopathology specimens demands that cytologists be adept at appropriately triaging material for ancillary studies. Moreover, familiarity with the results of these tests is equally important in order to suitably correlate findings with cytomorphology and provide accurate final diagnoses.

Lymph nodes are frequently biopsied to determine the etiology of lymphadenopathy, stage patients with known malignancy (e.g., lymphoma, carcinoma), determine if patients with known lymphoma have relapsed or progressed/transformed, as well as assess specific lymphoid neoplasms for prognostic or predictive biomarkers (e.g., CD20 or CD30 positivity for targeted therapy). Lymph nodes and related lymphoid tissues can be quickly, relatively cheaply, and reliably evaluated by percutaneous fine needle aspiration (FNA) and/or CNB with touch preparation compared to complete surgical excision (6). These minimally invasive techniques provide clinicians with a viable option to work-up patients for lymphoma who are unfit for surgery. Needle biopsy cytopreparations can be employed to assess palpable and deep-seated lymphadenopathy, and are beneficial in emergent conditions such as patients presenting with superior vena cava syndrome due to a bulky mediastinal tumor or spinal cord compression from paravertebral lymphadenopathy.

Although some studies have shown that CNB has higher sensitivity and negative predictive value than FNA when screening lymph nodes for lymphoma (7), combined FNA with CNB and ancillary studies is preferable to diagnose lymphoma (8,9). FNA provides good cellular material for flow cytometry and CNBs of reasonable size and number preserve tissue architecture and give the pathologist sufficient material to work with in order to accurately subtype and grade lymphoid tumors. Not surprisingly, needle biopsy of lymph nodes is typically recommended as the first-line of investigation in working up patients with lymphadenopathy for a primary diagnosis (10–13). Some authors recommend that a CNB should only be followed up by a secondary biopsy if there is a benign diagnosis yet the clinical presentation suggests malignant disease (14). Other authors feel that FNA and/or CNB of nodes should be followed up with an excisional lymph node biopsy anyway, to fully classify lymphomas (15). However, small biopsies can be a powerful diagnostic modality in the diagnosis of recurrent disease or to investigate for a large cell transformation from a small cell lymphoma, in addition to looking for response to therapy and/or biomarker changes with treatment (e.g., CD20 positivity after rituximab).

Several publications have shown that imprint cytology provides high sensitivity with high positive predictive value for several tissues including lymph nodes (16). Imprint cytology is also reliable in evaluating splenic tissue (17). In a study of 453 mediastinal nodal stations removed during mediastinoscopy that were evaluated by intraoperative imprint cytology for neoplastic cells, this technique had a reported sensitivity of 92.3%, specificity of 100%, accuracy of 98.4%, positive predictive value of 100%, and negative predictive value of 98.0% (18). However, not all studies have shown such promising outcomes. For example, in a study that included 100 lymph nodes evaluated by imprints, there was only 61% agreement with the histological diagnosis (19). The main diagnostic difficulties reported in this study were related to distinguishing between reactive changes and non-Hodgkin lymphoma (NHL), and distinguishing NHL from Hodgkin lymphoma (HL). Further diagnostic classification (e.g., subtyping of lymphomas and subclassification of Hodgkin lymphoma (HL)) in this study was also unreliable using imprints alone.

Bone marrow evaluation is another important and effective way of diagnosing and evaluating primary hematologic and metastatic neoplasms. Evaluating touch imprints are a standard practice in the examination of bone marrow at many medical centers (20,21). Bone marrow biopsy imprint preparations are particularly helpful with dry taps when an aspirate cannot be obtained (22,23). Touch imprints of bone marrow biopsies have been shown to be a reliable diagnostic tool for the evaluation of marrow cellularity and for the diagnosis of bone marrow involved by a neoplastic hematologic disease (24,25). In one study, bone marrow imprint cytology was able to detect metastatic cells in 96% of cases (26). In addition, fluorescence in-situ hybridization (FISH) on bone marrow imprints has been shown to markedly improve the identification of chromosomal abnormalities (27).

This chapter covers touch imprint cytology related to hematopathology. A plethora of benign and neoplastic hematopathology entities are discussed, adhering to the recent World Health Organization (WHO) classification for these tumors (Table 6.1). For each entity, this chapter highlights key diagnostic features, the differential diagnosis, and limitations to be aware of when interpreting imprints. Contemporary ancillary tests such as flow cytometry, immunohistochemistry, cytogenetics, and molecular studies are also discussed to ensure that material evaluated by TPs and imprints is appropriately triaged at the time of procurement.

NORMAL

Lymph Node

Lymph nodes have a capsule, cortex, and central medulla. The subcapsular portion contains the most follicles. The paracortex is that region between cortical follicles and the medulla. Follicles may be primary or secondary. Primary follicles are comprised of round aggregates of naïve B lymphocytes supported by a network of follicular dendritic cell (FDC) processes. Secondary follicles arise from primary follicles when they develop a central pale germinal center (GC) in response to antigenic stimulation of B-cells (Figure 6.1). The GC contains mostly B lymphocytes including centroblasts and centrocytes as well as scant T-cells, tingible-body macrophages (TBMs), and FDCs (CD21+, CD23+, CD35+, ER+). The GC is surrounded by an inner mantle zone and lighter outer marginal zone of B lymphocytes. Cytology preparations from reactive nodes with lymphoid follicles often contain lymphohistiocytic aggregates or follicular center fragments (Figure 6.2). The paracortex contains mostly mature T cells, some B immunoblasts, interdigitating dendritic cells

(S-100+, fascin+), plasmacytoid dendritic cells, histiocytes, and high endothelial venules. The medulla contains medullary cords and sinuses that drain material toward the hilum. These sinuses contain mostly macrophages (CD68+), and can become quite distended with sinus histiocytosis.

FNA smears of lymphoid tissue often show crush artifact in the form of lymphoid tangles. Neoplastic lymphoid cells tend to crush more easily. If well performed, TPs and imprints are usually free of such smear artifacts and tend to show better preserved cell cytology. Lymphoglandular bodies, also known as Söderstrom bodies, are commonly seen in the background of lymph node smears as well as TPs. However, they are not only characteristic of lymph nodes, but may be seen with other lymphoid tissues such as spleen, tonsils, and thymus. Lymphoglandular bodies are more common in lymphomas than benign lymph nodes, perhaps because neoplastic cells have more fragile cytopalsm. Depending on where a glass slide imprints tissue, these cytopreparations can contain any number of lymphoid cell types. A key feature when evaluating lymphoid cells is to determine the composition of lymphoid cells (e.g., monotonous vs polymorphous population) and their cell size. The main cell used for size reference is the histiocyte nucleus (or two red blood cells [RBCs]). A lymphoid cell of small size is less than the size of a histiocyte nucleus, one of intermediate size is the same size as a histiocyte nucleus, and a large lymphoid cell is greater than the size of a histiocyte nucleus (or >4 times the size of an RBC).

Mature lymphocytes are small cells with scant cytoplasm, round nuclei, and dark condensed chromatin. Centrocytes are intermediate-sized B lymphocytes with scant cytoplasm, cleaved nuclei, and inconspicuous nucleoli. Centroblasts are 3 to 4 times larger B lymphocytes with a narrow rim of basophilic cytoplasm, round nuclei, vesicular chromatin, and one to three prominent peripheral nucleoli. Mitotic figures in centroblasts are not uncommon. Immunoblasts are larger B lymphocytes characterized by having dark basophilic cytoplasm, a round nucleus, and a distinct central nucleolus. Plasmacytoid cells (sometimes called "plymphs") refer to lymphocytes with moderate amounts of cytoplasm and an eccentrically placed nucleus. Monocytoid B-cells (MBCs) are intermediate sized lymphocytes that resemble monocytes. They have abundant pale to clear cytoplasm, and bland cleaved nuclei with inconspicuous nucleoli. MBCs can be seen in several reactive (e.g., toxoplasma lymphadenitis, infectious mononucleosis) and neoplastic (e.g., marginal zone lymphoma) conditions (29). Dendritic cells have moderate to abundant cytoplasm, long cytoplasmic processes, pale oval nuclei that may be bi/multinucleated, and indistinct nucleoli (Figure 6.3). TBMs have abundant cytoplasm with intracytoplasmic apoptotic debris (Figure 6.4). Other infrequently encountered cell types may include neutrophils,

TABLE 6.1   WHO (2016) Classification of Mature Lymphoid, Histiocytic, and Dendritic Neoplasms

Mature B-Cell Neoplasms
  Chronic lymphocytic leukemia/small lymphocytic lymphoma
  Monoclonal B-cell lymphocytosis
  B-cell prolymphocytic leukemia
  Splenic marginal zone lymphoma
  Hairy cell leukemia
  Splenic B-cell lymphoma/leukemia, unclassifiable
      Splenic diffuse red pulp small B-cell lymphoma
      Hairy cell leukemia-variant
  Lymphoplasmacytic lymphoma
      Waldenström macroglobulinemia
  MGUS, IgM
  μ heavy-chain disease
  γ heavy-chain disease
  α heavy-chain disease
  MGUS, IgG/A
  Plasma cell myeloma
  Solitary plasmacytoma of bone
  Extraosseous plasmacytoma
  Monoclonal immunoglobulin deposition diseases
  Extranodal marginal zone lymphoma of MALT
  Nodal marginal zone lymphoma
      Pediatric nodal marginal zone lymphoma
  Follicular lymphoma
      In situ follicular neoplasia
      Duodenal-type follicular lymphoma
  Pediatric-type follicular lymphoma
  Large B-cell lymphoma with *IRF4* rearrangement
  Primary cutaneous follicle center lymphoma
  Mantle cell lymphoma
      In situ mantle cell neoplasia
  DLBCL, NOS
      Germinal center B-cell type
      Activated B-cell type
  T-cell/histiocyte-rich large B-cell lymphoma
  Primary DLBCL of the CNS
  Primary cutaneous DLBCL, leg type
  EBV⁺ DLBCL, NOS
  EBV⁺ mucocutaneous ulcer
  DLBCL associated with chronic inflammation
  Lymphomatoid granulomatosis
  Primary mediastinal (thymic) large B-cell lymphoma
  Intravascular large B-cell lymphoma
  ALK⁺ large B-cell lymphoma
  Plasmablastic lymphoma
  Primary effusion lymphoma
  HHV8⁺ DLBCL, NOS
  Burkitt lymphoma
  Burkitt-like lymphoma with 11q aberration
  High-grade B-cell lymphoma, with *MYC* and *BCL2* and/or *BCL6* rearrangements
  High-grade B-cell lymphoma, NOS
  B-cell lymphoma, unclassifiable, with features intermediate between DLBCL and classical Hodgkin lymphoma
Mature T and NK Neoplasms
  T-cell prolymphocytic leukemia
  T-cell large granular lymphocytic leukemia
  Chronic lymphoproliferative disorder of NK cells
  Aggressive NK-cell leukemia
  Systemic EBV⁺ T-cell lymphoma of childhood
  Hydroa vacciniforme–like lymphoproliferative disorder
  Adult T-cell leukemia/lymphoma
  Extranodal NK-/T-cell lymphoma, nasal type
  Enteropathy-associated T-cell lymphoma
  Monomorphic epitheliotropic intestinal T-cell lymphoma
  Indolent T-cell lymphoproliferative disorder of the GI tract
  Hepatosplenic T-cell lymphoma
  Subcutaneous panniculitis-like T-cell lymphoma

(continued)

TABLE 6.1   WHO (2016) Classification of Mature Lymphoid, Histiocytic, and Dendritic Neoplasms (*continued*)

Mycosis fungoides
Sézary syndrome
Primary cutaneous CD30+ T-cell lymphoproliferative disorders
   Lymphomatoid papulosis
   Primary cutaneous anaplastic large cell lymphoma
Primary cutaneous γδ T-cell lymphoma
Primary cutaneous CD8+ aggressive epidermotropic cytotoxic T-cell lymphoma
Primary cutaneous acral CD8+ T-cell lymphoma
Primary cutaneous CD4+ small/medium T-cell lymphoproliferative disorder
Peripheral T-cell lymphoma, NOS
Angioimmunoblastic T-cell lymphoma
Follicular T-cell lymphoma
Nodal peripheral T-cell lymphoma with TFH phenotype
Anaplastic large-cell lymphoma, ALK+
Anaplastic large-cell lymphoma, ALK−
   Breast implant–associated anaplastic large-cell lymphoma
Hodgkin Lymphoma
Nodular lymphocyte predominant Hodgkin lymphoma
CHL
   Nodular sclerosis CHL
   Lymphocyte-rich CHL
   Mixed cellularity CHL
   Lymphocyte-depleted CHL
PTLD
Plasmacytic hyperplasia PTLD
Infectious mononucleosis PTLD
Florid follicular hyperplasia PTLD
Polymorphic PTLD
Monomorphic PTLD (B- and T-/NK-cell types)
CHL PTLD
Histiocytic and Dendritic Cell Neoplasms
Histiocytic sarcoma
Langerhans cell histiocytosis
Langerhans cell sarcoma
Indeterminate dendritic cell tumor
Interdigitating dendritic cell sarcoma
Follicular dendritic cell sarcoma
Fibroblastic reticular cell tumor
Disseminated juvenile xanthogranuloma
Erdheim–Chester disease

ALK, anaplastic lymphoma kinase; CHL, classical Hodgkin lymphoma; CNS, central nervous system; DLBCL, diffuse large B-cell lymphoma; EBV, Epstein–Barr virus; GI, gastrointestinal; HHV8, human herpesvirus-8; MALT, mucosa-associated lymphoid tissue; MGUS, monoclonal gammopathy of undetermined significance; NK, natural killer; NOS, not otherwise specified; PTLD, posttransplant lymphoproliferative disorder; TFH, T follicular helper.

Source: Adapted from Ref. (28). Swerdlow SH, Campo E, Pileri SA, et al. The 2016 revision of the World Health Organization classification of lymphoid neoplasms. *Blood.* 2016;127:2375-2390.

eosinophils, plasma cells, mast cells, and sometimes endothelial cells. Nevus round-oval cells may be encountered in axillary nodes (30). Anthracotic pigment is a normal finding in hilar lymph nodes (Figure 6.5).

Spleen

The spleen (normally 150–200 g in adults) is the largest lymphoid tissue in the human body. It is composed of red pulp (75% of splenic volume) and white pulp, separated by a marginal zone. The red pulp contains many thin-walled venous sinusoids lined by littoral (endothelial) cells that are separated by splenic cords (of Billroth) containing macrophages. The function of the red pulp is to filter and ingest certain (e.g., old, damaged, antibody-coated) RBCs. The white pulp forms sheaths of lymphoid cells around arteries. This periarteriolar lymphoid sheath is composed of T-cells and B-cells forming lymphoid follicles, a surrounding mantle zone, and an outer marginal zone. Biopsy of the spleen is rare because there is a risk of serious hemorrhage. However, FNA is of lower risk and diagnostically useful.

Imprints can be obtained at the time of grossing the specimen (Figure 6.6). Because the spleen is usually very bloody, imprints are best performed after blotting away excess blood. White pulp disorders (e.g., lymphomas) tend to produce macroscopic nodules whereas red pulp disorders (e.g., leukemia, Gaucher disease, extramedullary hematopoiesis) (Figure 6.7) tend to diffusely enlarge the spleen. A variety of conditions can affect the spleen including cysts (e.g., epithelial, hydatid), infections (e.g., splenitis, granulomas, infectious mononucleosis, malaria), nonneoplastic disorders (e.g., congestive splenomegaly, amyloidosis, infarction, sickle cell disease), hematogenous neoplasms (e.g., lymphoma, hairy cell leukemia, myelofibrosis), and nonhematologic neoplasms (e.g., littoral cell angioma, metastases).

Bone Marrow

Bone marrow biopsies are usually obtained from the posterior superior iliac crest as it has a large amount of red marrow. They are performed to evaluate the bone marrow for hematologic conditions (e.g., anemia), involvement by malignancy (e.g., leukemia, lymphoma, metastatic disease) and/or determine postchemotherapy cellularity or post–bone marrow transplant engraftment. Trephine biopsy imprints are often prepared to accompany aspirated marrow smears. Normal bone marrow may also be encountered when evaluating osseous tumors and bone resection margins. Bone marrow cellularity is around 90% to 100% in the first years of life, but decreases with age while the amount of fat increases. In general, the long bones contain only white (fatty) marrow with no hematopoiesis. Normal marrow contains trilineage hematopoiesis (erythroid precursors, myeloid progenitors, and megakaryocytes) (Figure 6.8). The myeloid–monocytic lineage usually predominates. The presence of mitotically active cells is normal. Normal marrow imprints may occasionally also contain osteoblasts, multinucleated osteoclasts, adipocytes, and endothelial cells. Osteoblasts can resemble plasma cells. They have abundant blue-gray cytoplasm, an eccentric round nucleus, and one or more nucleoli, but unlike plasma cells their perinuclear clearing is separated from the nucleus, and their nucleus appears to protrude from one edge of the cell as opposed to abutting the normal contour of the cell (Figure 10.5). Hematopoietic stem cells (CD34+), hematogones (lymphoid progenitor cells), and plasma cells are normally infrequent (<1% of marrow cells). Mature lymphocytes may be present in low numbers, which may occasionally form lymphoid aggregates in a nonparatrabecular location.

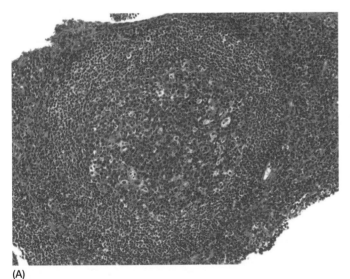

(A)

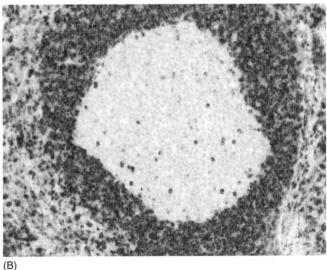

(B)

FIGURE 6.1 Benign lymph node. Core biopsy showing a reactive secondary lymphoid follicle with a central germinal center surrounded by mantle and marginal zones. BCL2 normally highlights mainly the marginal B-cells. ((A) H&E-stained core biopsy, low power; (B) BCL2 stain, low power.) H&E, hematoxylin and eosin.

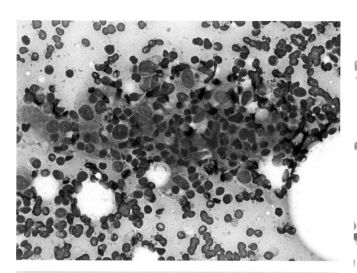

FIGURE 6.2 Benign lymph node. TP showing a lympho-histiocytic aggregate composed of mostly small and fewer larger mature lymphocytes, as well as several cohesive follicular dendritic cells. The dendritic cells have more abundant cytoplasm, vesicular nuclei, and a central nucleolus. Note the presence of background lymphoglandular bodies (DQ-stained TP, medium power). DQ, Diff-Quik; TP, touch preparation.

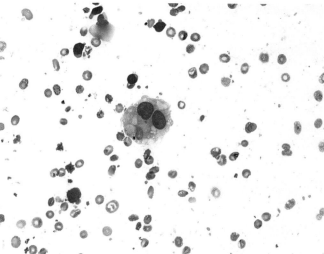

FIGURE 6.3 Follicular dendritic cell. The dendritic cell shown in the center of the image is much larger than mature lymphocytes. It is characterized by having abundant pale vacuolated cytoplasm, binucleation with vesicular chromatin, and small nucleoli. This cell mimics a Reed-Sternberg cell (DQ-stained cytopreparation, high power). DQ, Diff-Quik.

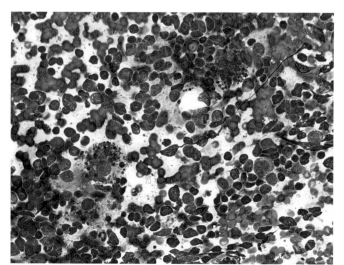

FIGURE 6.4 Benign lymph node. TP showing polymorphous lymphocytes mixed with several tingible-body macrophages (DQ-stained TP, medium power). DQ, Diff-Quik; TP, touch preparation.

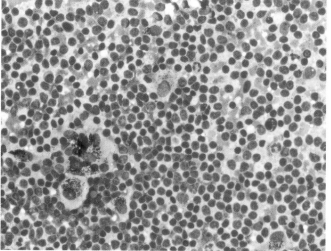

FIGURE 6.5 Benign hilar lymph node. TP showing a polymorphous lymphoid population admixed with scattered macrophages containing anthracotic pigment (DQ-stained TP, medium power). DQ, Diff-Quik; TP, touch preparation.

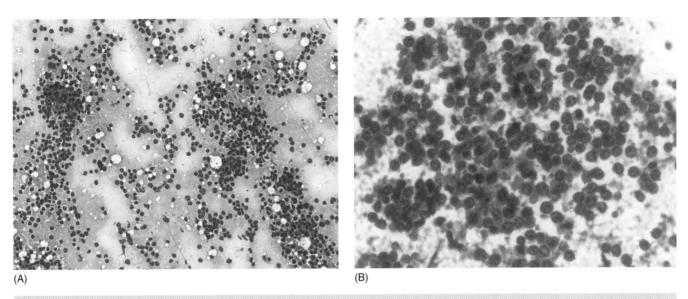

(A)

(B)

FIGURE 6.6 Benign spleen. TPs showing predominantly small lymphocytes derived from the white pulp. ((A) DQ-stained TP, low power; (B) H&E-stained imprint, high power.) DQ, Diff-Quik; H&E, hematoxylin and eosin; TP, touch preparation.

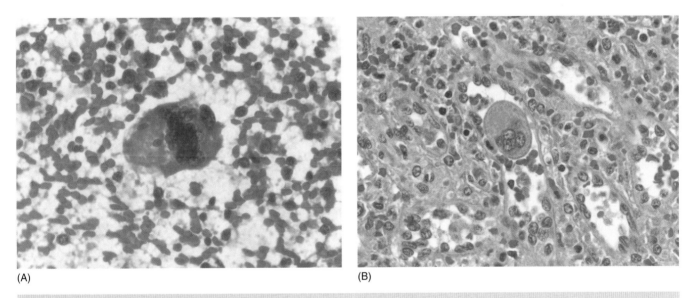

(A)

(B)

FIGURE 6.7 Spleen with extramedullary hematopoiesis. Megakaryocytes with abundant cytoplasm and multiple nuclei are shown. ((A) H&E-stained TP, high power; (B) H&E-stained splenectomy, high power.) H&E, hematoxylin and eosin; TP, touch preparation.

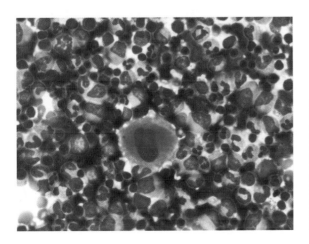

FIGURE 6.8 Normal bone marrow. TP showing trilineage hematopoiesis. Erythroid precursors are the smaller cells with dark blue cytoplasm, a high N:C ratio, and hyperchromatic nuclei. Myeloid-monocytic precursors have more cytoplasm and irregular nuclei showing varying stages of maturation. The megakaryocyte in the center is much larger, has abundant pale cytoplasm, and a multilobated nucleus (DQ-stained TP, high power). DQ, Diff-Quik; N:C, nuclear:cytoplasmic; TP, touch preparation.

BENIGN ENTITIES

Reactive Lymphoid Hyperplasia

Reactive lymphoid hyperplasia (RLH) due to antigenic stimulation is a common benign and often reversible cause of lymphadenopathy. Lymph node enlargement may be due to reactive follicular hyperplasia, diffuse paracortical expansion, and/or marked sinus histiocytosis. In general, there should be no cytologic or architectural atypia and no clonal process present (31,32). Reactive follicular hyperplasia reflects a B-cell response pattern, whereas paracortical hyperplasia or expanded interfollicular regions are mostly caused by a T-cell reaction. With follicular hyperplasia, enlarged follicles may vary in size and shape, and even coalesce. TPs from a node with reactive lymphoid follicles tend to produce follicle center fragments (i.e., lymphohistiocytic aggregates) (Figure 6.9). There may also be prominent GCs showing mixed small (centrocytes) and large (centroblasts) lymphocytes, as well as numerous TBMs (Figure 6.10). The presence of many conspicuous TBMs should raise the possibility of a rapidly proliferating high-grade lymphoma with a "starry sky" appearance (e.g., Burkitt lymphoma). Mitotic figures may be frequent with RLH. Imprints from areas with diffuse paracortical hyperplasia show a more evenly distributed polymorphous population of cells, including numerous small and fewer large lymphocytes (Figure 6.11). Immunoblasts in some cases may resemble Reed–Sternberg (RS) cells. Occasionally, there may be infrequent plasma cells, eosinophils, or mast cells.

The differential diagnosis of a heterogeneous lymphoid population includes other benign conditions (e.g., early stage cat scratch disease (CSD), Castleman disease) and lymphoma (marginal zone lymphoma, low-grade follicular lymphoma, T-cell rich B-cell lymphoma, HL, T-cell lymphoma), posttransplant lymphoproliferative disorder (PTLD), or partial lymph node involvement by malignancy. The differential diagnosis of increased plasma cells in a lymph node includes infection (e.g., HIV-related lymphadenopathy, syphilis, toxoplasmosis), Castleman disease (plasma cell variant), autoimmune-related lymphadenitis, IgG4-related lymphadenopathy, lymphoproliferative disorders with plasmacytic differentiation (e.g., marginal zone lymphoma, lymphoplasmacytic lymphoma, plasmablastic lymphoma, PTLD), and plasma cell neoplasia. Lymphadenopathy can occur in up to 80% of patients who have IgG4-related sclerosing disease, where there is an increase in IgG4$^+$ plasma cells and IgG4/IgG ratio (>40%) (33). Given the wide differential of RLH, specimen triage should include immunophenotyping by immunohistochemistry and/or flow cytometry to exclude a lymphoproliferative disorder. Even if ancillary studies confirm the diagnosis of RLH, in patients over 50 years of age follow-up is recommended because a large proportion of elderly patients may reveal a subsequent malignancy, usually lymphoma (34).

Granulomatous Lymphadenitis

Granulomatous inflammation involving lymph nodes can manifest with regional or generalized lymphadenopathy. The etiology may be infectious (e.g., mycobacterial, fungal), noninfectious and benign (e.g., sarcoidosis, foreign body reaction), or associated with malignancy. Sarcoidosis occurs most commonly in young female adults and African Americans, and is often associated with an elevated angiotensin-converting enzyme (ACE) blood level. Sarcoidosis typically involves the mediastinal lymph nodes. A CNB of peripheral nodes has been shown to provide high efficacy for diagnosing granulomas in sarcoidosis patients (35). Sarcoidosis is a diagnosis of exclusion. Also, the final diagnosis of sarcoidosis requires integration of pathology with clinical, laboratory, and radiologic findings. Neoplasms associated with granulomas that may be encountered include lymphoma (e.g., HL and NHL), squamous cell carcinoma, thyroid anaplastic carcinoma, lymphoepithelial carcinoma, and seminoma (36).

Granulomas are composed of cohesive epithelioid macrophages. They may occur with/without necrosis. In immunosuppressed patients (e.g., AIDS), there may be an associated suppurative pattern present. The cytomorphology of granulomatous lymphadenitis shows clusters of epithelioid histiocytes (macrophages) mixed with lymphocytes (Figures 6.12 and 6.13). Histiocytes are recognized as being round to elongated epithelioid shaped cells, which have a moderate amount of cytoplasm, and kidney bean or boomerang-shaped nuclei. They may sometimes contain nucleoli. Occasionally, there may also be multinucleated giant cells. The pattern of granulomas observed in cytology specimens do not appear to help distinguish tuberculosis (TB) from sarcoidosis (37). In sarcoidosis, however, there may be intracytoplasmic asteroid bodies (Figure 6.14), yellow-brown Hamazaki–Wesenberg inclusions, or concentrically laminated spherical Schaumann bodies. With any long-standing granuloma, there can be fibrosis and hyalinization, giving rise to hypocellular aspirates or imprints.

The differential diagnosis for necrotizing granulomas includes malignancy, CSD, Kikuchi lymphadenitis, autoimmune lymphadenitis (e.g., systemic lupus erythematosus), immunodeficiency-related chronic granulomatous disease, lymph node infarction, and trauma (e.g., prior FNA biopsy). The differential diagnosis for nonnecrotizing granulomas includes florid sinus histiocytosis, lipogranulomas, and metabolic storage disease (e.g., Gaucher disease). Nonnecrotizing granulomas can also be seen due to postchemotherapy effect for treated cancer. In one study of 1,275 cancer patients, nonnecrotizing granulomatous lymphadenopathy was identified in 12% of patients, of whom 8% had a concurrent diagnosis of cancer where the primary site of malignancy was primarily in or near the thorax (38). It is important to distinguish granulomas from other lymphocyte-rich specimens that contain similar appearing epithelial cell clusters such as thymoma (Figure 6.15), nasopharyngeal carcinoma, or lymphoepithelial carcinoma. Appropriate specimen triage for granulomatous lymphadenitis includes polarization microscopy to look for foreign material, ordering special stains for microorganisms, and submitting a portion of the sample for microbial culture. Immunostains using S100 and CD68 (KP1) can help confirm the presence of macrophages.

Dermatopathic Lymphadenopathy

Dermatopathic lymphadenopathy refers to nodal enlargement typically secondary to nearby exfoliative dermatitis caused by psoriasis, mycosis fungoides, or some other skin condition. It rarely occurs without clinical skin disease. Affected lymph nodes are characterized by nodular expansion of the interfollicular region due to S100 positive histiocytes (Figure 6.16) that may contain melanin pigment and/or fat. There may also be prominent postcapillary venules, Langerhans cells, dendritic cells, plasma cells, and eosinophils. The differential diagnosis includes RLH, conditions associated with pigment deposition (e.g., tattoo (Figure 6.17), prosthesis-related metallosis, nodal nevi inclusions, metastatic melanoma, and melanosis), HL, and mycosis fungoides. A Fontana–Masson special stain can be used to confirm melanin pigment. An iron stain will exclude hemosiderin deposition. It is not uncommon to find pelvic or inguinal lymph nodes in patients with cobalt–chromium or titanium hip implants with heavy metal microparticles or polyethylene particles associated with florid pigment-laden sinus histiocytosis. Melanosis is a rare manifestation of regressed melanoma, and when present, warrants a careful search for viable melanoma cells. In patients with cutaneous mycosis fungoides/Sézary syndrome, there may be only scattered or small groups of atypical lymphoid cells present in a background of more typical dermatopathic lymphadenopathy (39). Therefore, in such cases where mycosis fungoides is suspected immunophenotyping to detect an aberrant T-cell population and molecular studies to demonstrate a clonal TCR gene rearrangement are strongly recommended (40).

Rosai–Dorfman Disease

Sinus histiocytosis with massive lymphadenopathy (Rosai–Dorfman Disease) is a benign, self-limited condition that usually presents in young patients with massive, painless, bilateral cervical lymphadenopathy of unknown origin. Rarely, extranodal involvement may occur. The cytomorphology of this disease is characterized by a proliferation of histiocytes that have engulfed lymphocytes or other viable cells (emperipolesis) (Figures 6.18 and 6.19) (41). Histiocytes are easily recognized by their abundant vacuolated cytoplasm, round nuclei with large prominent nucleoli, and engulfed lymphocytes or sometimes plasma cells. In fixed material, a characteristic halo is often seen around engulfed cells, which helps to distinguish them from overlapping cells or tingible body debris. The background in these cytology samples usually contains reactive lymphocytes and plasma cells. The differential diagnosis includes RLH, hemophagocytosis, granulomatous lesions, HL, and Langerhans cell histiocytosis. The histiocytes in Rosai–Dorfman disease stain positively for CD68 and S100, but unlike in Langerhans cell histiocytosis they are negative for CD1a and Langerin.

Cat Scratch Disease

Lymphadenitis due to CSD is an acute, self-limiting infection caused by the Gram negative bacillus *Bartonella henselae*. It is common in children and young adults, and usually involves the axillary or head and neck lymph nodes. Localized, unilateral lymphadenopathy, often accompanied by fever, typically occurs 1 to 3 weeks after a cat scratch or bite. However, a history of animal exposure may not always be noted. Serologic studies for CSD have low sensitivity and specificity. The cytological features will depend on the phase of infection. In the initial phase, there is florid RLH (Figure 6.20). In subsequent phases, there are suppurative granulomas (Figure 6.21) with characteristic stellate microabscesses. Cytology preparations from infected nodes may show a reactive polymorphous lymphoid population with TBMs, increased plasmacytoid monocytes, dispersed epithelioid histiocytes, and sometimes suppurative granulomatous inflammation (42–44). The differential diagnosis in the initial phase is noninfectious RLH. In the later phases, the differential diagnosis includes an abscess, acute suppurative lymphadenitis due to other infections (e.g., TB, tularemia, lymphogranuloma venereum, yersiniosis), and Kikuchi necrotizing lymphadenitis. Special stains to identify pleomorphic coccobacilli and/or aggregates of curved bacilli include a modified silver/Steiner stain or Warthin–Starry stain. An immunostain for Bartonella is also commercially available (Figure 6.22) (45). Molecular studies (e.g., polymerase chain reaction (PCR)) may not always be available. Also, microbiology culture should be attempted but may be difficult due to the slow growth of this organism.

Acute Suppurative Lymphadenitis

Acute suppurative lymphadenitis usually presents with tender lymphadenopathy. The etiology is often related to infection including bacteria (e.g., *Staphylococcus* or *Streptococcus* spp.), actinomyces, or fungi. The cytological features typically show abscess material with abundant neutrophils and background granular debris. A careful search for intra- and extracellular organisms is necessary. The differential diagnosis includes other causes of infectious lymphadenopathy (e.g., CSD, tularemia, lymphogranuloma venereum), abscess, necrotizing lymphadenitis, Kikuchi lymphadenitis (where karyorrhectic debris mimics neutrophils), lymph node infarction, autoimmune-related lymphadenopathy, and malignancy (e.g., metastatic carcinoma with an inflammatory background). Special stains for microorganisms should be performed (e.g., Gram stain, AFB for mycobacteria, Grocott or Gomori's methenamine silver (GMS) for fungi, and Warthin–Starry or Steiner stain for bacteria associated with CSD). Microbial culture in this setting is important.

Mycobacterial Infection

Mycobacteria may cause lymphadenopathy as a result of a local (e.g., scrofula) or systemic infection. Hippocrates first coined the term "scrofula." Today, scrofula refers to a tuberculous infection of the cervicofacial lymph nodes. Lymphadenopathy may also occur in infants after bacille Calmette–Guerin (BCG) vaccination. Mycobacterial infection involving lymph nodes may be caused by *Mycobacterium tuberculosis* or atypical mycobacteria (e.g., *M. avium*, *M. intracellulare*, *M. fortuitum*, and *M. scrofulaceum*). In immunocompetent persons, the typical cytomorphology of mycobacterial infection includes caseating granulomatous inflammation. However, in patients who are immunocompromised (e.g., HIV-infected), there may also be suppurative necrotic inflammation, a mycobacterial spindle pseudotumor, or a specimen comprised entirely of necrosis (46).

Microscopic examination shows aggregates of epithelioid macrophages forming granulomas, multinucleated giant cells, and a dirty or granular background due to necrosis with/without acute inflammatory cells. Multinucleated giant cells of the Langhans type (peripherally placed nuclei) and foreign body type (randomly scattered nuclei) are more likely to be seen in TB than in sarcoidosis. The differential diagnosis includes acute suppurative or necrotizing lymphadenitis due to other infectious causes (e.g., CSD), Kikuchi lymphadenitis, autoimmune lymphadenitis, immunodeficiency, lymph node infarction, and malignancy with necrosis. Unlike fungal organisms that are usually conspicuous with routine cytology stains, it is rare to find mycobacteria without the use of special stains. Occasionally, mycobacteria may be seen as negative images (unstained microorganisms) with certain stains (e.g., air-dried Romanowsky-stained slides) (Figure 6.23). The finding of many unstained bacilli within macrophages resembles the tissue paper crinkled cytoplasm of Gaucher cells. Also, Whipple disease is characterized by many foamy macrophages. Ancillary tests for mycobacteria

include special stains for acid fast bacilli (AFB) (e.g., Ziehl–Neelsen stain, Kinyoun stain, Fite stain, Auramine-rhodamine stain), molecular testing (e.g., PCR), and/or microbial culture. With AFB stains, *M. tuberculosis* bacilli tend to be few in number, and are identified as slightly curved, slender rods measuring 2 to 4 μm in length. Microorganisms are easier to identify with atypical mycobacterial infection because they are typically much more numerous.

Fungal Infection

Fungal infections may result in lymphadenopathy. Common fungi implicated in lymphadenitis include *Cryptococcus neoformans*, *Histoplasma capsulatum*, and *Coccidioides immitis*. Pneumocystis and *Penicillium marneffei* are other opportunistic infections that may involve the lymph nodes of immunocompromised patients. The cytological features of fungal infection include acute and/or granulomatous inflammation, sometimes associated with necrosis. The differential diagnosis includes other infectious etiologies (e.g., TB, acute suppurative lymphadenitis) and noninfectious granulomatous disease. The key is to identify fungal organisms with their characteristic features (e.g., cryptococcal encapsulated yeast with narrow-based budding, small round to oval intracytoplasmic histoplasmosis). Calcified debris associated with old granulomas can sometimes mimic fungal organisms. Special histochemical stains such as GMS, Periodic acid-Schiff (PAS), and Fontana Masson stain for melanin are helpful to confirm the presence of fungal elements. At the time of specimen collection, triage should include submitting procured material for microbial culture.

Infectious Mononucleosis

Infectious mononucleosis is caused by Epstein–Barr virus (EBV) infection. Infected patients are usually teenagers or young adults, contagious, and present with a fever, fatigue, pharyngitis, tender cervical lymphadenopathy, splenomegaly, and sometimes hepatomegaly. Patients may have a positive Paul–Bunnell test, Monospot test, and EBV-specific serology. There is an associated leukocytosis with atypical CD8+ lymphocytes (Downey cells) present in peripheral blood smears. Lymph nodes from infected patients show a polymorphous lymphoid population of small lymphocytes admixed with plasma cells, and histiocytes. The characteristic finding is a prominent population of intermediate-to-large immunoblasts (Figure 6.24) (47,48). These cells have abundant cytoplasm, and can sometimes have pleomorphic or atypical nuclei with binucleation, resembling RS cells. Mitotic figures and infrequently necrosis may be encountered. The differential diagnosis includes RLH (e.g., drug-related hypersensitivity, postvaccinial lymphadenitis, other viral infection, autoimmune lymphadenitis, toxoplasma lymph-adenitis), lymphoma (e.g., lymphoblastic lymphoma, HL, immunoblastic diffuse large B-cell lymphoma (DLBCL)), and PTLD. Flow cytometry shows polyclonal B-cells and sometimes a reversed CD4:CD8 ratio. Immunohistochemistry is helpful to show that the RS-like cells are positive for CD20 and CD30 (variable) but are negative for CD15 and TdT. In-situ hybridization for EBV-encoded small RNA (EBER) is usually positive in infected B-cells.

HIV Lymphadenopathy

HIV-infected patients may present with lymphadenopathy due to HIV infection itself, coinfection (e.g., TB, bacillary angiomatosis), inflammatory processes (e.g., Castleman disease, immune reconstitution inflammatory syndrome), or malignancy (e.g., lymphoma, Kaposi sarcoma, metastases). Lymph node architecture evolves with HIV chronicity (49). Initially, nodes show hyperplastic geographic reactive follicles (pattern A), which are followed by follicle regression (pattern B), and ultimately end with a fibrotic node (pattern C). Warthin–Finkeldey-type giant cells (polykaryocytes) with multinucleated grape-like nuclei may be seen. Such cells may also be seen with measles and herpes simplex virus infection. The three patterns of HIV lymphadenitis are not easy to recognize by cytomorphology alone. The cytomorphology may be similar to RLH. The differential diagnosis includes Castleman disease. Immunohistochemistry for p24 can confirm HIV infection. Flow cytometry may be helpful to show that are CD8 are greater than CD4 lymphocytes and to exclude lymphoma.

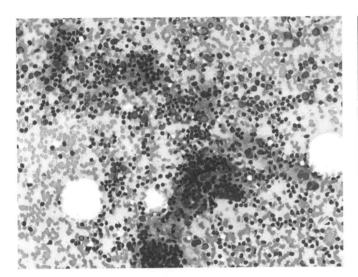

FIGURE 6.9 Reactive lymphoid hyperplasia. TP from a lymph node showing several lymphohistiocytic aggregates reflecting reactive follicular hyperplasia. The polymorphous appearance of this lymphoid population is due to a mixture of small centrocytes, larger centroblasts, occasional plasma cells, and follicular dendritic cells with abundant pale cytoplasm (DQ-stained TP, low power). DQ, Diff-Quik; TP, touch preparation.

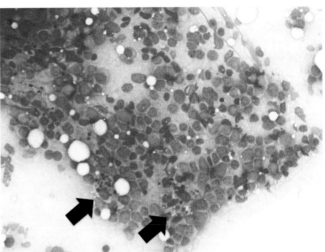

FIGURE 6.10 Reactive lymphoid hyperplasia. TP of a lymph node showing a polymorphous lymphoid population including several tingible-body macrophages (arrows), filled with apoptotic debris, derived from a reactive germinal center (DQ-stained TP, medium power). DQ, Diff-Quik; TP, touch preparation.

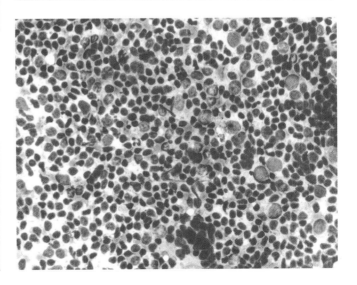

FIGURE 6.11 Reactive lymphoid hyperplasia. TP of a lymph node showing a polymorphous lymphoid population. Mature lymphocytes are the small cells with scant cytoplasm and dark nuclei. Centrocytes are intermediate-sized cells with scant cytoplasm and slightly cleaved nuclei. Centroblasts are the largest cells with a narrow rim of blue cytoplasm and round vesicular nuclei (DQ-stained TP, medium power). DQ, Diff-Quik; TP, touch preparation.

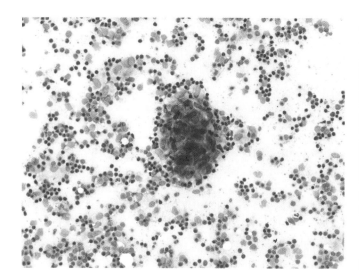

FIGURE 6.12 Granulomatous lymphadenitis. TP of a lymph node showing a central granuloma within a background of polymorphous lymphocytes and scattered single epithelioid histiocytes (DQ-stained TP, low power). DQ, Diff-Quik; TP, touch preparation.

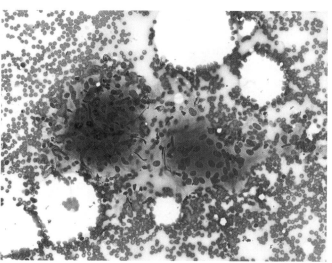

FIGURE 6.13 Granulomatous lymphadenitis. TP showing a well-formed nonnecrotizing granuloma (left) and large multinucleated histiocyte (right) with a clean background (DQ-stained TP, low power). DQ, Diff-Quik; TP, touch preparation.

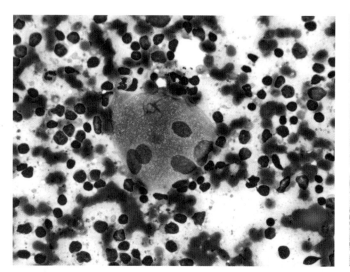

FIGURE 6.14 Granulomatous lymphadenitis. Multinucleated giant cell is shown containing a star-shaped asteroid body (DQ-stained TP, medium power). DQ, Diff-Quik; TP, touch preparation.

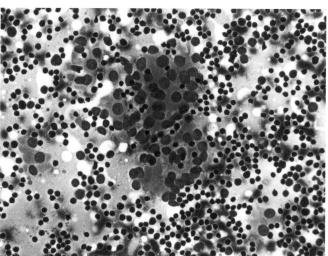

FIGURE 6.15 Lymphocyte-rich thymoma. Cohesive clusters of epithelial cells are shown with background lymphocytes that may be mistaken for granulomas (DQ-stained cytopreparation, medium power). DQ, Diff-Quik.

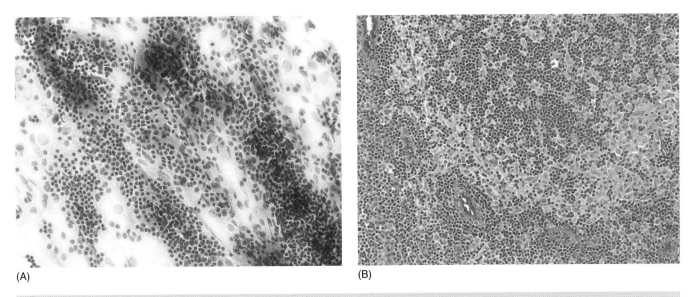

(A)

(B)

FIGURE 6.16 Dermatopathic lymphadenopathy. Touch imprint showing reactive lymphocytes admixed with abundant histiocytes and dendritic cells. The corresponding excised lymph node shows expansive interfollicular areas containing histiocytes and vascular proliferation. ((A) May–Grünwald–Giemsa stained touch preparation; (B) H&E-stained node excision, low power.) H&E, hematoxylin and eosin.

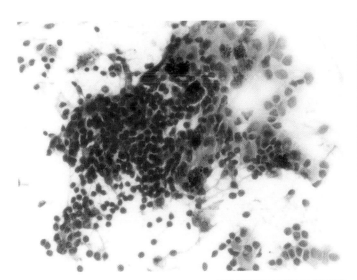

FIGURE 6.17 Lymphadenopathy with tattoo pigment. TP showing a lymphohistiocytic aggregate with pigment-laden macrophages (May–Grünwald–Giemsa stained TP, medium power). TP, touch preparation.

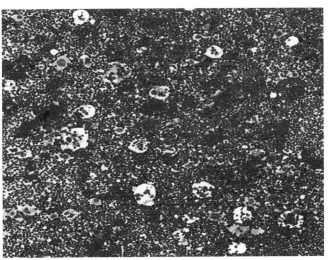

FIGURE 6.18 Rosai–Dorfman Disease. TP showing a dense polymorphous lymphoid population with scattered large histiocytes characterized by abundant clear cytoplasm and emperipolesis (Wright–Giemsa stained TP, low power). TP, touch preparation.

Image courtesy of Dr. Ronald Jaffe.

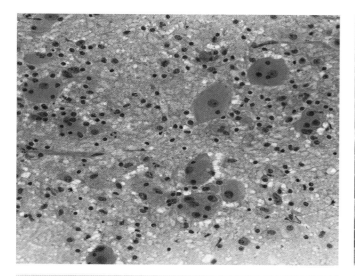

FIGURE 6.19 Rosai–Dorfman Disease. TP showing large histiocytes with abundant cytoplasm, round nuclei with prominent nucleoli, and engulfed lymphocytes and plasma cells (H&E-stained TP, low power). H&E, hematoxylin and eosin; TP, touch preparation.

Image courtesy of Dr. Ronald Jaffe.

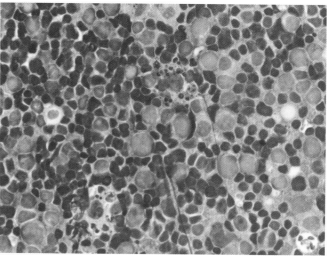

FIGURE 6.20 Cat scratch disease. Imprint of an excised lymph node from a patient with cat scratch disease shows a polymorphous lymphoid population with several monocytoid cells and tingible-body macrophages (Wright–Giemsa stained TP, high power). TP, touch preparation.

FIGURE 6.21 Cat scratch disease. Axillary lymph node showing suppurative granulomatous inflammation (H&E-stained excision, low power). H&E, hematoxylin and eosin.

FIGURE 6.22 Cat scratch disease. Numerous aggregates of microorganisms are highlighted using a commercially available monoclonal antibody to *Bartonella henselae* (Bartonella stain, high power).

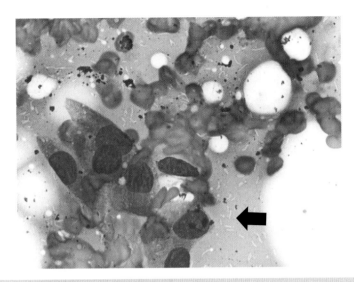

FIGURE 6.23 Atypical mycobacterial lymphadenopathy. Epithelioid macrophages are shown with negative staining of many mycobacteria (arrow) in the background. The negative image occurs due to the mycolic acid in the cell wall of the bacillus, which does not stain (Air-dried DQ-stained TP, oil magnification). DQ, Diff-Quik; TP, touch preparation.

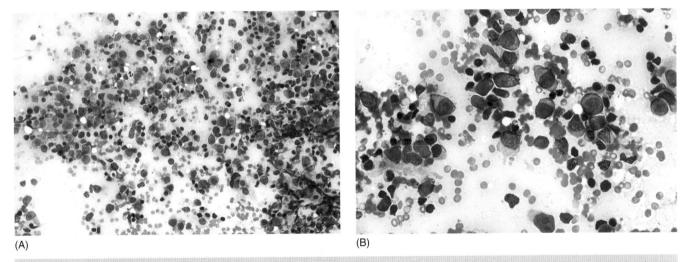

(A)

(B)

FIGURE 6.24 Infectious mononucleosis. TPs of a cervical lymph node from an 18-year-old female showing a predominant reactive immunoblastic population. Immunoblasts are characterized by having abundant blue cytoplasm, a high N:C ratio, and prominent central nucleoli. ((A) DQ-stained TP, low power; (B) DQ-stained TP, medium power.) DQ, Diff-Quik; N:C, nuclear:cytoplasmic; TP, touch preparation.

MALIGNANT ENTITIES

Lymphoblastic Lymphoma

Precursor lymphoid neoplasms include both B lymphoblastic leukemia/lymphoma (not otherwise specified [NOS] and with recurrent genetic abnormalities) and T lymphoblastic leukemia/lymphoma (formerly T-cell acute lymphoblastic lymphoma or T-ALL). Lymphoblastic lymphoma is more common in T-cells. This is an aggressive lymphoma that accounts for almost 50% of childhood NHL. T-cell lymphoblastic lymphomas classically present in young adolescent males with mediastinal (thymic) lymphadenopathy. These patients may develop superior vena cava syndrome, other compressive symptoms, and lymphomatous effusions, as well as hepatosplenomegaly, central nervous system (CNS), peripheral blood and bone marrow involvement. The cytomorphology includes small- to medium-sized lymphoblasts with scant cytoplasm, round nuclei, immature chromatin (i.e., finely granular), inconspicuous nucleoli, and mitoses (Figure 6.25) (50). Immunophenotyping by immunohistochemistry or flow cytometry shows that lymphoma cells are positive for T-cell markers (CD1a, CD2, CD3, CD4, CD5, CD7, CD8) or B-cell markers (CD19, CD79a, PAX5), as well as terminal deoxynucleotidyl transferase (TdT) and CD10. LCA may be negative. The differential diagnosis includes thymoma, particularly type B1 thymoma (lymphocyte rich), because thymic lymphocytes are also TdT positive. TdT may also stain Merkel cell carcinoma and infrequently small cell carcinoma. Molecular studies can be used to demonstrate TCR or Ig heavy chain gene rearrangement if needed.

Hodgkin Lymphoma

Classical Hodgkin Lymphoma

Classical Hodgkin lymphoma (CHL) includes four subtypes: nodular sclerosis, lymphocyte-rich (LRCHL), mixed cellularity, and lymphocyte-depleted HL. Most cases are derived from B-cells. HL has a bimodal age peak, presenting in both young adults and the elderly. Nodular sclerosis CHL is seen mostly in adolescents or young adults and is associated with a good prognosis. HIV infection is associated mainly with mixed cellularity and lymphocyte depleted CHL. Rarely, HL may occur as a result of transformation from a small cell lymphoma such as chronic lymphocytic leukemia/small lymphocytic lymphoma. Patients often present with painless cervical lymphadenopathy, but may also have enlarged mediastinal, axillary, and paraaortic lymph nodes. Nonaxial lymph node (e.g., mesenteric, Waldeyer ring) or primary extranodal involvement (e.g., spleen) occurs infrequently. Many patients have B symptoms (fever, night sweats, weight loss).

In one study where imprint material was reviewed from 34 HL cases, 76.5% were correctly diagnosed and 17.6% were suspected to be HL (51). Only two of the cases (6%) from this study were incorrectly diagnosed as reactive lesions because of an insufficient number of RS cells. Tumors from CHL cases typically contain a variable number (0.1%–10%) of large (15–45 μm) mononuclear Hodgkin and/or multinucleated RS cells associated with a mixed inflammatory background including nonneoplastic small T lymphocytes, eosinophils, neutrophils, histiocytes, and plasma cells (Figure 6.26). Samples may also contain fibroblasts, sclerotic tissue fragments, necrosis, or granulomas (52,53). Both aspirates and touch preparations derived from CHL of the nodular sclerosis type may be scant in cellularity due to dense sclerosis. In TPs, Hodgkin and RS cells may cluster together(Figures 1.8 and 6.27), particularly in the rare syncytial variant of nodular sclerosing CHL, and this could be mistaken for metastatic carcinoma (52). These large mononuclear and binucleated RS cells have abundant cytoplasm and prominent eosinophilic, sometimes oblong, macronucleoli (Figure 6.28).

The differential diagnosis of CHL includes RLH, viral lymphadenitis with large cells (EBV or HIV-related lymphadenopathy), various NHLs (e.g., T-cell rich DLBCL, anaplastic large cell lymphoma), and nasopharyngeal carcinoma. RS-like cells can be seen in a variety of benign and neoplastic lesions in the absence of HL (54). Ancillary studies are therefore required to distinguish CHL from these aforementioned entities. Hodgkin and RS cells are positive for CD30 (Golgi and membranous staining) (Figure 6.29), CD15, MUM-1, LMP1, fascin, and EBER. They may be weakly PAX5 positive. They are typically negative for LCA, CD20 (a minority of cases may be positive), OCT-2, BOB.1, EMA, and anaplastic lymphoma kinase (ALK). Of note, CD30 immunoreactivity may also be seen in CD8+ T-cells, virus-infected T-cells, EBV-infected B-cells such as with infectious mononucleosis and EBV-positive DLBCL, mediastinal (thymic) large B-cell lymphoma (weak staining), anaplastic large cell lymphoma, decidua, and embryonal carcinoma. Flow cytometry may show an increase in CD4+ T-cells. In contrast, RLH typically shows an increase in CD8+ T-cells. In older patients with a monotonous or atypical small lymphoid population in the background, flow cytometry can also help determine if HL arose as a transformation from a small cell lymphoma. RS cells may contain Ig gene rearrangements in many cases, and may rarely have clonal TCR gene rearrangements.

In some cases, it may be difficult to make a definitive diagnosis due to overlapping features. For such cases, it may be best to render a diagnosis of B-cell lymphoma, unclassifiable, with features intermediate between DLBCL (especially primary mediastinal large B-cell lymphoma) and CHL (55). These "grey zone" lymphomas usually involve the mediastinum in young men and are more aggressive. They often have many pleomorphic Hodgkin-like cells and necrosis. CD45 and B-cell markers (e.g., CD20) are also more likely to be positive in these cases than in CHL.

Nodular Lymphocyte Predominant Hodgkin Lymphoma

Nodular lymphocyte predominant Hodgkin lymphoma (NLPHL) is less common than CHL and occurs mainly in young men. Although it has an indolent behavior, the recurrence rate of this monoclonal B-cell neoplasm is higher than CHL. NLPHL typically involves peripheral lymph nodes. Affected nodes are replaced with expansive nodules composed of small B lymphocytes and sparse lymphocyte predominant (LP) cells, previously called L&H (lymphocytic & histiocytic) or popcorn tumor cells. L&H cells are large cells that have a round or multilobulated nucleus, finely granular chromatin, and distinct nucleoli (Figure 6.30). There may also be admixed epithelioid histiocytes, dendritic cells, scant eosinophils, and plasma cells. Some cases can have varied growth patterns, including nodes with more diffuse areas and/or regions with numerous T cells. Some cases may evolve into a diffuse T-cell–rich proliferation lacking any FDCs, which would be consistent with a T-cell histiocyte-rich large B-cell lymphoma. Not surprisingly, cases of NLPHL are commonly misdiagnosed in cytology specimens as benign reactive lymphoid tissue (56). This is largely because of their polymorphous appearance and due to the fact that scant mononucleate L&H cells are not easy to recognize. Moreover, classic RS-like cells are not usually seen. NLPHL can be differentiated from CHL with adequate immunostaining (57). LP cells are positive for LCA (variable), CD79a, CD20, PAX5, OCT-2, BOB.1, J chain, IgD, and EMA (variable) but are negative for CD30, CD15, and fascin. Flow cytometry may show an increase in CD4+ and CD8+ (double positive) T-cells.

Non-Hodgkin Lymphoma

NHL includes a diverse group of lymphomas that vary in cell type (i.e., mostly B-cell NHL and infrequently T-cell or null cell NHL) and cell size (e.g., small, intermediate and large cell lymphomas) (Table 6.2). The role of cytology in primary diagnosis, subclassification, and grading of patients with lymphoma is controversial. Nevertheless, cytodiagnosis of NHL has been shown to be a reliable method with high sensitivity (58). Imprint cytology, in particular, has been shown to reveal certain morphologic details such as plasmacytoid features (Figure 6.31) in various lymphomas that are often not discernible in tissue sections (59). In one study, large cell lymphoma and large cell transformation could be reliably diagnosed by FNA as long as greater than 40% large cells were present (60). Several commonly encountered lymphomas are discussed below. In general, the cytological features of these lymphomas include an abnormal population of atypical lymphoid cells with lymphoglandular bodies (cytoplasmic fragments) (Figure 6.32). It is important to be aware that apoptotic debris, platelets, stain artifact, and ultrasound gel may mimic lymphoglandular bodies. Moreover, although lymphoglandular bodies are often accepted as being diagnostic of lymphoid tissue (61), they may exceptionally also be encountered in some nonlymphoid malignancies (e.g., small cell carcinoma, non–small cell carcinoma, melanoma, seminoma, and ganglioneuroblastoma) (62). Lymphoglandular bodies can also be seen in HL and with reactive lymphadenitis. The number of lymphoglandular bodies seen is likely to be higher in May–Grünwald–Giemsa than H&E-stained slides, and also higher in FNA smears compared to imprints (63). Immunophenotyping, determined by immunohistochemistry and/or flow cytometry, is essential for subtyping NHL. FISH or molecular abnormalities are also necessary, as they may help identify characteristic translocations.

TABLE 6.2 Differential Diagnosis of NHL Based on Cell Size

Predominantly Small Cell Population
- CLL/SLL
- Mantle cell lymphoma
- Follicular lymphoma
- Marginal zone lymphoma
- Lymphoplasmacytic lymphoma
- T-cell lymphomas

Intermediate (Medium) Cell Population
- Lymphoblastic lymphoma
- Burkitt lymphoma
- Mantle cell lymphoma, blastoid variant
- T-cell lymphomas

Predominantly Large Cell Population
- Diffuse large B cell lymphoma
- Plasmablastic lymphoma
- Anaplastic large cell lymphoma

CLL, chronic lymphocytic leukemia; NHL, Non-Hodgkin lymphoma; SLL, small lymphocytic lymphoma.

Follicular Lymphoma

Follicular lymphoma is the most common small cell lymphoma. This NHL originates from germinal/follicular center B-cells. It occurs predominantly in older adults. Patients usually present with generalized, painless, waxing lymphadenopathy. Many have bone marrow involvement. Follicular lymphoma can also occur in almost any extranodal site (e.g., spleen, liver, intestines, skin). Follicular lymphoma is an indolent lymphoma, but up to 25% to 30% of patients may transform to a large B-cell lymphoma (e.g., DLBCL, Burkitt, B-cell ALL) with a more poor prognosis and rapid disease progression. Involved nodes are effaced by neoplastic follicles comprised of both small cleaved cells without nucleoli (centrocytes) and larger non-cleaved cells with multiple nucleoli (centroblasts). TPs from areas with a follicular growth pattern tend to show patches of lymphocytes created by imprints of the lymphoid follicles (Figure 6.33). In cytology samples, centrocytes are monomorphic small lymphocytes with scant cytoplasm and nuclear irregularities or clefts in their nuclei creating bilobed or buttock-like cells (Figure 6.34). These B-cells typically have prominent chromocenters or clumps of chromatin within their nuclei. Centroblasts are larger cells (three times the size of mature lymphocytes) with moderate cytoplasm, large noncleaved nuclei with open chromatin, and can have one to three peripheral nucleoli. Rare cases may show signet ring cell features (64). Pediatric-type follicular lymphoma, which may occur in adults, is characterized by large expansile highly proliferative follicles within lymph nodes that have prominent blastoid follicular center cells. Necrosis and TBMs are typically not present. Sometimes nonneoplastic follicles and follicles only partially colonized by follicular lymphoma cells may be present.

Grading of follicular lymphoma is based on the average number of intrafollicular centroblasts per 40× high power field (HPF) (where grade 1 = 0–5, grade 2 = 6–15, and grade 3 > 15 centroblasts/HPF). At least 10 HPFs within different follicles need to be evaluated. Grade 1 and 2 constitute low grade. Grading is possible, but can be difficult in cytology samples (65). In particular, grade 3 with many centroblasts (Figure 6.35) is difficult to reliably differentiate from DLBCL. On average, there should be less than 10% centroblasts in grade 1, close to 25% in grade 2, and 50% in grade 3. A Ki67 labeling index may help with grading follicular lymphoma. Grade 1-2 follicular lymphomas tend to have a Ki67 index of less than 20%. The immunophenotype of follicular lymphoma shows that lymphoma cells are positive for CD20, CD19, CD79a, CD10, BCL2, BCL6, and surface Ig, but are negative for CD5. CD10 may be lost in higher grade lymphomas and those with a diffuse growth pattern. Pediatric-type follicular lymphoma, primary cutaneous follicular lymphomas, and predominantly diffuse follicular lymphoma with 1p36 deletion may lack the *BCL2* rearrangement, but may show some BCL2 protein expression. On occasion, flow cytometric studies may demonstrate indolent follicular lymphoma-like B cells (so-called in situ follicular lymphoma) that must not be over-interpreted as follicular lymphoma (66). In around 85% of cases cytogenetics will show the hallmark t(14;18)(q32;q21) rearrangement involving the *BCL2* and *IgH* genes.

Small Lymphocytic Lymphoma/Chronic Lymphocytic Leukemia

SLL/CLL accounts for around 7% of NHL and manifests mainly in older adults. Patients present with leukemia (CLL) and/or disease (SLL) involving the bone marrow, lymph nodes, or other extranodal sites (e.g., spleen, liver). Most cases are of B-cell origin. These lymphomas have a diffuse growth pattern comprised of small round mature lymphocytes. TPs tend to be cellular and because of their diffuse growth pattern imprints of these lymphomas often show an even spread of lymphocytes (Figure 6.36). The monomorphic small lymphocytes are characterized by having clumped chromatin (soccer ball-like appearance) and scant, eccentrically placed cytoplasm giving some cells a plasmacytoid appearance (Figure 6.37). In tissue sections, pale stained pseudofollicles or proliferation centers may be present that contain prolymphocytes, which are slightly larger lymphocytes with abundant cytoplasm and prominent nucleoli. Large, confluent and/or highly proliferative proliferation centers are adverse prognostic indicators.

Lymphoma cells are positive for CD20 (dim), CD19, CD79a, CD5, CD23, and lymphocyte enhancer–binding factor 1 (LEF1), but are negative for CD10, cyclin D1, and FMC7. CD5 negative cases may rarely occur, often in patients who are older that present with more advanced disease and lower absolute lymphocyte counts than CD5+ B-cell CLL. Positivity for CD38 or ZAP70 portends a worse prognosis. FISH for 17p (TP53 locus) and 11q (ATM) deletions and mutational status of the *IgVH* gene also provide prognostic information. *NOTCH1*, *SF3B1*, and *BIRC3* are also recognized as mutations of potential clinical relevance. Cytogenetics may show trisomy 12 or chromosome 13q14 deletion. While CLL/SLL is an indolent lymphoma, some cases may transform to a high-grade neoplasm via prolymphocytic transformation (Figure 6.38), or to a large cell lymphoma such as DLBCL (Richter's syndrome) (Figure 6.39), or rarely to CHL. In patients suspected of transformation, it may be important to perform a CNB rather than just FNA (67). A high Ki-67 labeling index is a valuable adjunct to recognize those patients at risk of an accelerated clinical course with possible transformation (68).

Marginal Zone Lymphoma

Marginal zone lymphoma accounts for about 10% of B-cell lymphomas. These are indolent lymphomas. They include nodal, extranodal (mucosa-associated lymphoid tissue, i.e., MALT-lymphoma) and splenic marginal zone lymphoma. Extranodal lymphoma is the more common type, with half of these comprising gastric lymphomas. Gastric MALT lymphoma is associated with *Helicobacter pylori* gastritis. MALT lymphoma of the salivary gland is associated with Sjögren's syndrome. Similarly, patients with Hashimoto's thyroiditis are at risk of developing MALT lymphoma of the thyroid gland. These lymphomas are characterized by a perifollicular (marginal zone) heterogeneous proliferation comprised of small lymphocytes, monocyte-like centrocytes with abundant pale cytoplasm, and larger immunoblast-like centroblasts. In mucosal tissue, the B-cells infiltrate epithelium to form lymphoepithelial lesions. Cytology samples are characterized by having a polymorphous population of small- to intermediate-sized lymphocytes, plasma cells, and FDCs (Figure 6.40). Some of the cells may have plasmacytic differentiation (Figure 6.41). The differential diagnosis includes RLH. Correlation with serum protein electrophoresis is helpful to exclude lymphoplasmacytic lymphoma. Immunophenotyping shows that lymphoma cells are positive for CD20 but are negative for CD5, CD10, CD23, and BCL6. Cytogenetics shows t(11;18)(q21;q21) or trisomy 3. Given that there is phenotypic overlap (CD5 and CD10 negative) with lymphoplasmacytic lymphoma and CD5-negative mantle cell lymphoma (MCL), excluding the presence of a *MYD88* mutation seen in lymphoplasmacytic lymphoma and excluding a *CCND1* translocation in a CD5-negative MCL can aid in making a diagnosis.

Mantle Cell Lymphoma

Mantle cell lymphoma (MCL) comprises up to 10% of NHL. It occurs more commonly in elderly men. This is the most aggressive type of small B-cell lymphoma. Patients usually present with advanced stage, experience rapid clinical progression, and often relapse. There is frequent extranodal spread to the peripheral blood, bone marrow, and gastrointestinal tract (e.g., lymphomatous polyposis). The cytologic features include a monomorphic population of small- to medium-sized lymphocytes with irregular box-like nuclear contours and fine chromatin (Figure 6.42). Mitotic figures are common. A small cell variant has been described that consists of small round lymphocytes with more clumped chromatin mimicking SLL/CLL. The blastoid and pleomorphic morphologic variants behave aggressively. In the blastoid variant lymphoma cells resemble lymphoblasts with finely dispersed chromatin and multiple small nucleoli. The blastoid variant also has an increased mitotic rate (at least 20–30 mitoses/10 HPF) or high Ki67 labeling index (e.g.,

≥30%). The pleomorphic variant contains many larger cells with pale cytoplasm and more irregular nuclear contours (Figure 6.43). Immunophenotyping shows that lymphoma cells are positive for CD20 (bright), CD19, CD5, cyclin D1 (BCL1) (Figure 6.44), BCL2, FMC7, CD43, and SOX11 but are negative for CD10, CD23, and BCL6. Rare cases may be negative for CD5 or cyclin D1. These can be identified by SOX11 immunohistochemistry and the identification of other (e.g., *CCND2*) translocations (69,70). High expressions of p53 and MYC aberrations are associated with an aggressive clinical course. Cytogenetics shows t(11;14)(q13;q32) causing overexpression of the *PRAD/BCL-1* gene that encodes cyclin D1. Rarely, cases may show composite MCL and CLL/SLL.

Lymphoplasmacytic Lymphoma

Lymphoplasmacytic lymphoma is a rare subtype of B-cell NHL. This indolent lymphoma occurs mostly in older adults. Patients frequently have a serum paraprotein (usually monoclonal IgM spike) and Waldenström's macroglobulinemia. Lymphoma may involve the bone marrow and extramedullary tissues (e.g., lymph nodes, spleen, and liver). Infiltrates are characterized by small lymphocytes showing plasmacytoid or plasma cell differentiation. Cytology specimens typically show a polymorphous population with small- to intermediate-sized lymphocytes, plasmacytoid lymphocytes, plasma cells, and mast cells. Lymphoma cells may have cytoplasmic (Russell) or nuclear (Dutcher) inclusions due to immunoglobulin. Immunophenotyping shows that lymphoma cells are positive for CD20, CD79a, CD38 (variable), and surface IgM but are negative for CD5, CD10, and CD23. Uncommon phenotypes may show CD5 or CD10 expression. The differential diagnosis includes RLH and marginal zone lymphoma. This lymphoma may transform to DLBCL with RS-like cells or immunoblasts. The majority of cases of lymphoplasmacytic lymphoma will have *MYD88* L265P mutations.

Burkitt Lymphoma

Burkitt lymphoma is a rapidly proliferating highly aggressive lymphoma. The three clinical variants are endemic, sporadic, and immunodeficiency-associated Burkitt lymphoma. Endemic Burkitt lymphoma is seen mostly in Africa where it presents in children, involving their jaws and facial bones. The sporadic form occurs throughout the world and usually involves the gastrointestinal tract, retroperitoneum, kidneys, ovaries, or breast. Immunodeficiency-associated Burkitt lymphoma is primarily associated with AIDS. The CSF may be involved in 20% to 30% patients with Burkitt lymphoma. These lymphomas are frequently associated with EBV infection. The diagnosis relies on finding a monotonous infiltrate of intermediate-sized lymphocytes. Lymphoma cells have round nuclei with finely clumped or dispersed chromatin and multiple, centrally located nucleoli. Burkitt cells typically have scant basophilic cytoplasm with discrete vacuoles (Figure 6.45), best seen on Romanowsky-stained smears. The abovementioned cellular features of Burkitt cells are best perceived in imprints (71). Immunodeficiency-associated Burkitt lymphoma may have a more pleomorphic appearance. Often, abundant apoptosis and numerous TBMs are also present (Figure 6.46), which create a "starry sky" appearance in surgical tissue sections. Florid granulomas may be seen, which are associated with a good prognosis.

The differential diagnosis includes DLBCL including plasmablastic lymphoma, lymphoblastic lymphoma, blastoid MCL, and nonhematologic round cell tumors (e.g., Ewing sarcoma). For intermediate cases with overlapping morphological (Figure 6.47) and genetic features, the 2008 WHO diagnosis used was B-cell lymphoma, unclassifiable, with features intermediate between DLBCL and Burkitt lymphoma (BCLU); formerly called Burkitt-like lymphoma (72). According to the newer (2016) WHO classification, such intermediate cases are best placed into the category "high-grade B-cell lymphomas with/without *MYC* and *BCL2* or *BCL6* translocations (i.e., double/triple hit lymphoma)," or if they lack a *MYC* and *BCL2* and/or *BCL6* rearrangement they can be placed in the category of "high-grade B-cell lymphoma, not otherwise specified (HGBL, NOS)" (28). Immunophenotyping shows that Burkitt lymphoma cells are positive for CD20, CD10, and BCL6 but are negative for CD5, CD23, BCL2, and TdT. The rate of proliferation for Burkitt lymphoma, as determined by Ki-67 staining, should be ≥95%. Cytogenetics shows activation of the c-*MYC* oncogene via several rearrangements including t(8;14) in 80%, t(2;8) in 15%, and t(8;22) in 5% of cases. *MYC* translocations can also been seen in DLBCL, follicular lymphoma, and multiple myeloma. Burkitt-like lymphoma with 11q aberration is a newer entity with a follicular growth pattern that closely resembles Burkitt lymphoma, but lacks a *MYC* rearrangement. Up to 70% of Burkitt lymphoma cases may also have *TCF3* or *ID3* mutations.

Diffuse Large B-Cell Lymphoma

DLBCL is the most common subtype of B-cell NHL, which comprises about 25% to 30% of B-cell NHL. DLBCL occurs mainly in older adults. Underlying immunodeficiency (e.g., HIV infection) is a risk factor. Afflicted patients present with rapidly progressive lymphadenopathy or extranodal disease (e.g., skin, CNS, gastrointestinal tract, bone, testis) at diagnosis. DLBCL is an aggressive lymphoma. They commonly arise de novo (primary DLBCL), but may occur (secondary DLBCL) due to progression or transformation from a less aggressive lymphoma (e.g., CLL/SLL, follicular lymphoma, marginal zone lymphoma, HL).

These lymphomas are defined by having large B-cells (usually three to five times larger than a RBC, or with nuclei at least two times the size of a mature lymphocyte). They usually exhibit a diffuse growth pattern. Lymphoma cells may resemble centroblasts or immunoblasts. Those that resemble centroblasts (centroblastic variant) have scant cytoplasm, oval-round nuclei with fine vesicular chromatin, and two to four predominantly membrane-bound nucleoli (Figure 6.48). Those resembling immunoblasts (immunoblastic variant) have more cytoplasm and large nuclei with one central nucleolus (Figure 6.49). Greater than 90% of cells must resemble immunoblasts to diagnose the immunoblastic variant. DLBCL tumor cells may also have plasmacytic differentiation. Sometimes tumor cells are more anaplastic (anaplastic variant), which can be associated with neutrophils. Such tumors may mimic T-cell anaplastic large cell lymphoma, HL, anaplastic carcinoma (particularly if they show clustering and are EMA+), or sarcoma. Other rare morphologic variants include DLBCL with spindle-shaped or signet ring cells. Tumor cells tend to be fragile, and hence frequently get distorted or crushed in cytology preparations. TBMs can be seen in high-grade variants.

DLBCL is composed of a heterogeneous group of B-cell lymphoproliferative malignancies (Table 6.1). Many cases are diagnosed as DLBCL, NOS. The differential diagnosis of DLBCL incudes poorly differentiated carcinoma (including nasopharyngeal carcinoma), myeloid sarcoma, melanoma, seminoma/dysgerminoma, and thymoma. Immunophenotyping shows that lymphoma cells are positive for CD20, CD19, CD79a, PAX5, CD10 (variable), CD30 and ALK (anaplastic variant), and CD5 (10%), but are negative for CD138 and TdT. The CD5+ DLBCL variant has a poorer prognosis. DLBCL may be of germinal center B-cell (GCB) type (CD10+, BCL6+, MUM1−) or activated (non-GC) B-cell (ABC) type (CD10−, BCL6−, MUM1+). The ABC subtype is associated with worse outcomes when treated with standard chemoimmunotherapy. The distinction of GCB vs ABC subtype is therefore important. Hans proposed an algorithm using a small set of immunohistochemical stains (CD10, BCL6, and MUM1/IRF4) for this purpose (73). Several mutational changes (e.g., *BCL2*, *BCL6*, c-*MYC*) and elevated Ki-67 expression are also associated with poor outcomes. Coexpression of MYC and BCL2 represents a double-expressor lymphoma that has a worse outcome. DLBCL may be difficult to diagnose with flow cytometry because of their increased tumor cell fragility and/or poor cell viability (i.e., necrosis). IgH and IgL are clonally rearranged, but may be difficult to document in T-cell rich cases due to the paucity of large B-cells.

T-Cell/Histiocyte-Rich Large B-Cell Lymphoma

This variant of DLBCL is characterized by scant numbers of scattered large, atypical B-cells associated with a background of abundant small T-cells (CD3+, CD5+) and variable numbers of histiocytes (CD68+) (Figure 6.50). This lymphoma may involve lymph nodes or extranodal sites. Unlike CHL, eosinophils or plasma cells are not present. Immunophenotyping shows that the large lymphoma cells are positive for B-cell markers, BLC6, BCL2 (variable), and EMA but are negative for CD15, CD30, and CD138. Due to the scarcity of large B-cells, T-cell-rich B-cell lymphoma (TCRBCL) is particularly difficult to diagnose in cytology samples (74).

Primary DLBCL of the CNS

Primary DLBCL of the CNS (PCNSL) accounts for 2% to 3% of all brain tumors. They typically occur in elderly males. Up to 20% to 40% of patients may present with multiple brain lesions. Extraneural dissemination is rare. Morphologically tumor cells mostly resemble centroblasts. Apart from the lymphoma cells, crush preparations may also show intermingled reactive small lymphocytes, macrophages, microglial cells, and reactive astrocytes (Figure 6.51A). Tumor cells tend to grow in perivascular spaces (Figure 6.51B) and expand into tumors characterized by a diffuse growth pattern. Necrosis is common in patients treated with high dose corticosteroids.

Primary Cutaneous DLBCL (Leg Type)

This primary cutaneous DLBCL is composed of large B-cells that arise mainly in the lower legs. It accounts for only 4% of primary skin lymphomas. Most patients are elderly woman. Skin nodules usually present on one or both legs and often disseminate to extracutaneous sites. Morphologically they are composed of a diffuse sheet of monotonous large round cells. In most cases, there are cells with a centroblastic and immunoblastic appearance. The tumor cells typically do not infiltrate the epidermis. The differential diagnosis includes cutaneous follicle center lymphoma, the most common primary cutaneous B-cell lymphoma, and nonhematological malignancies (e.g., melanoma, Merkel cell carcinoma, epithelioid sarcoma) (75). Immunophenotyping shows that lymphoma cells are positive for B-cell markers, BCL2 (variable), BCL6, and MUM1 (variable) but are negative for CD10, CD30, and CD138. EBV is negative in primary cutaneous DLBCL.

EBV-Positive DLBCL

EBV-positive DLBCL, NOS (formerly EBV+ DLBCL of the elderly) may occur in immunocompetent patients of any age that do not have a prior lymphoma. This category of lymphoma does not include EBV+ B-cell lymphomas that can be given a more specific diagnosis (e.g., lymphomatoid granulomatosis, EBV+ mucocutaneous ulcer). The majority of patients have extranodal disease. Some cases contain mostly large cells while others can be more polymorphous,

where few large B-cells are admixed with background inflammatory cells (small T-cells, plasma cells, and histiocytes). The large cells typically have moderate cytoplasm and nuclei with prominent nucleoli. These large RS-like cells can mimic HL. These lymphomas often have characteristic geographic necrosis. The neoplastic cells are positive for CD20 (variable), CD79a, MUM1, and CD30 (weak and variable) but are negative for CD10, CD15, and BCL6. EBV infection of the large atypical cells can be demonstrated by positive LMP-1 immunohistochemistry and in-situ hybridization for EBER. Of note, EBV-positivity can be seen in other lymphomas (e.g., HL, Burkitt lymphoma, plasmablastic lymphoma, lymphomatoid granulomatosis, PEL, PTLD), nonneoplastic lymphoproliferations (e.g., infectious mononucleosis), and certain lymphoepithelial carcinomas (e.g., gastric, nasopharyngeal).

DLBCL Associated With Chronic Inflammation

This EBV-associated DLBCL occurs in the setting of long-standing (e.g., >10 years) chronic inflammation. They typically arise in body cavities, but may go on to invade adjacent structures. The best-known example is pyothorax-associated lymphoma (PAL). Other sites of involvement include the bone, joints, and periarticular soft tissue. In most cases, the tumor cells have centroblastic and/or immunoblastic morphology and are associated with extensive necrosis. A subset of cases may have plasmacytic differentiation, showing loss of B-cell markers and expression of CD138 and MUM1. Some cases may also coexpress T-cell markers and CD30.

Primary Mediastinal (Thymic) Large B-Cell Lymphoma

Primary mediastinal large B-cell lymphoma (PMBL) usually arises in young adult women. They may present with superior vena cava syndrome. This lymphoma is of thymic B-cell origin and unrelated to EBV infection. It involves the thymus and may spread to involve the mediastinal nodes and invade adjacent structures (pleura, lung, pericardium, thoracic wall). There is usually no generalized lymphadenopathy, as this lymphoma is often confined to the thorax. With advanced disease lymphoma may disseminate to extranodal sites (e.g., liver, adrenal and very rarely to bone marrow). Histopathology shows a diffuse growth pattern with medium to large cells and compartmentalizing alveolar fibrosis (Figure 6.52). Cytology samples include large tumor cells that vary from having abundant cytoplasm with round to oval nuclei, to cells with RS-like multilobated, and sometimes pleomorphic nuclei. They have small nucleoli. A high mitotic activity is not uncommon. FNA samples are often nondiagnostic or may have only scant cellularity due to dense sclerosis. Therefore, a core biopsy may be required.

In a study evaluating intraoperative touch imprints of anterior mediastinal neoplasms, the correct diagnosis was obtained on touch imprints alone in 76% to 81% of cases versus 67% to 86% based on frozen sections alone (76). The most common error in interpreting imprints and frozen sections in this study was distinguishing thymic epithelial tumors (thymoma and thymic carcinoma) from lymphoma. This is not surprising, because there are many similar appearing entities that may arise in this anatomic location. The differential diagnosis of PMBL includes nodular sclerosis CHL, conventional DLBCL, lymphoblastic lymphoma, anaplastic large-cell lymphoma, mediastinal grey zone lymphoma (with combined features of PMBL and CHL), lymphocyte-rich thymoma, lymphoid-rich tumors (e.g., lymphoepithelial carcinoma, seminoma), Castleman disease (hyaline vascular variant), sclerosing mediastinitis, and sclerotic soft tissue tumors. The neoplastic cells of PMBL are positive for B-cell markers (CD19, CD20, CD79a, PAX5, MUM1), CD10 (25%), BCL6 (50%–60%), and CD30 (weak) but are negative for CD15 and Ig expression. They usually harbor an Ig heavy/light-chain gene rearrangement, rarely a c-MYC abnormality, and can have a unique gain in chromosome 9p.

ALK-Positive Large B-Cell Lymphoma

ALK-positive large B-cell lymphoma (ALK+ LBCL) is a rare B-cell lymphoma characterized by large immunoblast-like or plasmablast-like cells associated with an intravascular (sinusoidal) growth pattern and extensive necrosis. Some cases may have pseudo-acinar and/or pseudo-papillary formations, RS-like cells, plasmacytic features, and prominent neutrophil infiltrates. Because these tumor cells may have abundant cytoplasm, epithelioid morphology, and demonstrate cohesion they may be mistaken for carcinoma (77). The differential diagnosis also includes CD30-positive ALK+ T/null anaplastic large cell lymphoma. The neoplastic cells in ALK+ LBCL are positive for CD45 (weak), ALK1, plasma cell markers (CD38, CD138, MUM1), CD30 (weak and focal), EMA, and Napsin A but are negative for CD20, CD79a, CD3, and AE1/3. Most patients present with advanced disease and experience an aggressive clinical course.

Primary Effusion Lymphoma

Primary effusion lymphoma (PEL) is a large cell lymphoma that typically presents as a serous effusion (pleural, pericardial, and peritoneal) without a detectable tumor mass (classic PEL). Most cases occur in young males with HIV infection. These lymphomas are associated with Kaposi sarcoma herpesvirus/human herpesvirus-8 (KSHV/HHV8). Coexistent EBV positivity may be seen in the majority of cases. The spectrum of HHV8-associated lymphomas has expanded to now include large B-cell lymphomas arising in HHV8-associated multicentric Castleman disease, as well as extracavitary lymphomas (solid PEL) without serous effusions (78). Reported extranodal sites include the gastrointestinal tract, spleen, liver, skin, soft tissue, and rarely other locations. Solid PEL is virtually indistinguishable from classic PEL on the basis of morphology and phenotype. Solid PEL also occurs in HIV-infected patients, and often in males who experience an aggressive clinical course. Neoplastic cells are large with a wide range of morphology including cells with immunoblastic, plasmacytoid, centroblastic, anaplastic, and rarely RS-like features. The neoplastic cells are positive for CD45, plasma cell markers (CD138, MUM1), T-cell markers (rare), CD30, EMA, and LNA1 (HHV8) but are negative for pan-B-cell markers (CD19, CD20, CD79a), natural killer (NK) markers, and BCL6. The overall survival in these patients is generally very poor.

Plasmablastic Lymphoma

Plasmablastic lymphoma (PBL) is an aggressive rare B-cell lymphoma characterized by a diffuse proliferation of plasmablasts. Plasmablasts morphologically resemble B immunoblasts but immunophenotypically mimic plasma cells. PBL of oral mucosa type is usually associated with HIV males, arises in extranodal sites (e.g., jaw), and has minimal plasmacytic differentiation. PBL with plasmacytic differentiation, on the other hand, is associated with transplants and autoimmune disease, and does not involve the oral cavity. PBL has heterogeneous cytologic findings including atypical lymphocytes ranging from intermediate to large cells with scant to moderate cytoplasm, slight nuclear pleomorphism, vesicular chromatin, and one or many prominent nucleoli (79,80). Multinucleated cells, mitotic figures, TBMs and necrosis may be seen. The differential diagnosis includes other lymphomas with plasmablastic differentiation (e.g., ALK+ B-cell lymphoma, PEL, EBV+ DLBCL), immunoblastic DLBCL, Burkitt lymphoma, plasmacytoma, and other poorly differentiated malignancies (e.g., carcinoma, melanoma). The neoplastic cells are positive for CD45, CD20 (weak-to-negative), CD79a, CD10 (variable), plasma cell markers (CD138, MUM1), CD30 (variable), CD56 (variable), and EMA but are negative for PAX5 and LNA1 (HHV8). The Ki-67 proliferation index usually exceeds 90%. EBV markers show a latency pattern 1 (LMP– and EBER+). Myeloma can be differentiated because these patients may have a paraprotein and plasma cell neoplasms are more often CD56+, cyclinD1+, and EBV-negative. c-MYC rearrangements occur in up to 50% of cases and are associated with an aggressive course.

"Double/Triple Hit" High-Grade B-cell Lymphoma

Double-hit lymphoma is an aggressive B-cell lymphoma defined by concurrent rearrangement of MYC and BCL2, or less likely *BCL6*. Triple-hit lymphoma is when all three of these rearrangements are present. According to the 2016 WHO classification, these neoplasms belong to the category "high-grade B-cell lymphoma, with MYC and BCL2 and/or BCL6 rearrangements" (28). They present in elderly patients who have widespread lymphadenopathy or who manifest with an extranodal mass. Rarely, they may arise in an effusion. These lymphomas are associated with an aggressive clinical course and poor outcome. Histologically they exhibit heterogeneous morphology with a GCB-cell immunophenotype and high proliferation index (81). Tumors are composed of medium to large B-cells, few small lymphocytes, and sometimes there is associated apoptosis (Figure 6.53) with increased macrophages creating a "starry sky" appearance that resembles Burkitt lymphoma. The large cells may have deeply basophilic cytoplasm with vacuoles and segmented nuclei (Figure 6.54) (82). Ancillary studies are required to confirm their B-cell phenotype and delineate *MYC/BCL2/BCL6* aberrations. Therefore, whenever a high-grade large cell lymphoma is identified onsite during immediate evaluation or during intraoperative consultation, it is important to collect several (at least three) unstained imprints that can be used for potential FISH studies. Flow cytometry shows that most cases are positive for CD10, may underexpress CD45, CD20, and/ or CD19, and lack surface light chain (83).

T/NK-Cell Disorders

The T-cell lymphomas comprise about 10% of NHLs. T-cell lymphoblastic lymphoma is covered in section "Lymphoblastic Lymphoma." Apart from the cutaneous lymphomas, common mature T- or NK-cell neoplastic entities include peripheral T-cell lymphoma (NOS), adult T-cell leukemia/lymphoma, extranodal NK/T cell lymphoma (nasal type), anaplastic large cell lymphoma (ALK positive/negative), Sézary syndrome, angioimmunoblastic T-cell lymphoma, and enteropathy-associated T-cell lymphoma. T-/NK-cell lymphomas may be found in peripheral blood, bone marrow, lymph nodes, and extranodal sites, often the skin. Lymph node cytology coupled with ancillary techniques is employed to stage and follow-up patients with cutaneous lymphomas (84,85). This can be diagnostically challenging, because such nodes often have concomitant dermatopathic lymphadenopathy changes, related to nearby skin lesions. Imprint cytology of T/NK lymphoid lesions correlates well with their histopathology (86). T-/NK-cell lymphomas are classified largely based on their clinical features, since most of these subtypes do not have a specific immunoprofile. Immunophenotyping is helpful to demonstrate loss of pan-T-cell markers (e.g., CD2, CD3, CD5, CD7), loss of both CD4 and CD8, or expression of both CD4 and CD8 (double positive). PCR for T-cell receptor gene rearrangement can help prove clonality. The majority (90%) of peripheral T-cell lymphomas have rearrangements of T-alpha, beta, and gamma.

Peripheral T-Cell Lymphoma (NOS)

This is an aggressive, heterogeneous group of peripheral T-cell lymphomas (PTCL) that do not fit into one of the specified WHO defined entities. They mostly involve adults who present with nodal or extranodal disease and B symptoms. They have a broad cytology spectrum ranging from polymorphous to monomorphous lymphoid populations (Figure 6.55) (87). Several of the larger lymphoma cells have irregular, hyperchromatic nuclei, prominent nucleoli, and numerous mitotic figures. Specimens often also contain plasma cells, histiocytes, eosinophils, and RS-like cells. The differential diagnosis therefore includes HL. PTCL, NOS is characterized by an aberrant T-cell phenotype and T-cell receptor genes may be clonally rearranged.

Anaplastic Large Cell Lymphoma

Anaplastic large cell lymphoma (ALCL) occurs mainly in children and young adults. These lymphomas usually present in lymph nodes and/or extranodal sites. Up to 40% of patients have mediastinal involvement. ALCL is also a rare complication associated with breast implants. In these cases, it usually presents as an accumulation of seroma fluid between the implant and surrounding fibrous capsule, about 10 years after the implant was inserted. ALCL is characterized by large pleomorphic lymphoid cells with abundant cytoplasm, horseshoe or doughnut-shaped nuclei, and multiple often tubular-shaped nucleoli (88). Some cells can have wreath-like or multiple nuclei. So-called "hallmark" cells have an indented nucleus with a paranuclear (eosinophilic) Golgi region (Figure 6.56). ALCL may be mistaken for anaplastic carcinoma or sarcoma. The small cell and lymphohistiocytic variants of ALCL are harder to recognize because the cells are not large or anaplastic. Lymph nodes may have sclerosis and eosinophilia, making them hard to differentiate from CHL. Neutrophil-rich ALCL may mimic lymphadenitis. Cytology samples may rarely have a tigroid background, mimicking the cytologic appearance of seminoma (89). ALCL displaying spindle cells can even mimic sarcoma (90). Lymphoma cells are positive for T-cell markers (CD2, CD4, ±CD3), CD30 (strong and diffuse), ALK, and EMA (majority). As the neoplastic cells may be few, with flow cytometry they may fall outside of the lymphocyte gate. Patients with ALCL that are positive for ALK or t(2;5) are mostly children, and usually have a better prognosis than those that are ALK-negative. The ALK-negative neoplasms occur mostly in elderly men.

Angioimmunoblastic T-Cell Lymphoma

Angioimmunoblastic T-cell lymphoma (AITL) is an EBV-associated neoplasm that presents with generalized lymphadenopathy in adults. It is grouped with follicular T-cell lymphoma in the 2016 WHO classification under nodal T-cell lymphomas. AITL is characterized by a polymorphous population of lymphocytes admixed with fragments containing arborizing high endothelial venules and FDCs (91). The lymphoid cells have abundant clear cytoplasm and minimal cytologic atypia. Occasionally, RS-like cells may be seen. There are often also eosinophils (Figure 6.57), plasma cells, and histiocytes present. The neoplastic T-cells are positive for T-cell markers (CD2, CD3, CD4, CD5), CD10, CXCL13, and PD-1. The associated B-cells (immunoblasts) are polytypic and EBV-positive. In some cases, these atypical B-cell blasts simulate Hodgkin–RS cells, which may mimic CHL. Secondary B-cell neoplasms (CHL, DLBCL, plasmacytoma) can occur in these cases.

Extranodal NK/T Cell Lymphoma (Nasal Type)

This aggressive NK/T-cell lymphoma often occurs in Asians and individuals from Central and South America. NK/T-cell lymphoma is associated with EBV infection. It typically involves extranodal sites, especially the upper aerodigestive tract (e.g., nasal cavity). This lymphoma was previously called lethal midline granuloma due to the extensive midfacial destruction these lesions caused. Tumors are characterized by angiocentric proliferation and necrosis (92). Their cytomorphology shows a broad spectrum with small, large, and anaplastic cells (Figure 6.58). In TPs stained with Giemsa, cytoplasmic granules may be detected. There may also be plasma cells and eosinophils present. NK cells are positive for CD56, T-cell markers (CD2, cytoplasmic CD3, CD7, CD8), CD16, perforin, granzyme B, TIA-1, and in situ hybridization for EBER. CD56 is not specific for NK/T-cell cells and can be seen in other lymphomas, neuroendocrine tumors, Merkel cell carcinoma, various sarcomas (e.g., rhabdomyosarcoma, desmoplastic small cell tumor, mesenchymal chondrosarcoma), endometrial stromal tumor, neurothekeoma, and certain blastomas (e.g., neuroblastoma, retinoblastoma).

Posttransplant Lymphoproliferative Disorders

PTLD can occur following solid organ (e.g., kidney, lung) or bone marrow transplantation. The frequency of occurrence correlates with the degree of immunosuppression. The majority (80%) of PTLD cases are of host origin and associated with EBV infection. Most body sites can be involved, including the allograft. They may regress with reduced immunosuppression. According to the WHO, there are four subtypes of PTLD (93):

- **Early lesions:** These polyclonal lesions are nonneoplastic. They contain mostly plasma cells (plasmacytic hyperplasia) or immunoblasts (infectious mononucleosis-like). This category also includes florid follicular hyperplasia PTLD.

- **Polymorphic PTLD:** These are neoplastic lesions. They contain a polymorphous population of cells including lymphocytes with plasma cells. While they may show polytypic light chain expression by flow cytometry, they do have clonal immunoglobulin gene rearrangements.
- **Monomorphic PTLD (B- and T-/NK-cell types):** These lesions are classified according to the B-cell or T-cell lymphoma they resemble. The most common lymphoma seen is DLBCL.
- **CHL PTLD:** This is the least common form of PTLD.

Cytology samples obtained from the aforementioned polymorphous proliferations show a heterogeneous lymphoid population. However, there are usually increased plasma cells or immunoblast-like cells present. Monomorphic PTLD specimens show features of the B-cell lymphoma they resemble. RS-like cells may be seen in all of the subtypes of PTLD (Figure 6.59). The differential diagnosis includes infectious mononucleosis. Light chain restriction may not be seen with immunophenotyping. Therefore, molecular testing is often required to prove clonality. In-situ hybridization for EBV infection using EBER is helpful, as only 20% of cases are negative.

Plasma Cell Neoplasia

Plasma cell neoplasms include plasmacytoma (osseous and extraosseous), plasma cell (multiple) myeloma, and conditions related to tissue immunoglobulin deposition (e.g., primary amyloidosis). They can involve the bone marrow, bone (lytic lesions), or arise in extramedullary sites (e.g., upper respiratory tract, lung, skin). Primary plasmacytoma of lymph nodes is rare. Tumors are composed of an abnormal intermediate-to-large plasma cell population. The morphologic features of myeloma are similar to solitary plasmacytoma. Mature plasma cells are characterized by having eccentric nuclei, clumped chromatin, and paranuclear clearing (Figures 6.60 and 6.61). Atypical cytomorphology includes binucleation, nuclear atypia, and plasmablastic features (e.g., higher nuclear:cytoplasmic (N:C) ratio, prominent nucleoli) (Figure 6.62). The presence of Mott cells, Russell bodies, and Dutcher Bodies provide helpful diagnostic clues. Plasma cell neoplasms can occasionally be associated with amyloidosis (Figure 6.63), as well as crystal storage histiocytosis (Figure 6.64) resulting from the storage of crystalline immunoglobulin inclusions in reactive histiocytes (94).

Immunophenotyping by immunohistochemistry or flow cytometry shows the following positive markers: (CD45, CD79a, CD138, CD38, CD56, monotypic cytoplasmic kappa/lambda and sometimes Cyclin-D1), and negative markers: (CD19, CD20, CD3, CD30, surface immunoglobulin) (95). Kappa and lambda immunostains can be challenging to interpret due to high background staining. Cytokeratin expression as well as EMA, CD31, and CD117 may be seen in some cases. Also, it is important to be aware that CD138 may stain certain carcinomas and sarcoma. Unlike certain similar appearing lymphomas (e.g., plasmablastic lymphoma), plasma cell neoplasms are unrelated to EBV infection. The differential diagnosis includes benign lymphoplasmacytic proliferations (e.g., IgG4-related sclerosing disease), B-cell lymphomas with plasmacytic differentiation (e.g., lymphoplasmacytic lymphoma, plasmablastic lymphoma, primary effusion lymphoma), and nonlymphoid conditions with plasmacytoid appearing cells (e.g., melanoma, mesothelioma, lobular carcinoma of the breast).

Myeloid Neoplasms

Table 6.3 summarizes the various forms of acute myeloid leukemia (AML) according to the WHO (96). AML is characterized by myeloblasts (immature myeloid cells). Myeloblasts are large round to oval cells (10–20 µm) with a high N:C ratio and single nucleus characterized by immature chromatin and one or more prominent nucleoli (Figure 6.65). They may have cytoplasmic granules and sometimes Auer rods. Promyelocytes seen with acute promyelocytic leukemia and AML with maturation are larger than myeloblasts. Blasts with monocytic differentiation typically have more abundant cytoplasm with vacuoles and cleaved or lobulated nuclei that resemble monocytes (Figure 6.66).

TABLE 6.3 WHO (2016) Classification of Myeloid Neoplasms and Acute Leukemia

Myeloproliferative Neoplasms
- CML, *BCR-ABL1*[+]
- CNL
- PV
- PMF
- ET
- Chronic eosinophilic leukemia, NOS
- Myeloproliferative neoplasms, unclassifiable

Mastocytosis

Myeloid/lymphoid neoplasms with eosinophilia and rearrangement of *PDGFRA, PDGFRB,* or *FGFR1,* or with *PCM1-JAK2*

MDS/MPN
- CMML
- aCML, *BCR-ABL1*[-]
- JMML
- MDS/MPN with ring sideroblasts and thrombocytosis (MDS/MPN-RS-T)
- MDS/MPN, unclassifiable

MDS

Myeloid neoplasms with germ line predisposition

AML
- AML with recurrent genetic abnormalities
- AML with myelodysplasia-related changes
- Therapy-related myeloid neoplasms
- AML, NOS
- AML with minimal differentiation
- AML without maturation
- AML with maturation
- Acute myelomonocytic leukemia
- Acute monoblastic/monocytic leukemia
- Pure erythroid leukemia
- Acute megakaryoblastic leukemia
- Acute basophilic leukemia
- Acute panmyelosis with myelofibrosis
- Myeloid sarcoma
- Myeloid proliferations related to Down syndrome

Blastic plasmacytoid dendritic cell neoplasm

Acute leukemias of ambiguous lineage
- Acute undifferentiated leukemia
- Mixed phenotype acute leukemia

B-lymphoblastic leukemia/lymphoma

T-lymphoblastic leukemia/lymphoma

AML, acute myeloid leukemia; aCML, atypical chronic myeloid leukemia; CML, chronic myeloid leukemia; CMML, chronic myelomonocytic leukemia; CNL, chronic neutrophilic leukemia; ET, essential thrombocythemia; JMML, juvenile myelomonocytic leukemia; MDS, myelodysplastic syndromes; MPN, myeloproliferative neoplasms; NOS, not otherwise specified; PMF, primary myelofibrosis; PV, polycythemia vera.

Source: Adapted from Ref. (96). Arber DA, Orazi A, Hasserjian R, et al. The 2016 revision to the World Health Organization classification of myeloid neoplasms and acute leukemia. *Blood*. 2016;127:2391-2405.

Monocytic differentiation may be encountered with acute monoblastic and monocytic leukemia, as well as acute myelomonocytic leukemia. Lymphoblasts are also large cells with a high N:C ratio, but have only scant basophilic cytoplasm and more granular chromatin than myeloblasts (Figure 6.67). The nuclei of lymphoblasts may sometimes be pulled to one side creating a "hand-mirror" appearance.

Myeloid Sarcoma

Myeloid sarcoma (formerly called granulocytic sarcoma or chloroma) is an extramedullary tumor of myeloblasts. These tumors may occur de novo as the first indication of imminent AML, or they may coincide with a new diagnosis of AML, or represent relapse in a patient with previously diagnosed AML. They may also represent blastic transformation of myeloproliferative neoplasms and myelodysplastic syndromes. Myeloid sarcoma is more common in males and presents in patients of median age 56 years (range, 1 month–89 years). They can involve many sites of the body such as skin, mucous membranes, orbits, CNS, nodes, bone, gonads, and internal organs (97). They may also manifest with serous effusions. Multiple sites may be involved in 10% or less of cases. Treatment is generally similar to that of AML, which may include systemic chemotherapy and possible stem cell transplantation.

A diagnosis of myeloid sarcoma is challenging in cytology samples, especially if a tumor occurs prior to a diagnosis of AML. Moreover, adequate cellularity containing blasts is required (Figures 6.68 and 6.69). Peripheral blood or normal bone marrow contamination containing circulating blasts may confound the picture. Lymphoglandular bodies, typically suggestive of lymphoma, can occur (98). The presence of maturing cells such as promyelocytes in acute promyelocytic leukemia can resemble abundant neutrophils and hence may mimic infection. Abundant mixed granulocytes may mask scant blasts (e.g., AML with increased eosinophils). The differential diagnosis includes lymphomas (e.g., Burkitt, DLBCL, lymphoblastic, blastic MCL, plasmablastic lymphoma), small round cell tumors, poorly differentiated carcinoma, melanoma, histiocytic sarcoma, and other hematopoietic entities (e.g., extramedullary hematopoiesis, myeloproliferative neoplasms that are not in blast transformation).

Supportive ancillary studies including immunohistochemistry and flow cytometry are essential, and are most helpful in cases with high blast cellularity. Blasts are positive for early hematopoietic antigens (CD34, HLA-DR). Immunoreactivity is typically further based on blast differentiation such as granulocytic differentiation (MPO, CD117, CD13, CD33), monoblastic differentiation (CD68, CD43, CD163, CD56, CD14, lysozyme) or a mixed pattern of immunoreactivity suggestive of myelomonoblastic leukemia (Figure 6.70). Immunostains can also be used to identify erythroid differentiation (glycophorin A, hemoglobin, CD71) or megakaryoblastic differentiation (factor VIII, CD31, CD41, CD61). Sometimes if a patient has AML with a known genetic abnormality it may help to perform molecular testing in order to identify the same abnormality, especially if there are only scant blasts present.

Histiocytic and Dendritic Cell Neoplasms

This rare group of neoplasms includes histiocytic sarcoma, Langerhans cell histiocytosis and sarcoma, interdigitating and FDC sarcoma, fibroblastic reticular cell tumor, disseminated juvenile xanthogranuloma, and Erdheim–Chester disease. These tumors need to be differentiated from granulomatous and xanthogranulomatous inflammation, malakoplakia, and nonhematopoietic spindle cell tumors.

Langerhans Cell Histiocytosis

Langerhans cell histiocytosis is a clonal neoplasm that occurs mostly in children. It can present with unifocal (single lytic bone lesion in eosinophilic granuloma) or multifocal (involvement of bone, skin, and lungs) disease. Those with monosystemic disease have a good prognosis whereas children under 2 years of age and with multisystemic disease have a poor prognosis. Patients with Hand-Schüller-Christian disease (multifocal unisystem disease) have exophthalmos, diabetes insipidus, and bone defects. Those with Letterer–Siwe disease (multifocal multisystem disease) have rapidly progressing disease with Langerhans cell proliferation in many tissues.

Cytology samples demonstrate a prominent population of Langerhans cells (Figure 6.71). Tumor cells are characterized by nuclei with grooves or indentations. Nuclear grooves tend to be rather distinct in imprint slides (99). Tumor cell nuclei lack prominent nucleoli. Mitotic activity can be variable. Although infrequently performed, electron microscopy shows Birbeck granules (tennis racket–shaped cytoplasmic inclusions) within the Langerhans cells. These specimens typically also contain many eosinophils, histiocytes, and occasional neutrophils (100). In some cases, there may be eosinophilic abscesses rich in Charcot–Leyden crystals. Langerhans cell sarcoma should be considered in cases that exhibit marked cytologic atypia. The differential diagnosis for eosinophilia in lymph nodes includes infections (e.g., parasites, fungi), drug and allergic reactions, Kimura disease, inherited disorders (e.g., Omenn syndrome), hypereosinophilic syndrome, collagen vascular disease, HL, and T-cell lymphoma. Langerhans cells are positive for CD1a and Langerin, and may also be S100 and CD68 positive. Mutually exclusive somatic mutations in mitogen-activated protein kinase (MAPK) pathway genes have been identified in around 75% of cases, including recurrent *BRAF-V600E* and *MAP2K1* mutations.

FDC Sarcoma

These neoplasms are derived from FDCs. They can present at any age, but are usually seen in patients of mean age 44 years. They can occur with Castleman disease. Only the inflammatory variant of FDC sarcoma is EBV-related. Patients typically manifest with lymphadenopathy (e.g., neck) or extranodal tumors. Intra-abdominal tumors are particularly aggressive, where over 90% are likely to metastasize. They tend to metastasize to lymph nodes, lung, and liver.

The histopathology of FDC sarcoma shows spindled cells with diffuse, fascicular, whorled, or storiform growth. The syncytia of dendritic cells often have admixed lymphocytes present. Uncommon features include the presence of epithelioid cells, clear cells, oncocytic cells, fluid-filled cysts, osteoclast giant cells, myxoid stroma, necrosis, and hemorrhage. The inflammatory variant has increased lymphoplasmacytic cells. Cytology samples tend to be cellular and composed of single or interwoven sheets of spindled to ovoid cells (Figure 6.72). Single cells may be seen interconnected to neighboring single cells via thread-like cytoplasmic processes (101). These cells have moderate cytoplasm, indistinct cell borders, oval-elongated nuclei with pleomorphism, vesicular chromatin, small distinct nucleoli, and nuclear pseudo-inclusions. There may be bi-/multinucleation, and tumor cells may resemble RS cells.

The differential diagnosis includes other histiocytic/dendritic tumors (e.g., Langerhans cell sarcoma, interdigitating dendritic cell sarcoma), other spindle/epithelioid tumors (e.g., melanoma, neural tumors, thymoma, nasopharyngeal carcinoma), spindle cell neoplasms (e.g., soft tissue sarcoma, gastrointestinal stromal tumor (GIST)), granulomatous inflammation, HL, and spindle cell variant of DLBCL. A diagnosis of FDC sarcoma based on cytology alone is challenging. Therefore, immunohistochemistry is necessary to confirm the diagnosis. Follicular dendritic tumor cells are positive for follicular dendritic markers (CD21, CD35, CD23, clusterin) and D2-40, variably positive for EMA (50%), CD45, CD68, S100 (10%), actin, vimentin, and fascin, but are negative for CD1a, keratin, HMB45, and vascular markers.

Metastases

Lymph nodes are a common site of metastases. Metastatic disease can safely be diagnosed by CNB with Touch preparation being rapidly performed onsite (16). For example, a biopsy of supraclavicular lymph node metastases can be easily and quickly obtained in the evaluation of thoracic malignancies for staging and diagnostic purposes (102). Virchow's node (i.e., left supraclavicular lymph node) is a common site of metastases for gastrointestinal tumors or other visceral malignancies. Sarcomas usually metastasize hematogenously, hence they are rarely seen in lymph nodes. However, sarcomas that do metastasize to lymph nodes include Ewing sarcoma/primitive neuroectodermal tumor (PNET), synovial sarcoma, epithelioid sarcoma, clear cell sarcoma (melanoma of soft parts), angiosarcoma, rhabdomyosarcoma, and FDC sarcoma.

Lymph nodes can be readily sampled by FNA and/or CNB. In one study, ultrasound-guided core biopsy in the head and neck region looking for metastatic squamous cell carcinoma was shown to be of higher accuracy than FNA (103). Nevertheless, FNA alone is a safe alternative when a smaller needle is desired, such as when a lymph node is located near a blood vessel. Two well-directed 14 G core biopsy samples appear to be adequate to reliably make a diagnosis of metastatic carcinoma (104). If a CNB can be successfully obtained, an excisional biopsy may not be necessary (105). CNB typically provides large enough samples of tissue suitable for comprehensive genomic analyses (106). Onsite assessment of a CNB TP permits appropriate triage of tissue for ancillary studies. Following specimen adequacy evaluation, additional biopsy cores/passes can be diverted for immunohistochemistry and/or molecular testing with decreased turnaround times. Imprint cytology is particularly valuable for the intraoperative evaluation of sentinel nodes (107), and for the detection of tumor metastases in bone marrow (108). Confirming a metastatic carcinoma on imprint cytology is also helpful in order to avoid decalcification of the specimen so that uncompromised FISH studies and other molecular studies can be performed.

The majority of metastatic carcinomas likely to be encountered will be of non-small cell type, including metastatic adenocarcinoma or squamous cell carcinoma. Touch imprints in these cases typically show clusters of hyperchromatic cells at low magnification (Figure 3.10; Figures 6.73 and 6.74). A lymphoid background may not always be present if a node is completely replaced by tumor. Other conditions to be aware of where epithelioid cells are intermixed with lymphoid cells include granulomatous inflammation, thymoma, nasopharyngeal carcinoma, seminoma, and lymphoepithelioma-like carcinomas. Metastatic carcinomas that demonstrate a discohesive pattern, such as signet ring cell type or poorly differentiated tumors (Figure 6.75), may be harder to recognize. Metastases that mimic lymphoma or leukemia include small round cell tumors (e.g., small cell carcinoma), basaloid squamous cell carcinoma, Merkel cell carcinoma (Figure 6.76), and small cell variants of various tumors (e.g., melanoma, sarcoma). With small cell carcinoma there is typically more clustering of tumor cells and nuclear molding than occurs with lymphoma. However, background apoptotic debris seen with neuroendocrine tumors may mimic lymphoglandular bodies. Paranuclear blue bodies are a helpful feature of small cell carcinoma (Figure 6.77) (109). Finally, with increasing use of neoadjuvant therapy for breast carcinoma, it is important to be aware that extramedullary hematopoiesis may be encountered within lymph nodes (110). In these cases, hematopoietic precursors (e.g., megakaryocytes) in lymph nodes may potentially be misdiagnosed as metastatic carcinoma.

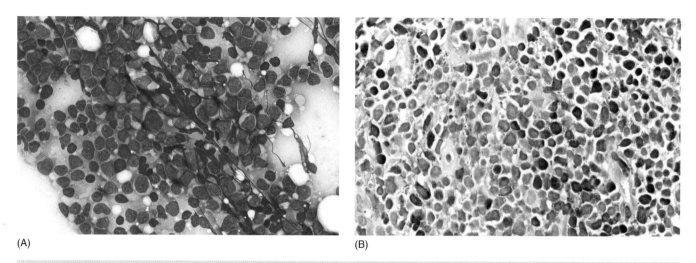

(A)   (B)

FIGURE 6.25 T-Lymphoblastic lymphoma. (A) TP from a neck lymph node of a 28-year-old female showing medium-sized lymphoblasts with a very high N:C ratio, irregular nuclear contours, and finely dispersed condensed nuclear chromatin. (B) Lymphoblasts are TdT-positive supporting the diagnosis. ((A) DQ-stained TP, high power; (B) TdT stain; medium power.) DQ, Diff-Quik; N:C, nuclear:cytoplasmic; TdT, terminal deoxynucleotidyl transferase; TP, touch preparation.

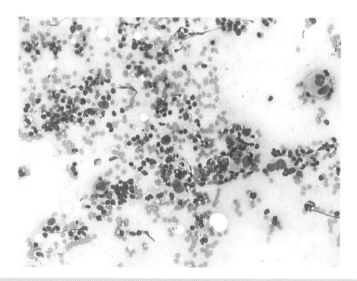

FIGURE 6.26 Classical Hodgkin lymphoma. TP of a lymph node showing scattered mononuclear Hodgkin cells and multinucleated RS cells. The background contains small lymphocytes, some eosinophils, and scant neutrophils (DQ-stained TP, low power). DQ, Diff-Quik; TP, touch preparation.

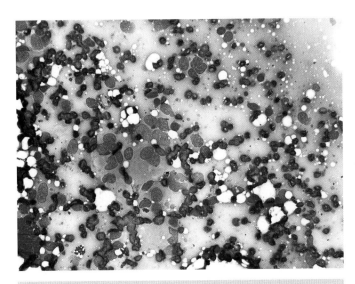

FIGURE 6.27 Classical Hodgkin lymphoma. TP showing a predominance of Hodgkin and RS cells (DQ-stained TP, medium power). DQ, Diff-Quik; RS, Reed–Sternberg; TP, touch preparation.

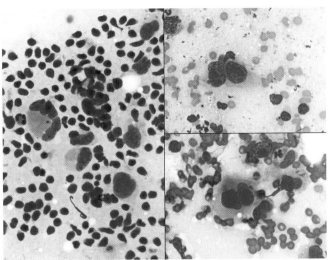

FIGURE 6.28 Classical Hodgkin lymphoma. Diagnostic RS cells are large cells characterized by having abundant cytoplasm, multiple nuclei (usually binucleated) with round contours, pale chromatin, and prominent macronucleoli present in separate nuclear lobes. The mononuclear variants are termed Hodgkin cells (DQ-stained TP, high power). DQ, Diff-Quik; RS, Reed–Sternberg; TP, touch preparation.

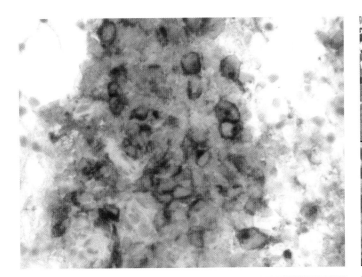

FIGURE 6.29 Classical Hodgkin lymphoma. RS cells demonstrate typical membrane and paranuclear dot-like CD30 staining (CD30 stain high power). RS, Reed–Sternberg.

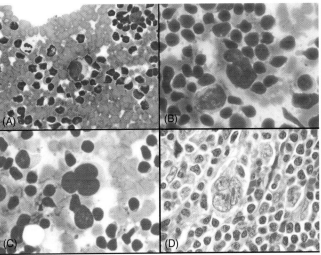

FIGURE 6.30 Nodular lymphocyte predominant Hodgkin lymphoma. Composite image showing large LP cells with popcorn-shaped nuclei. ((A–C) DQ-stained TP, high power; (D), H&E-stained section, oil magnification.) DQ, Diff-Quik; H&E, hematoxylin and eosin; LP, lymphocyte predominant; TP, touch preparation.

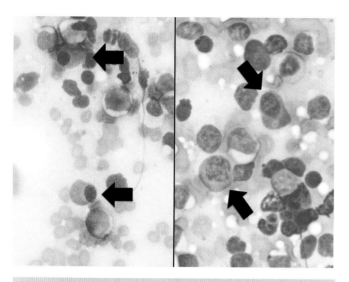

FIGURE 6.31 Non-Hodgkin B-cell lymphomas with plasmacytoid features. TPs showing plasmacytoid lymphocytes (arrows) characterized by moderate baso-philic cytoplasm and an eccentric nucleus with clumped chromatin resembling mature plasma cells (DQ-stained TP, medium power). DQ, Diff-Quik; TP, touch preparation.

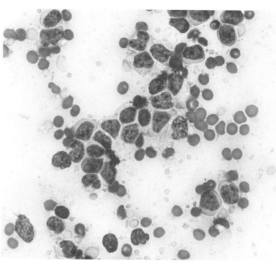

FIGURE 6.32 Non-Hodgkin B-cell lymphoma. TP from a bone biopsy showing atypical small-sized lymphocytes associated with lymphoglandular bodies (DQ-stained TP, medium power). DQ, Diff-Quik; TP, touch preparation.

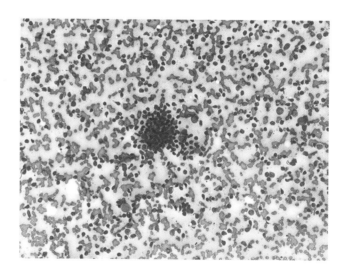

FIGURE 6.33 Follicular lymphoma. TP of this lymph node shows a polymorphous population of lymphocytes containing several small centrocytes and scant large centroblasts. This appearance mimics a reactive process. Therefore, immuno-phenotyping was necessary to confirm the diagnosis of this low-grade lymphoma (DQ-stained TP, low power). DQ, Diff-Quik; TP, touch preparation.

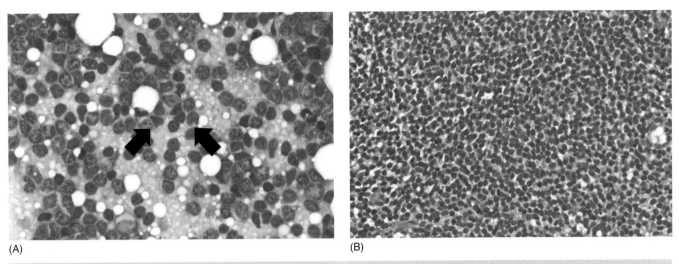

(A)

(B)

FIGURE 6.34 Follicular lymphoma. TP showing a predominant population of small lymphocytes. Note that some of these cells have nuclear irregularities including clefts in their nuclei (arrows). ((A) DQ-stained TP, medium power; (B) H&E-stained core biopsy, medium power.) DQ, Diff-Quik; H&E, hematoxylin and eosin; TP, touch preparation.

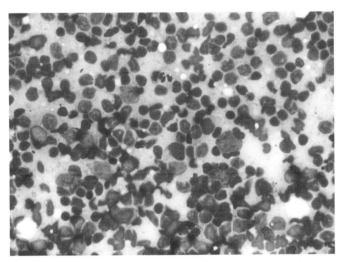

FIGURE 6.35 Follicular lymphoma. TP of this lymph node shows an increased number of larger centroblasts in keeping with a high-grade follicular lymphoma (DQ-stained TP, medium power). DQ, Diff-Quik; TP, touch preparation.

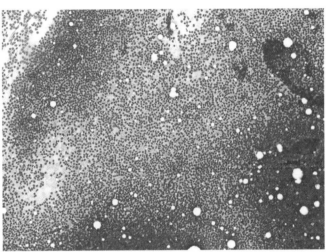

FIGURE 6.36 SLL/CLL. Hypercellular TP of an axillary node showing an even imprint of predominantly small lymphocytes (DQ-stained TP, low power). CLL, chronic lymphocytic leukemia; DQ, Diff-Quik; SLL, small lymphocytic lymphoma; TP, touch preparation.

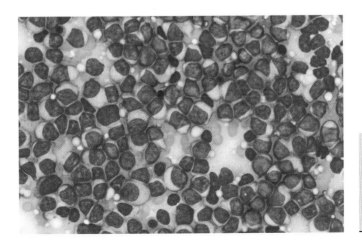

FIGURE 6.37 SLL/CLL. These monomorphic round lymphoma cells are characterized by scant cytoplasm and nuclei with distinct clumped chromatin that lack obvious nucleoli (DQ-stained TP, high power). CLL, chronic lymphocytic leukemia; DQ, Diff-Quik; SLL, small lymphocytic lymphoma; TP, touch preparation.

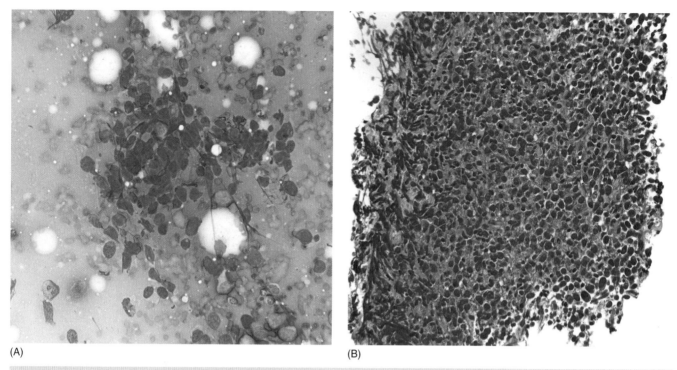

(A)   (B)

FIGURE 6.38 SLL/CLL with prolymphocytoid transformation. TP showing increased larger prolymphocytes with coarse chromatin and prominent central nucleoli. ((A) DQ-stained TP, medium power; (B) H&E-stained core biopsy, medium power.) CLL, chronic lymphocytic leukemia; DQ, Diff-Quik; H&E, hematoxylin and eosin; SLL, small lymphocytic lymphoma; TP, touch preparation.

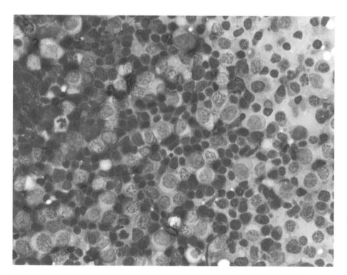

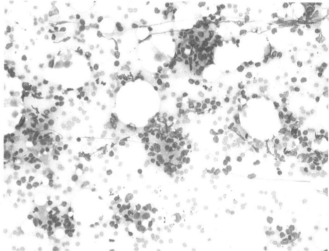

FIGURE 6.39 SLL/CLL with Richter transformation. TP showing many large atypical lymphocytes with background smaller CLL cells. The larger lymphoma cells retain their CLL phenotype (DQ-stained TP, medium power). CLL, chronic lymphocytic leukemia; DQ, Diff-Quik; SLL, small lymphocytic lymphoma; TP, touch preparation.

FIGURE 6.40 Marginal zone lymphoma. TP showing polymorphous small- and intermediate-sized lymphocytes and aggregates of lymphoid cells containing follicular dendritic cells that have more moderate cytoplasm (DQ-stained TP, low power). DQ, Diff-Quik; TP, touch preparation.

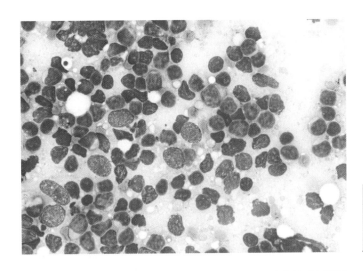

FIGURE 6.41 Marginal zone lymphoma. TP showing mixed small centrocytes, immunoblast-like cells, and centroblasts with plasmacytoid features (DQ-stained TP, high power). DQ, Diff-Quik; TP, touch preparation.

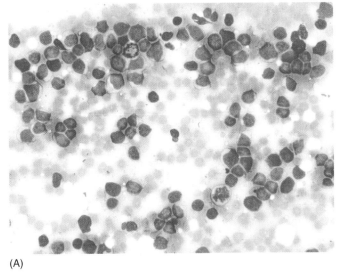

(A)

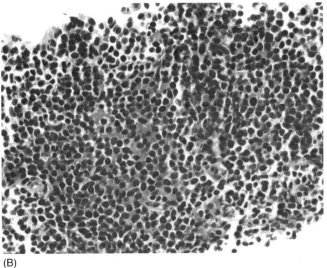

(B)

FIGURE 6.42 Mantle cell lymphoma. Monotonous population of small lymphocytes characterized by box-shaped nuclei with dispersed chromatin and inconspicuous nucleoli. Note the presence of mitotic figures indicating the aggressive nature of this lymphoma. ((A) DQ-stained TP, medium power; (B) H&E-stained core biopsy, medium power.) DQ, Diff-Quik; H&E, hematoxylin and eosin; TP, touch preparation.

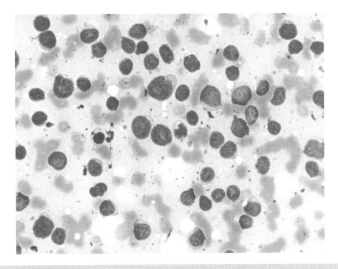

FIGURE 6.43 Mantle cell lymphoma, pleomorphic variant. TP showing pleomorphic lymphocytes that were immunophenotypically proven to be mantle cell lymphoma (DQ-stained TP, high power). DQ, Diff-Quik; TP, touch preparation.

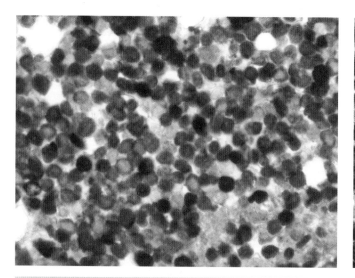

FIGURE 6.44   Mantle cell lymphoma. Lymphoma cells demonstrate strong and diffuse cyclin D1 immunoreactivity (CyclinD1 stain, high power).

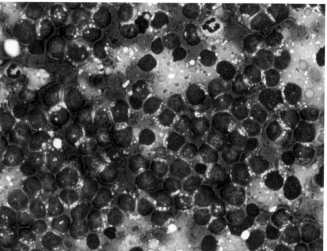

FIGURE 6.45   Burkitt lymphoma. Touch imprint of an abdominal tumor showing many medium-sized lymphocytes with deeply basophilic cytoplasm containing clear lipid vacuoles (DQ-stained TP, high power). DQ, Diff-Quik; TP, touch preparation.

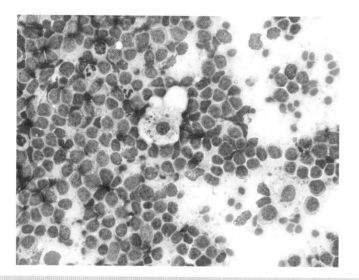

FIGURE 6.46   Burkitt lymphoma. TP showing abundant lymphoma cells associated with a central tingible-body macrophage (DQ-stained TP, medium power). DQ, Diff-Quik; TP, touch preparation.

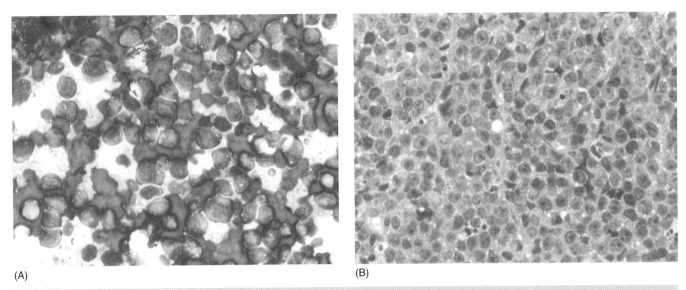

(A)

(B)

FIGURE 6.47 B-cell lymphoma, unclassifiable, with features intermediate between DLBCL and Burkitt lymphoma. The TP and corresponding core biopsy of this mesenteric mass show tumor cells resembling Burkitt lymphoma. However, there are also several larger cells present with central macronucleoli. Immunophenotyping showed that these monoclonal B-cells strongly co-expressed CD10 and BCL2. ((A) DQ-stained TP, high power; (B) H&E-stained core biopsy, high power.) DLBCL, diffuse large B-cell lymphoma; DQ, Diff-Quik; H&E, hematoxylin and eosin; TP, touch preparation.

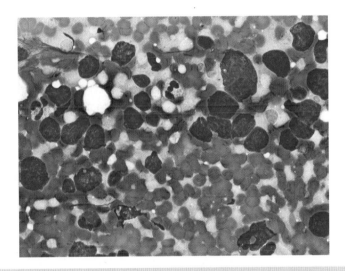

FIGURE 6.48 Diffuse large B-cell lymphoma, centroblastic variant. This cytology specimen obtained from a neck lymph node of a 61-year-old man shows large atypical lymphocytes with pleomorphic nuclei and multiple nucleoli. Note that the fragile cytoplasm is stripped from these cells, which accounts for the background lymphoglandular bodies (DQ-stained TP, high power). DQ, Diff-Quik; TP, touch preparation.

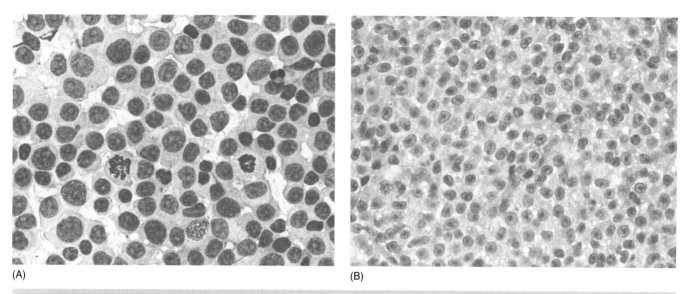

FIGURE 6.49 Diffuse large B-cell lymphoma, immunoblastic variant. Most of the lymphoma cells shown have a moderate amount of cytoplasm and slightly pleomorphic nuclei with a central macronucleolus. ((A) DQ-stained TP, high power; (B) H&E-stained core biopsy, high power.) DQ, Diff-Quik; H&E, hematoxylin and eosin; TP, touch preparation.

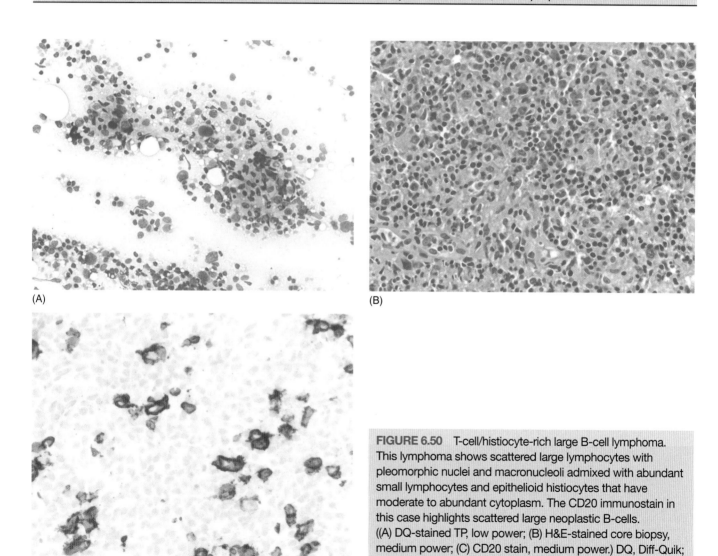

FIGURE 6.50 T-cell/histiocyte-rich large B-cell lymphoma. This lymphoma shows scattered large lymphocytes with pleomorphic nuclei and macronucleoli admixed with abundant small lymphocytes and epithelioid histiocytes that have moderate to abundant cytoplasm. The CD20 immunostain in this case highlights scattered large neoplastic B-cells. ((A) DQ-stained TP, low power; (B) H&E-stained core biopsy, medium power; (C) CD20 stain, medium power.) DQ, Diff-Quik; H&E, hematoxylin and eosin; TP, touch preparation.

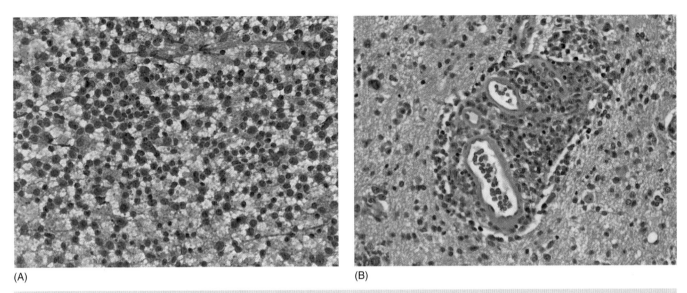

(A)   (B)

FIGURE 6.51 Primary DLBCL of the central nervous system. (A) Intraoperative cytopreparation showing a predominant population of atypical lymphoid cells. (B) Brain biopsy showing an accumulation of tumor cells within the perivascular space. ((A) H&E-stained crush preparation, low power; (B) H&E-stained core biopsy, low power.) DLBCL, diffuse large B-cell lymphoma; H&E, hematoxylin and eosin.

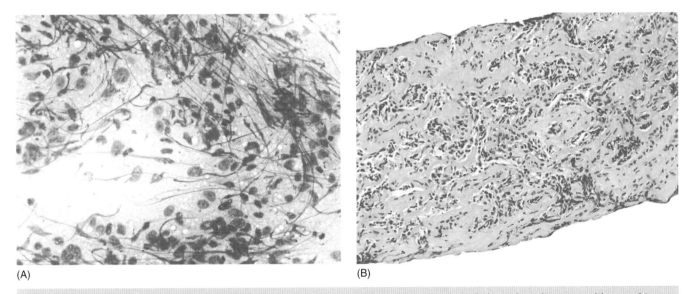

(A)   (B)

FIGURE 6.52 Primary mediastinal large B-cell lymphoma. TP showing small to mostly large lymphocytes with round to oval nuclei containing distinct nucleoli. Note the distortion artifact of fragile lymphocytes caused by rough manipulation of the firm core. The corresponding core biopsy shows dense fibrosis with proliferating lymphocytes confined to alveolar compartments. ((A) DQ-stained TP, medium power; (B) H&E-stained core biopsy, low power.) DQ, Diff-Quik; H&E, hematoxylin and eosin; TP, touch preparation.

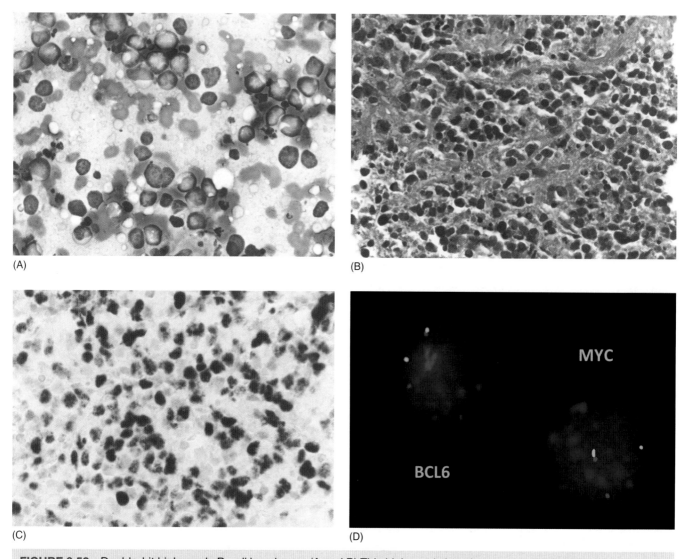

(A)

(B)

(C)

(D)

FIGURE 6.53 Double-hit high-grade B-cell lymphoma. (A and B) This high-grade lymphoma contains variably sized lymphocytes with pleomorphic nuclei and increased apoptosis. Ancillary studies confirmed concurrent *MYC* and *BCL6* rearrangements. (C) MYC immunohistochemistry shows strong nuclear staining in most of the tumor cells. (D) FISH is positive for the *MYC* gene rearrangement. FISH is also positive for the *BCL6* gene rearrangement along with an extra 5' (telomeric) signal for *BCL6*. ((A) DQ-stained TP, high power; (B) H&E-stained core biopsy, high power; (C) MYC immunohistochemistry, high power; (D) FISH performed on TPs and images courtesy of Mary Ann West.) DQ, Diff-Quik; FISH, fluorescence in situ hybridization; H&E, hematoxylin and eosin; TP, touch preparation.

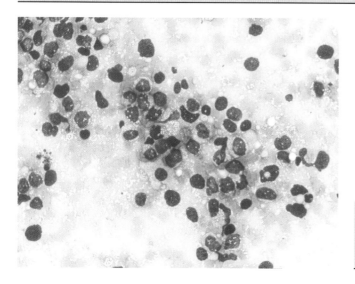

FIGURE 6.54 Double-hit high-grade B-cell lymphoma. TP showing large lymphoma cells with many small cytoplasmic vacuoles and irregular nuclei (DQ-stained TP, medium power). DQ, Diff-Quik; TP, touch preparation.

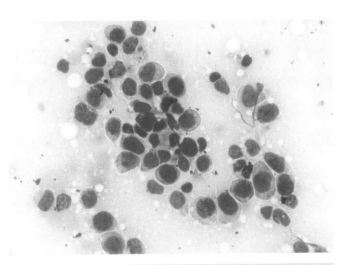

FIGURE 6.55 Peripheral T-cell lymphoma (NOS). TP of a groin lymph node in a 54-year-old man showing small-, intermediate-, and large-sized atypical lymphocytes. A combination of immunohistochemistry and flow cytometry was required to demonstrate an aberrant T-cell immuno-phenotype (DQ-stained TP, high power). DQ, Diff-Quik; NOS, not otherwise specified; TP, touch preparation.

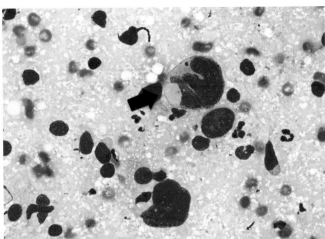

FIGURE 6.56 Anaplastic large cell lymphoma, ALK negative. This nodal lymphoma has atypical T-lymphocytes including several large anaplastic cells. Note the hallmark cell in the center of this image that has an eosinophilic paranuclear Golgi region (arrow) indenting the nucleus (DQ-stained TP, high power). ALK, anaplastic lymphoma kinase; DQ, Diff-Quik; TP, touch preparation.

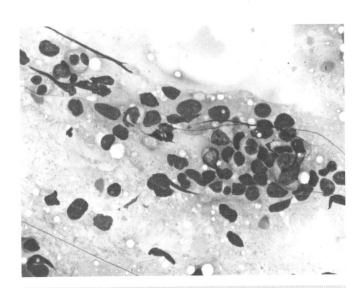

FIGURE 6.57 Angioimmunoblastic T-cell lymphoma. TP showing atypical lymphocytes admixed with eosinophils (DQ-stained TP, high power). DQ, Diff-Quik; TP, touch preparation.

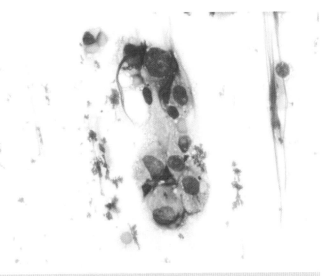

FIGURE 6.58 Extranodal NK/T-cell lymphoma, nasal type. TP of a chest wall lymphoma showing large atypical lymphocytes with abundant vacuolated cytoplasm. Azurophilic granules are not evident with this stain. Immunophenotyping confirmed these were NK-cells (DQ-stained TP, high power). DQ, Diff-Quik; NK, natural killer; TP, touch preparation.

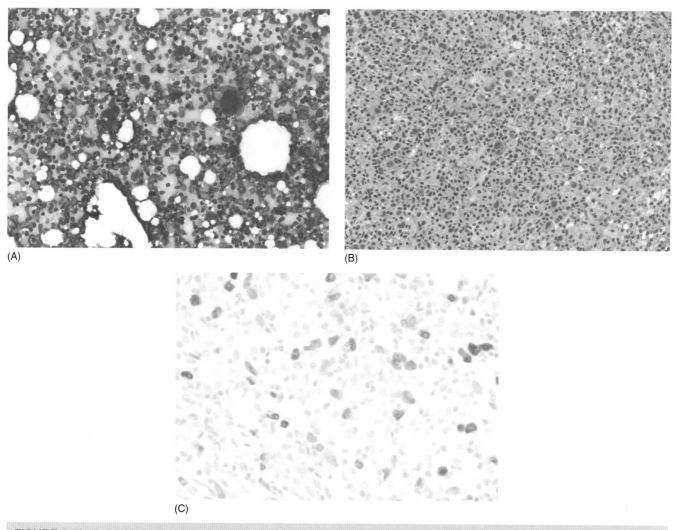

(A)

(B)

(C)

FIGURE 6.59 Hodgkin lymphoma-like PTLD. The (A) TP and (B) corresponding core biopsy show several scattered large RS cells with prominent nucleoli. The background shows a cellular polymorphous lymphoid population. (C) Many of the cells are EBV-infected. ((A) DQ-stained TP, low power; (B) H&E-stained core biopsy, low power; (C) EBER in situ hybridization, low power.) DQ, Diff-Quik; EBER, EBV-encoded small RNA; EBV, Epstein–Barr virus; H&E, hematoxylin and eosin; PTLD, posttransplant lymphoproliferative disorder; RS, Reed–Sternberg; TP, touch preparation.

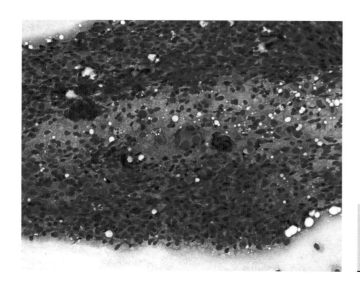

FIGURE 6.60 Plasmacytoma of bone. TP showing numerous plasma cells with an occasional large multi-nucleated tumor cell (DQ-stained TP, low power). DQ, Diff-Quik; TP, touch preparation.

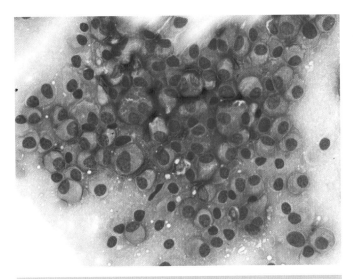

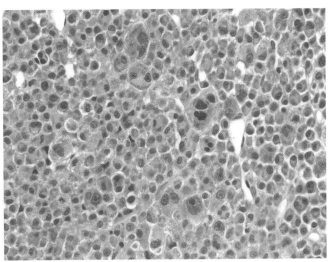

FIGURE 6.61 Plasmacytoma of bone. TP showing numerous mononuclear and binucleated plasma cells. Note that many of the plasma cells have abundant cytoplasm, eccentrically located nuclei, clumped chromatin ("clockface" pattern), absent nucleoli, and paranuclear clearing (DQ-stained TP, medium power). DQ, Diff-Quik; TP, touch preparation.

FIGURE 6.62 Plasmacytoma of bone. This biopsy shows a mixture of mature small plasma cells and larger pleomorphic forms with irregular nuclei and prominent nucleoli. Nuclear pleomorphism rarely occurs in reactive plasma cells (H&E-stained core biopsy, medium power). H&E, hematoxylin and eosin.

(A)

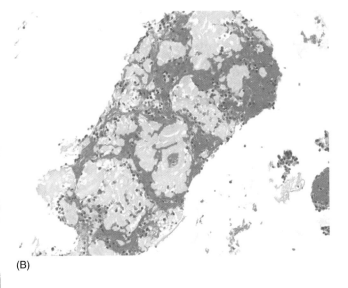

(B)

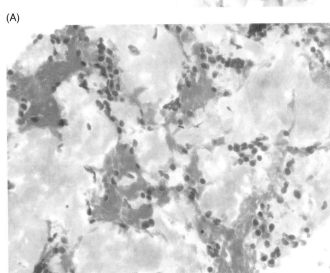

(C)

FIGURE 6.63 Plasma cell neoplasia associated with amyloid. (A) TP showing amorphous waxy, clumps of pink amyloid. (B) Amyloid deposition seen associated with mature neoplastic plasma cells. (C) Congo red, shown here, staining amyloid a salmon-pink color, is a useful stain to confirm the diagnosis and demonstrates apple-green birefringence under polarized light. ((A) DQ-stained TP, low power; (B) H&E-stained cell block, low power; (C) Congo red stained cell block, medium power.) DQ, Diff-Quik; H&E, hematoxylin and eosin; TP, touch preparation.

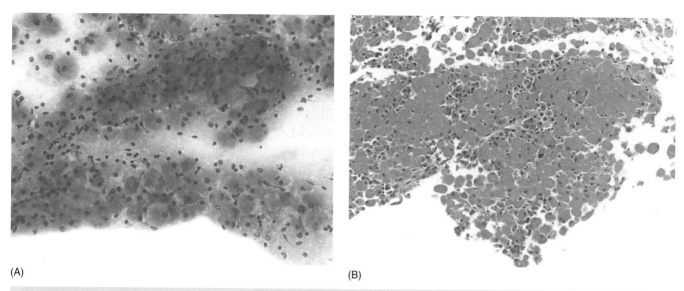

(A)

(B)

FIGURE 6.64 Plasma cell neoplasia associated with crystal storage histiocytosis. (A) Abundant histiocytes are shown stuffed with intracytoplasmic crystalline material admixed with scant mature neoplastic plasma cells. ((A) DQ-stained TP, low power; (B) H&E-stained cell block, low power.) DQ, Diff-Quik; H&E, hematoxylin and eosin; TP, touch preparation.

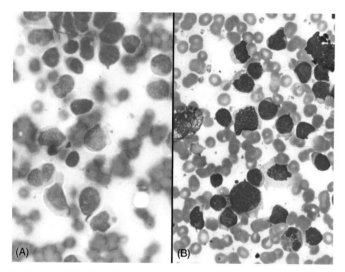

(A)   (B)

FIGURE 6.65 Blasts. (A) Myeloblasts and (B) lymphoblasts are both characterized by high N:C ratios and immature chromatin. Immunophenotyping is often required to reliably distinguish these blasts. ((A) and (B) DQ-stained TP, high power.) DQ, Diff-Quik; N:C, nuclear:cytoplasmic; TP, touch preparation.

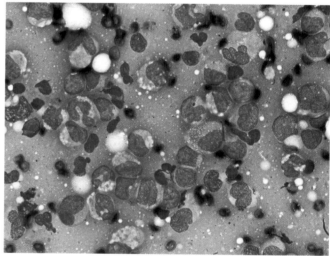

FIGURE 6.66 Myeloid sarcoma with monocytic differentiation. TP is shown from a patient who relapsed with acute myelomonocytic leukemia. Note that blasts with monocytic differentiation have abundant vacuolated cytoplasm and lobulated nuclei (DQ-stained TP, high power). DQ, Diff-Quik; TP, touch preparation.

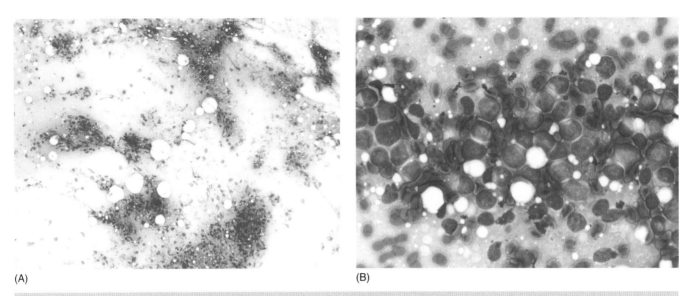

(A)   (B)

FIGURE 6.67 Myeloid sarcoma. TP showing blasts that mimic lymphoma. Compared to mature lymphocytes these blasts have fine reticular (immature) chromatin. ((A) DQ-stained TP, low power; (B) DQ-stained cytology preparation, high power.) DQ, Diff-Quik; TP, touch preparation.

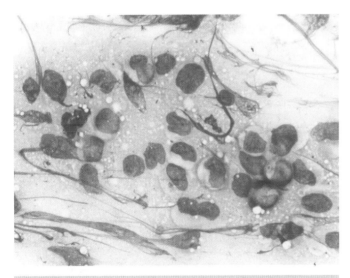

FIGURE 6.68 Myeloid sarcoma with monocytic differentiation. TP from a patient with acute monocytic leukemia (AML M5b) who relapsed one year after bone marrow transplantation, where some of the blasts can be seen with cleaved nuclei (DQ-stained TP, high power). DQ, Diff-Quik; TP, touch preparation.

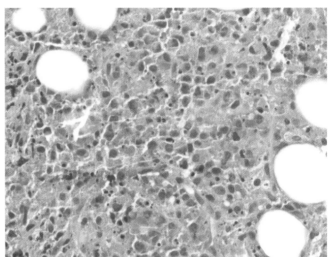

FIGURE 6.69 Myeloid sarcoma involving soft tissue. Core biopsy showing abundant blasts infiltrating fibrofatty tissue (H&E-stained core biopsy, medium power). H&E, hematoxylin and eosin.

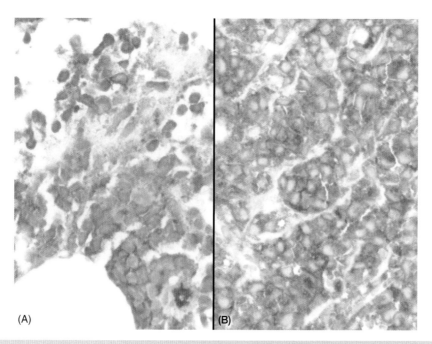

(A)

(B)

FIGURE 6.70 Myeloid sarcoma. Myeloblasts are shown with (A) CD34 and (B) CD33 immunoreactivity. ((A) and (B) Immunohistochemistry, medium power.)

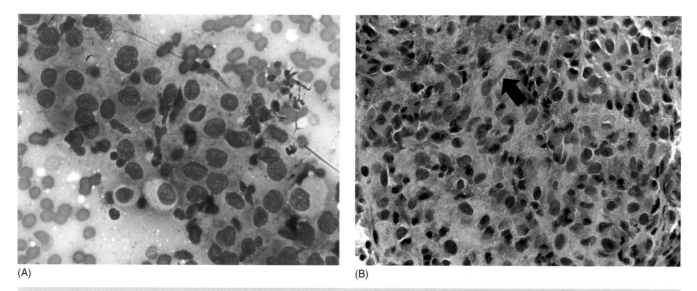

(A)

(B)

FIGURE 6.71 Langerhans cell histiocytosis (eosinophilic granuloma). (A) TP from a frontal sinus tumor in a 21-year-old male shows Langerhans cells with moderate cytoplasm and nuclear grooves. (B) The corresponding biopsy shows Langerhans cells admixed with abundant eosinophils. Note the Charcot–Leyden crystal (arrow) derived from eosinophil granules. ((A) DQ-stained TP, high power; (B) H&E-stained core biopsy, high power.) DQ, Diff-Quik; H&E, hematoxylin and eosin; TP, touch preparation.

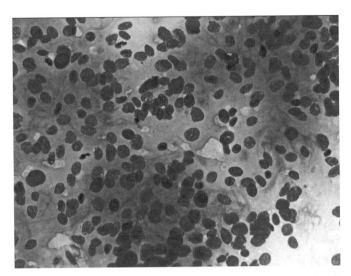

FIGURE 6.72 Follicular dendritic cell sarcoma. A syncytial fragment of tumor cells is shown formed by dendritic cells that have indistinct cytoplasm without individual cell borders. The tumor cells have oval-elongated pleomorphic nuclei and indistinct nucleoli (DQ-stained TP, high power). DQ, Diff-Quik; TP, touch preparation.

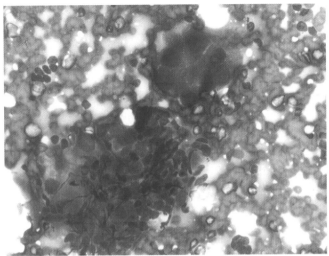

FIGURE 6.73 Metastatic ovarian clear cell carcinoma. This TP of a node shows clusters of tumor cells with abundant finely vacuolated cytoplasm and enlarged nuclei present among crushed small lymphocytes (DQ-stained TP, low power). DQ, Diff-Quik; TP, touch preparation.

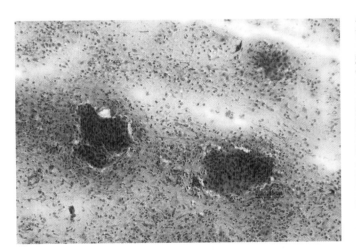

FIGURE 6.74 Metastatic squamous cell carcinoma of tonsil. This intraoperative imprint shows clusters of poorly differentiated carcinoma with background necrosis (H&E-stained imprint preparation, low power). H&E, hematoxylin and eosin.

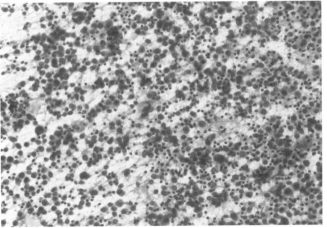

FIGURE 6.75 Metastatic poorly differentiated carcinoma. This intraoperative imprint of a lymph node shows predominantly discohesive epithelioid tumor cells with scant small lymphocytes in the background (H&E-stained imprint preparation, low power). H&E, hematoxylin and eosin.

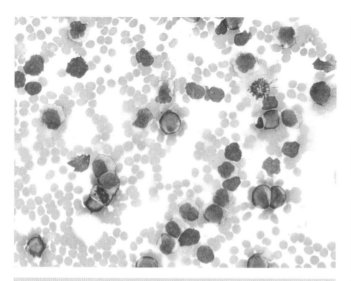

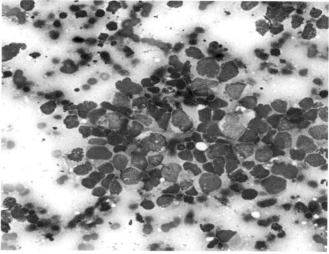

FIGURE 6.76 Metastatic Merkel cell carcinoma. These tumor cells resemble lymphoma. However, the tumor cells show focal cohesion and have a moderate amount of cytoplasm. Immunophenotyping is necessary to confirm the diagnosis (DQ-stained cytopreparation, medium power). DQ, Diff-Quik.

FIGURE 6.77 Metastatic small cell carcinoma. These tumor cells resemble lymphoma. However, the tumor cells show clustering, have a small amount of cytoplasm, and contain characteristic paranuclear blue bodies (DQ-stained cytopreparation, medium power). DQ, Diff-Quik.

Image courtesy of Dr. Sara Monaco.

REFERENCES

1. Ultmann JE, Koprowska I, Engle RL Jr. A cytological study of lymph node imprints. *Cancer.* 1958;11:507-524.
2. Feinberg MR, Bhaskar AG, Bourne P. Differential diagnosis of malignant lymphomas by imprint cytology. *Acta Cytol.* 1980;24:16-25.
3. Dunphy CH. *Frozen Section Library: Lymph Nodes.* New York, NY: Springer; 2012:7-26.
4. Katz RL. Pitfalls in the diagnosis of fine-needle aspiration of lymph nodes. *Monogr Pathol.* 1997;39:118-133.
5. Pambuccian SE, Bardales RH. Essentials in cytopathology In: Rosenthal DL, ed. *Lymph Node Cytopathology.* New York, NY: Springer; 2011.
6. de Kerviler E, Benet C, Brière J, de Bazelaire C. Image-guided needle biopsy for diagnosis and molecular biology in lymphomas. *Best Pract Res Clin Haematol.* 2012;25:29-39.
7. Ryu YJ, Cha W, Jeong WJ, et al. Diagnostic role of core needle biopsy in cervical lymphadenopathy. *Head Neck.* 2015;37: 229-233.
8. Amador-Ortiz C, Chen L, Hassan A, et al. Combined core needle biopsy and fine-needle aspiration with ancillary studies correlate highly with traditional techniques in the diagnosis of nodal-based lymphoma. *Am J Clin Pathol.* 2011;135:516-524.
9. Metzgeroth G, Schneider S, Walz C, et al. Fine needle aspiration and core needle biopsy in the diagnosis of lymphadenopathy of unknown aetiology. *Ann Hematol.* 2012;91:1477-1484.
10. Skelton E, Jewison A, Okpaluba C, et al. Image-guided core needle biopsy in the diagnosis of malignant lymphoma. *Eur J Surg Oncol.* 2015;41:852-858.
11. He Y, Ji X, Xie Y, et al. Clinical application of ultrasound-guided core needle biopsy with multiple punches in the diagnosis of lymphoma. *World J Surg Oncol.* 2015;13:126.
12. Oh KH, Woo JS, Cho JG, et al. Efficacy of ultrasound-guided core needle gun biopsy in diagnosing cervical lymphadenopathy. *Eur Ann Otorhinolaryngol Head Neck Dis.* 2016;133:401-404.
13. Allin D, David S, Jacob A, et al. Use of core biopsy in diagnosing cervical lymphadenopathy: a viable alternative to surgical excisional biopsy of lymph nodes? *Ann R Coll Surg Engl.* 2016;5:1-3.
14. Groneck L, Quaas A, Hallek M, et al. Ultrasound-guided core needle biopsies for workup of lymphadenopathy and lymphoma. *Eur J Haematol.* 2016;97:379-386.
15. Frederiksen JK, Sharma M, Casulo C, Burack WR. Systematic review of the effectiveness of fine-needle aspiration and/or core needle biopsy for subclassifying lymphoma. *Arch Pathol Lab Med.* 2015;139:245-251.
16. Kubik MJ, Bovbel A, Goli H, et al. Diagnostic value and accuracy of imprint cytology evaluation during image-guided core needle biopsies: review of our experience at a large academic center. *Diagn Cytopathol.* 2015;43:773-779.
17. Kobayashi TK, Tamagaki T, Yoneyama C, et al. Imprint cytology of Gaucher's disease presenting as a splenic mass. A case report with molecular approaches. *Acta Cytol.* 1998;42:419-424.
18. Jakubiak M, Pankowski J, Obrochta A, et al. Fast cytological evaluation of lymphatic nodes obtained during transcervical extended mediastinal lymphadenectomy. *Eur J Cardiothorac Surg.* 2013;43:297-301.
19. Molyneux AJ, Attanoos RL, Coghill SB. The value of lymph node imprint cytodiagnosis: an assessment of interobserver agreement and diagnostic accuracy. *Cytopathology.* 1997;8: 256-264.
20. Tilak V, Das S, Bundhun S. Value of bone marrow imprint smears in early diagnosis of bone marrow pathologies. *J Clin Diagn Res.* 2014;8:FC01-3.

21. Chandra S, Chandra H. Comparison of bone marrow aspirate cytology, touch imprint cytology and trephine biopsy for bone marrow evaluation. *Hematol Rep*. 2011;3:e22.

22. Crisan D, Farkas DH. Bone marrow biopsy imprint preparations: use for molecular diagnostics in leukemias. *Ann Clin Lab Sci*. 1993;23:407-422.

23. Hazarika B. Touch imprint matters ... *Blood*. 2013;121:2585.

24. Varma N, Dash S, Sarode R, Marwaha N. Relative efficacy of bone marrow trephine biopsy sections as compared to trephine imprints and aspiration smears in routine hematological practice. *Indian J Pathol Microbiol*. 1993;36:215-226.

25. Aboul-Nasr R, Estey EH, Kantarjian HM, et al. Comparison of touch imprints with aspirate smears for evaluating bone marrow specimens. *Am J Clin Pathol*. 1999;111:753-758.

26. Chandra S, Chandra H, Saini S. Bone marrow metastasis by solid tumors-probable hematological indicators and comparison of bone marrow aspirate, touch imprint and trephine biopsy. *Hematology*. 2010;15:368-372.

27. Gong X, Lu X, Wu X, et al. Role of bone marrow imprints in haematological diagnosis: a detailed study of 3781 cases. *Cytopathology*. 2012;23:86-95.

28. Swerdlow SH, Campo E, Pileri SA, et al. The 2016 revision of the World Health Organization classification of lymphoid neoplasms. *Blood*. 2016;127:2375-2390.

29. Camacho FI, García JF, Sánchez-Verde L, et al. Unique phenotypic profile of monocytoid B cells: differences in comparison with the phenotypic profile observed in marginal zone B cells and so-called monocytoid B cell lymphoma. *Am J Pathol*. 2001;158:1363-1369.

30. Zaharopoulos P, Hudnall SD. Nevus-cell aggregates in lymph nodes: fine-needle aspiration cytologic findings and resulting diagnostic difficulties. *Diagn Cytopathol*. 2004;31:180-184.

31. Stani J. Cytologic diagnosis of reactive lymphadenopathy in fine needle aspiration biopsy specimens. *Acta Cytol*. 1987;31:8-13.

32. Monaco SE, Khalbuss WE, Pantanowitz L. Benign non-infectious causes of lymphadenopathy: a review of cytomorphology and differential diagnosis. *Diagn Cytopathol*. 2012;40:925-938.

33. Cheuk W, Chan JK. Lymphadenopathy of IgG4-related disease: an underdiagnosed and overdiagnosed entity. *Semin Diagn Pathol*. 2012;29:226-234.

34. Yu GH, McGrath CM. Follow-up of morphologically reactive lymphoid proliferations in fine-needle aspirates of elderly patients. *Diagn Cytopathol*. 2000;23:249-252.

35. Boussouar S, Medjhoul A, Bernaudin JF, et al. Diagnostic efficacy of ultrasound-guided core-needle biopsy of peripheral lymph nodes in sarcoidosis. *Sarcoidosis Vasc Diffuse Lung Dis*. 2015;32:188-193.

36. Khurana KK, Stanley MW, Powers CN, Pitman MB. Aspiration cytology of malignant neoplasms associated with granulomas and granuloma-like features: diagnostic dilemmas. *Cancer*. 1998;84:84-91.

37. Kaur G, Dhamija A, Augustine J, et al. Can cytomorphology of granulomas distinguish sarcoidosis from tuberculosis? Retrospective study of endobronchial ultrasound guided transbronchial needle aspirate of 49 granulomatous lymph nodes. *Cytojournal*. 2013;10:19.

38. DePew ZS, Gonsalves WI, Roden AC, et al. Granulomatous inflammation detected by endobronchial ultrasound-guided transbronchial needle aspiration in patients with a concurrent diagnosis of cancer: a clinical conundrum. *J Bronchology Interv Pulmonol*. 2012;19:176-181.

39. Galindo LM, Garcia FU, Hanau CA, et al. Fine-needle aspiration biopsy in the evaluation of lymphadenopathy associated with cutaneous T-cell lymphoma (mycosis fungoides/Sézary syndrome). *Am J Clin Pathol*. 2000;113:865-871.

40. Bakels V, Van Oostveen JW, Geerts ML, et al. Diagnostic and prognostic significance of clonal T-cell receptor beta gene rearrangements in lymph nodes of patients with mycosis fungoides. *J Pathol*. 1993;170:249-255.

41. Mallick S, Ghosh R, Iyer VK, et al. Cytomorphological and morphometric analysis of 22 cases of Rosai-Dorfman disease: a large series from a tertiary care centre. *Acta Cytol*. 2013;57:625-632.

42. Stastny JF, Wakely PE Jr, Frable WJ. Cytologic features of necrotizing granulomatous inflammation consistent with cat-scratch disease. *Diagn Cytopathol*. 1996;15:108-115.

43. Kojima M, Nakamura S, Koshikawa T, et al. Imprint cytology of cat scratch disease. A report of eight cases. *APMIS*. 1996;104:389-394.

44. Donnelly A, Hendricks G, Martens S, et al. Cytologic diagnosis of cat scratch disease (CSD) by fine-needle aspiration. *Diagn Cytopathol*. 1995;13:103-106.

45. Caponetti GC, Pantanowitz L, Marconi S, et al. Evaluation of immunohistochemistry in identifying Bartonella henselae in cat-scratch disease. *Am J Clin Pathol*. 2009;131:250-256.

46. Michelow P, Omar T, Field A, Wright C. The cytopathology of mycobacterial infection. *Diagn Cytopathol*. 2016;44:255-262.

47. Kardos TF, Kornstein MJ, Frable WJ. Cytology and immunocytology of infectious mononucleosis in fine needle aspirates of lymph nodes. *Acta Cytol*. 1988;32:722-726.

48. Stanley MW, Steeper TA, Horwitz CA, et al. Fine-needle aspiration of lymph nodes in patients with acute infectious mononucleosis. *Diagn Cytopathol*. 1990;6:323-329.

49. Caponetti G, Pantanowitz L. HIV-associated lymphadenopathy. *Ear Nose Throat J*. 2008;87:374-375.

50. Bhaker P, Das A, Rajwanshi A, et al. Precursor T-lymphoblastic lymphoma: speedy diagnosis in FNA and effusion cytology by morphology, immunochemistry, and flow cytometry. *Cancer Cytopathol*. 2015;123:557-565.

51. Funamoto Y, Nagai M, Haba R, et al. Diagnostic accuracy of imprint cytology in the assessment of Hodgkin's disease in Japan. *Diagn Cytopathol*. 2005;33:20-25.

52. Luboshitzky R, Dharan M, Nachtigal D, et al. Syncytial variant of nodular sclerosing Hodgkin's disease presenting as a thyroid nodule. A case report. *Acta Cytol*. 1995;39:543-546.

53. Kardos TF, Vinson JH, Behm FG, et al. Hodgkin's disease: diagnosis by fine-needle aspiration biopsy. Analysis of cytologic criteria from a selected series. *Am J Clin Pathol*. 1986;86:286-291.

54. Iacobuzio-Donahue CA, Clark DP, Ali SZ. Reed-Sternberg-like cells in lymph node aspirates in the absence of Hodgkin's disease: pathologic significance and differential diagnosis. *Diagn Cytopathol*. 2002;27:335-339.

55. Jaffe ES, Stein H, Swerdlow SH, et al. B-cell lymphoma, unclassifiable, with features intermediate between diffuse large B-cell lymphoma and classical Hodgkin lymphoma. In: Swerdlow SH, Campo E, Harris NL, et al., eds. *WHO Classification of Tumours of Haematopoietic and Lymphoid Tissue*. 4th ed. Switzerland: WHO Press; 2008:267-268.

56. Subhawong AP, Ali SZ, Tatsas AD. Nodular lymphocyte-predominant Hodgkin lymphoma: cytopathologic correlates on fine-needle aspiration. *Cancer Cytopathol*. 2012;120:254-260.

57. Zhang JR, Raza AS, Greaves TS, Cobb CJ. Fine-needle aspiration diagnosis of Hodgkin lymphoma using current WHO classification—re-evaluation of cases from 1999-2004 with new proposals. *Diagn Cytopathol*. 2006;34:397-402.

58. Xing J, Monaco SE, Pantanowitz L. Utility and effectiveness of fine needle aspiration and core needle biopsy with touch imprint for diagnosing and subclassifying lymphoma. *J Am Soc Cytopathol*. 2015;4:S50.

59. Koo CH, Rappaport H, Sheibani K, et al. Imprint cytology of non-Hodgkin's lymphomas based on a study of 212 immunologically characterized cases: correlation of touch imprints with tissue sections. *Hum Pathol*. 1989; 20(12 suppl 1):1-137.

60. Gong JZ, Williams DC Jr, Liu K, Jones C. Fine-needle aspiration in non-Hodgkin lymphoma: evaluation of cell size by cytomorphology and flow cytometry. *Am J Clin Pathol*. 2002;117:880-888.

61. Thunnissen FB, Kroese AH, Ambergen AW, et al. Which cytological criteria are the most discriminative to distinguish carcinoma, lymphoma, and soft-tissue sarcoma? A probabilistic approach. *Diagn Cytopathol*. 1997;17:333-338.

62. Flanders E, Kornstein MJ, Wakely PE Jr, et al. Lymphoglandular bodies in fine-needle aspiration cytology smears. *Am J Clin Pathol*. 1993;99:566-569.

63. Francis IM, Das DK, al-Rubah NA, Gupta SK. Lymphoglandular bodies in lymphoid lesions and non-lymphoid round cell tumours: a quantitative assessment. *Diagn Cytopathol*. 1994;11:23-27.

64. Wang J, Katz RL, Stewart J, et al. Fine-needle aspiration diagnosis of lymphomas with signet ring cell features: potential pitfalls and solutions. *Cancer Cytopathol*. 2013;121:525-532.

65. Klopčič U, Lavrenčak J, Gašljević G, et al. Grading of follicular lymphoma in cytological samples. *Cytopathology*. 2016;27:390-397.

66. Pillai RK, Surti U, Swerdlow SH. Follicular lymphoma-like B cells of uncertain significance (in situ follicular lymphoma) may infrequently progress, but precedes follicular lymphoma, is associated with other overt lymphomas and mimics follicular lymphoma in flow cytometric studies. *Haematologica*. 2013; 98:1571-1580.

67. Jain N, Keating MJ. Richter transformation of CLL. *Expert Rev Hematol*. 2016;9:793-801.

68. Shin HJ, Caraway NP, Katz RL. Cytomorphologic spectrum of small lymphocytic lymphoma in patients with an accelerated clinical course. *Cancer*. 2003;99:293-300.

69. Zhang YH, Liu J, Dawlett M, et al. The role of SOX11 immunostaining in confirming the diagnosis of mantle cell lymphoma on fine-needle aspiration samples. *Cancer Cytopathol*. 2014;122: 892-897.

70. Narurkar R, Alkayem M, Liu D. SOX11 is a biomarker for cyclin D1-negative mantle cell lymphoma. *Biomark Res*. 2016;4:6.

71. Leoncini L, Raphael M, Stein H, et al. Burkitt lymphoma. In: Swerdlow SH, Campo E, Harris NL, et al., eds. *WHO Classification of Tumours of Haematopoietic and Lymphoid Tissue*. 4th ed. Switzerland: WHO Press; 2008:262-264.

72. Bellan C, Stefano L, Giulia de F, et al. Burkitt lymphoma versus diffuse large B-cell lymphoma: a practical approach. *Hematol Oncol*. 2010;28:53-56.

73. Hans CP, Weisenburger DD, Greiner TC, et al. Confirmation of the molecular classification of diffuse large B-cell lymphoma by immunohistochemistry using a tissue microarray. *Blood*. 2004;103:275-282.

74. Das DK, Pathan SK, Mothaffer FJ, et al. T-cell-rich B-cell lymphoma (TCRBCL): limitations in fine-needle aspiration cytodiagnosis. *Diagn Cytopathol*. 2012;40:956-963.

75. Plaza JA, Kacerovska D, Stockman DL, et al. The histomorphologic spectrum of primary cutaneous diffuse large B-cell lymphoma: a study of 79 cases. *Am J Dermatopathol*. 2011;33: 649-655.

76. Kornstein MJ, Max LD, Wakely PE Jr. Touch imprints in the intraoperative diagnosis of anterior mediastinal neoplasms. *Arch Pathol Lab Med*. 1996;120:1116-1122.

77. Lin O, Koreishi A, Brandt SM, et al. ALK⁺ large B-cell lymphoma: a rare variant of aggressive large B-cell lymphoma mimicking carcinoma on cytology specimens. *Diagn Cytopathol*. 2013;41: 404-407.

78. Pantanowitz L, Wu Z, Dezube BJ, Pihan G. Extracavitary primary effusion lymphoma of the anorectum. *Clin Lymphoma Myeloma*. 2005;6:149-152.

79. Lin O, Gerhard R, Zerbini MC, Teruya-Feldstein J. Cytologic features of plasmablastic lymphoma. *Cancer*. 2005;105:139-144.

80. Reid-Nicholson M, Kavuri S, Ustun C, et al. Plasmablastic lymphoma: cytologic findings in 5 cases with unusual presentation. *Cancer*. 2008;114:333-341.

81. Pillai RK, Sathanoori M, Van Oss SB, Swerdlow SH. Double-hit B-cell lymphomas with BCL6 and MYC translocations are aggressive, frequently extranodal lymphomas distinct from BCL2 double-hit B-cell lymphomas. *Am J Surg Pathol*. 2013;37:323-332.

82. Elkins CT, Wakely PE. Cytopathology of "double-hit" non-Hodgkin lymphoma. *Cancer Cytopathol*. 2011;119:263-271.

83. Roth CG, Gillespie-Twardy A, Marks S, et al Flow cytometric evaluation of double/triple hit lymphoma. *Oncol Res*. 2016;23: 137-146.

84. Pai RK, Mullins FM, Kim YH, Kong CS. Cytologic evaluation of lymphadenopathy associated with mycosis fungoides and Sezary syndrome: role of immunophenotypic and molecular ancillary studies. *Cancer*. 2008;114:323-332.

85. Vigliar E, Cozzolino I, Picardi M, et al. Lymph node fine needle cytology in the staging and follow-up of cutaneous lymphomas. *BMC Cancer*. 2014;14:8.

86. Singh S, Gupta N, Tekta GR. Imprint cytology facilitating the diagnosis of primary cutaneous anaplastic large cell lymphoma of iliac fossa. *J Cytol*. 2012;29:267-269.

87. Yao JL, Cangiarella JF, Cohen JM, Chhieng DC. Fine-needle aspiration biopsy of peripheral T-cell lymphomas. A cytologic and immunophenotypic study of 33 cases. *Cancer*. 2001;93:151-159.

88. Das P, Iyer VK, Mathur SR, Ray R. Anaplastic large cell lymphoma: a critical evaluation of cytomorphological features in seven cases. *Cytopathology*. 2010;21:251-258.

89. Sakr H, Cruise M, Chahal P, et al. Anaplastic lymphoma kinase positive large B-cell lymphoma: literature review and report of an endoscopic fine needle aspiration case with tigroid backgrounds mimicking seminoma. *Diagn Cytopathol*. 2016;45:148-155.

90. Vij M, Dhir B, Verma R, et al. Cytomorphology of ALK⁺ anaplastic large cell lymphoma displaying spindle cells mimicking a sarcomatous tumor: report of a case. *Diagn Cytopathol*. 2011;39:775-779.

91. Ng WK, Ip P, Choy C, Collins RJ. Cytologic findings of angioimmunoblastic T-cell lymphoma: analysis of 16 fine-needle aspirates over 9-year period. *Cancer*. 2002;96:166-173.

92. Cho EY, Gong G, Khang SK, et al. Fine needle aspiration cytology of CD56-positive natural killer/T-cell lymphoma of soft tissue. *Cancer*. 2002;96:344-350.

93. Swerdlow SH, Webber SA, Chadburn A, Ferry JA. Post-transplant lymphoproliferative disorders. In: Swerdlow SH, Campo E, Harris NL, et al., eds. *WHO Classification of Tumours of Haematopoietic and Lymphoid Tissue*. 4th ed. Switzerland: WHO Press; 2008:343-349.

94. Jones D, Bhatia VK, Krausz T, Pinkus GS. Crystal-storing histiocytosis: a disorder occurring in plasmacytic tumors expressing immunoglobulin kappa light chain. *Hum Pathol*. 1999;30:1441-1448.

95. Lorsbach RB, Hsi ED, Dogan A, Fend F. Plasma cell myeloma and related neoplasms. *Am J Clin Pathol*. 2011;136:168-182.

96. Arber DA, Orazi A, Hasserjian R, et al. The 2016 revision to the World Health Organization classification of myeloid neoplasms and acute leukemia. *Blood*. 2016;127:2391-2405.

97. Pantanowitz L, Thompson L. Myeloid sarcoma. *Ear Nose Throat J*. 2005;84:470-471.

98. Singhal RL, Monaco SE, Pantanowitz L. Cytopathology of myeloid sarcoma: a study of 16 cases. *J Am Soc Cytopathol*. 2015;4:98-103.

99. Tamiolakis D, Barbagadaki S, Proimos E, et al. Touch imprint cytological diagnosis of nodal Langerhans cell histiocytosis. *B-ENT*. 2009;5:115-118.

100. Kakkar S, Kapila K, Verma K. Langerhans cell histiocytosis in lymph nodes. Cytomorphologic diagnosis and pitfalls. *Acta Cytol*. 2001;45:327-332.

101. Yang GC, Wang J, Yee HT. Interwoven dendritic processes of follicular dendritic cell sarcoma demonstrated on ultrafast papanicolaou-stained smears: a case report. *Acta Cytol*. 2006;50: 534-538.

102. Stigt JA, Boers JE, Boomsma MF. Ultrasound-guided tissue core biopsies in Supraclavicular lymph nodes in patients with suspected thoracic malignancies. *Respiration*. 2015;90:412-415.

103. Saha S, Woodhouse NR, Gok G, et al. Ultrasound guided Core Biopsy, Fine Needle Aspiration Cytology and Surgical Excision Biopsy in the diagnosis of metastatic squamous cell carcinoma in the head and neck: an eleven year experience. *Eur J Radiol*. 2011;80:792-795.

104. Macaskill EJ, Purdie CA, Jordan LB, et al. Axillary lymph node core biopsy for breast cancer metastases—how many needle passes are enough? *Clin Radiol.* 2012;67:417-419.

105. Forghani MN, Memar B, Jangjoo A, et al. The effect of excisional biopsy on the accuracy of sentinel lymph node mapping in early stage breast cancer: comparison with core needle biopsy. *Am Surg.* 2010;76:1232-1235.

106. Bohelay G, Battistella M, Pagès C, et al. Ultrasound-guided core needle biopsy of superficial lymph nodes: an alternative to fine-needle aspiration cytology for the diagnosis of lymph node metastasis in cutaneous melanoma. *Melanoma Res.* 2015;25:519-527.

107. Lumachi F, Marino F, Zanella S, et al. Touch imprint cytology and frozen-section analysis for intraoperative evaluation of sentinel nodes in early breast cancer. *Anticancer Res.* 2012;32:3523-3526.

108. Kjurkchiev G, Valkov I. Role of touch imprint and core biopsy for detection of tumor metastases in bone marrow. *Diagn Cytopathol.* 1998;18:323-324.

109. De Las Casas LE, Gokden M, Mukunyadzi P, et al. A morphologic and statistical comparative study of small cell carcinoma and non-Hodgkin's lymphoma in fine-needle aspiration biopsy material from lymph nodes. *Diagn Cytopathol.* 2004;31:229-234.

110. Prieto-Granada C, Setia N, Otis CN. Lymph node extramedullary hematopoiesis in breast cancer patients receiving neoadjuvant therapy: a potential diagnostic pitfall. *Int J Surg Pathol.* 2013;21:264-246.

CHAPTER 7

Genitourinary System

Anil V. Parwani and Liron Pantanowitz

INTRODUCTION

Touch imprint cytology can be a helpful ancillary tool when evaluating benign or malignant lesions or neoplasms of the genitourinary system, either during an intraoperative evaluation such as margin assessment, or during an adequacy or diagnostic assessment during a fine-needle aspiration (FNA) procedure. Studies have demonstrated that implementation of touch preparations to evaluate samples collected by image-guided core needle biopsy can lead to improved diagnostic yield and rapid result reporting. To date, there have been a limited number of studies specifically focused on the genitourinary system. Nevertheless, knowledge of imprint cytomorphology has been gained with metastatic genitourinary lesions. Initial assessment of a lesion by touch imprint cytology can also help appropriately triage samples for ancillary studies. A disadvantage of touch preparations is their inability to easily distinguish an in situ lesion from invasive carcinoma. The focus of this chapter is to present the touch imprint cytomorphology of normal structures commonly encountered in the genitourinary system, as well as highlight some commonly encountered benign and malignant entities.

NORMAL

Normal Kidney

Each kidney is composed of an external cortical zone (cortex), inner medullary zone (medulla), and a renal pelvis that opens into the ureter. Touch imprints of normal kidney may show a variety of normal kidney elements such as glomeruli, proximal, and distal tubules (Figure 7.1). The architectural patterns of these structures evaluated by touch imprint cytology are similar to that seen on histopathological evaluation. A normal kidney touch imprint may show increased cellularity if obtained from an area with multiple glomeruli and tubules. Glomeruli form compact, rounded, cohesive

three-dimensional (3D) balls of cells with a lobular structure associated with thin-walled blood-filled capillaries (Figure 7.2A and 7.2B). The presence of glomeruli can help favor a benign or reactive condition. Glomeruli may be mistaken for a neoplasm due to clustering (forming aggregates), increased cellularity, and smearing artifact. The differential diagnosis of a glomerulus includes papillary renal cell carcinoma (PRCC), which will often show more pronounced cellular atypia with true fibrovascular cores. Glomeruloid bodies in a Wilms tumor can also be a mimic. Renal tubules are composed of cuboidal epithelium and tend to form more two-dimensional (2D) clusters. Proximal renal tubules have larger and more eosinophilic cells (Figure 7.3A and 7.3B) than distal tubules (Figure 7.4). Both tubules have bland nuclear features. The finding of benign tubules is usually indicative of a nondiagnostic specimen. Proximal tubular cells may mimic an oncocytic (granular) renal neoplasm (e.g., oncocytoma) and distal tubules can mimic PRCC. However, malignancies tend to be more cellular and exhibit some atypia. Occasionally, touch imprints may contain urothelial cells from the renal pelvis. The presence of superficial umbrella cells in such cases (Figure 7.5) can be alarming.

Normal Urothelium

Normal urothelium may be encountered anywhere along the urothelial tract from the renal pelvis down to the ureters, urinary bladder, and urethra. Normal urothelium is composed of superficial umbrella cells, intermediate cells, and basal cells. Urothelial cells are typically rounded and have sharply defined cytoplasm (Figure 7.6). Umbrella cells are larger cells, about the same size as mature squamous epithelial cells, and are often multinucleated (Figure 7.7). Umbrella cell nuclei are also slightly larger, whereas basal cell nuclei are usually more hyperchromatic. In situations where there is inflammation, reactive urothelial cells may be encountered (Figure 7.8). Occasionally, in touch preparations there may be squamous cells identified either as a normal component, such as from the trigone of the bladder or terminal part of the urethra, or in situations where there is squamous metaplasia. Benign columnar cells may arise from periurethral glands, areas with cystitis glandularis (Figure 7.9), or from contamination (e.g., prostate or seminal vesicle).

Normal Prostate

Imprint cytology has been reported for the evaluation of prostatic capsule involvement by prostate cancer (1) and to interpret prostate core needle biopsies (2). It is uncommon to encounter normal prostate in touch prep specimens. Normal prostatic parenchyma is composed of prostatic glands and associated stroma. Normal prostatic glands form flat sheets of benign epithelial cells with round nuclei and inconspicuous nucleoli (Figure 7.10A and 7.10B) Micro-acini may sometimes be observed (Figure 7.11). Inflammation including macrophages may be present in conditions like prostatitis. Occasionally, seminal vesicle may be encountered in touch preps characterized by lipofuscin pigment (Figure 7.12) and cells with marked variability in nuclear size and shape (Figure 7.13), a feature that may mimic malignancy (3). Intranuclear cytoplasmic inclusions, nuclear folding, and prominent nucleoli may be observed in some cases. Seminal vesicle secretions often cause a background "parched earth" appearance (Figure 7.14).

Normal Testis

The testicular parenchyma is composed of numerous seminiferous tubules. They contain germ cells that differentiate into spermatozoa, supporting Sertoli cells and Leydig (interstitial) cells. Testicular touch preparation of a normal testis biopsy should show germ cells in varying stages of spermatogenesis. Complete maturation of germ cells is represented by the presence of spermatogonia (intermediate-sized cells with a high nuclear to cytoplasmic ratio containing single, oval-to-round, darkly stained nuclei with even chromatin), spermatocytes (slightly larger cells with nuclei containing more coarse or thread-like chromatin), spermatids (small-sized cells with minimal cytoplasm, darkly stained small, and oval nuclei), and spermatozoa (sperm) (Figure 7.15A and 7.15B). Spermatozoa tails are a helpful feature (Figure 7.16), but may not always be distinct with a Pap stain. Sertoli cells have cytoplasm with poorly delineated cell borders and a vesicular, oval nucleus, with smooth contours and a distinct, large nucleolus. Intracytoplasmic crystalloids of Charcot–Böttcher may be seen in some Sertoli cells (Figure 7.17). Male infertility is traditionally evaluated by tissue core biopsies of the testes. Touch preparations of these biopsies are a helpful adjunct to biopsy because of its ability to clearly evaluate all stages of spermatogenesis (4,5).

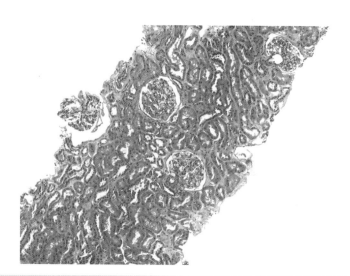

FIGURE 7.1 Normal kidney. This core biopsy illustrates the key elements that could be encountered in a TP including glomeruli as well as distal and proximal tubules. The glomerulus consists of podocytes, mesangial cells, and capillary endothelial cells. Proximal tubules have a larger diameter and taller tubular cells that are more eosinophilic than distal tubules (H&E-stained, medium power). H&E, hematoxylin and eosin; TP, touch preparation.

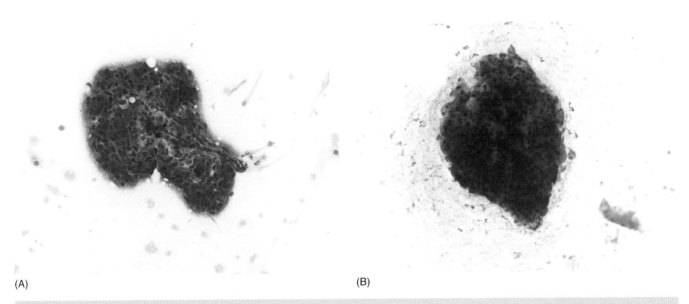

(A)

(B)

FIGURE 7.2   Normal glomerulus. These TPs demonstrate intact glomeruli. ((A) DQ-stained TP, medium power; (B) Pap-stained TP, medium power.) DQ, Diff-Quik; TP, touch preparation.

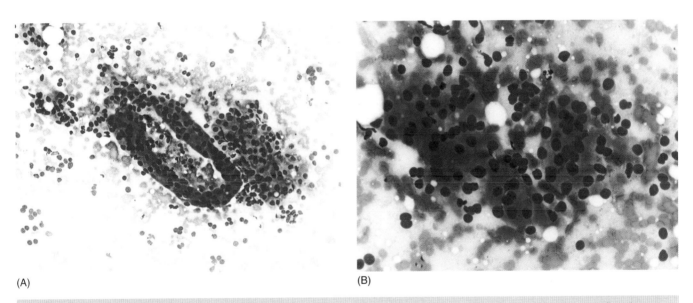

(A)

(B)

FIGURE 7.3   Normal proximal convoluted tubule. Tubules may form (A) 3D tubular structures or (B) imprint as flat sheets. Their cells have abundant granular cytoplasm that may not always have distinct cell borders. ((A) DQ-stained TP, medium power; (B) DQ-stained TP, high power.) DQ, Diff-Quik; TP, touch preparation.

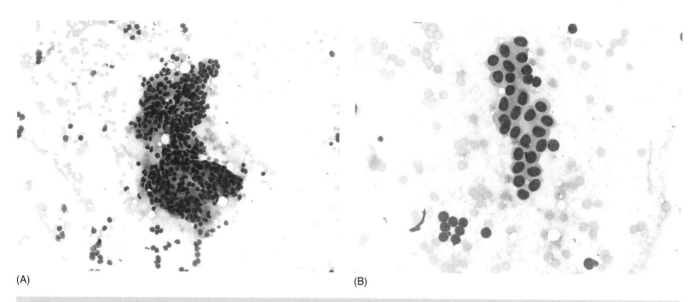

(A)   (B)

FIGURE 7.4   Normal distal convoluted tubule. Note that these tubular cells have scant cytoplasm that is not granular. They resemble tubular segments from the loop of Henle. ((A) and (B) DQ-stained TP, medium power.) DQ, Diff-Quik; TP, touch preparation.

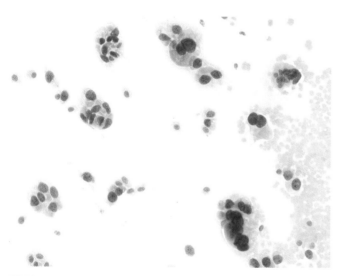

FIGURE 7.5   Normal renal pelvis urothelium. This TP shows predominantly large, multinucleated umbrella cells (Pap-stained TP, medium power). TP, touch preparation.

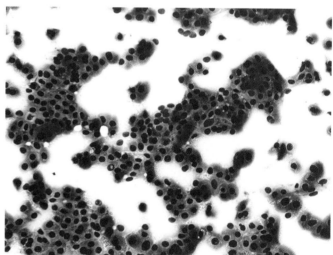

FIGURE 7.6   Normal bladder urothelium. Touch imprint showing benign basal-intermediate urothelial cells. These cuboidal cells have homogeneous dense cytoplasm, a low nuclear:cytoplasmic ratio, and uniform central round to oval nuclei with smooth nuclear contours and indistinct nucleoli (DQ-stained TP, medium power). DQ, Diff-Quik; TP, touch preparation.

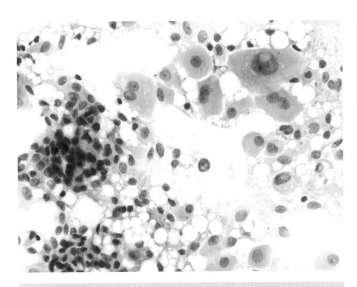

FIGURE 7.7 Benign umbrella cells. This touch imprint shows a cluster of large umbrella cells to the right. Some of these cells have a single nucleus and others are multinucleated. Umbrella cells are always benign, but may coexist with urothelial tumors (Pap-stained TP, medium power). TP, touch preparation.

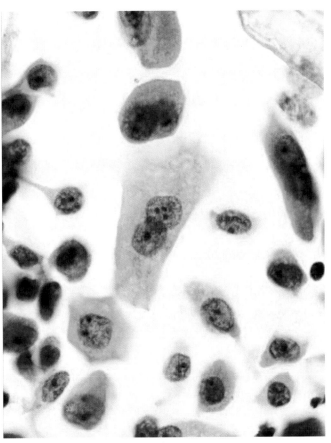

FIGURE 7.8 Reactive urothelial cells. The nuclei of these cells contain nucleoli with regular nuclear contours (Pap-stained TP, high power). TP, touch preparation.

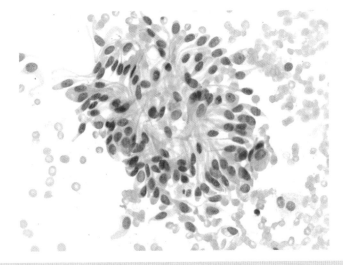

FIGURE 7.9 Benign glandular cells associated with cystitis glandularis. These glandular cells show elongated cytoplasm with basally located bland nuclei (Pap-stained TP, medium power). TP, touch preparation.

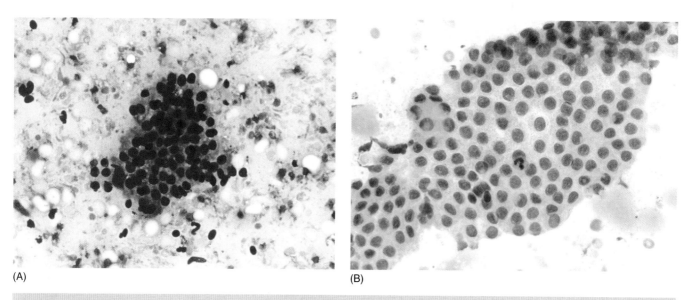

(A)   (B)

FIGURE 7.10 Benign prostate gland. These touch imprint preparations show cohesive sheets of benign epithelial cells with bland round nuclei that are evenly distributed. ((A) DQ-stained TP, medium power; (B) Pap-stained TP, medium power.) DQ, Diff-Quik TP, touch preparation.

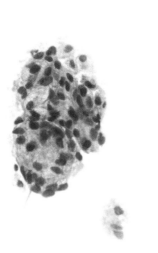

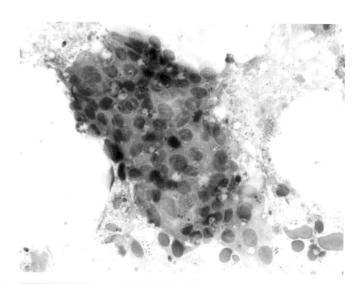

FIGURE 7.11 Benign prostate gland. Touch imprint showing a group of benign epithelial cells forming microacini (Pap-stained TP, medium power). TP, touch preparation.

FIGURE 7.12 Benign seminal vesicle. This TP shows a flat sheet of bland epithelial cells with characteristic intracytoplasmic yellow lipofuscin pigment (Pap-stained TP, medium power). TP, touch preparation.

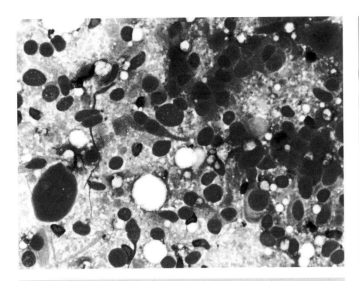

FIGURE 7.13 Benign seminal vesicle. Note the heterogeneity of nuclear size and shapes in this cytology imprint. Several of the nuclei have a smudgy appearance (DQ-stained TP, medium power). DQ, Diff-Quik; TP, touch preparation.

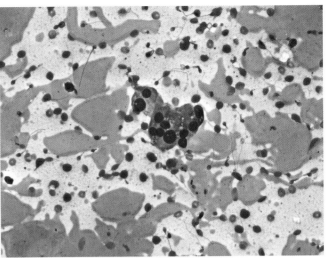

FIGURE 7.14 Benign seminal vesicle. The background material in this TP shows thick secretions and scattered sperm (DQ-stained TP, medium power). DQ, Diff-Quik; TP, touch preparation.

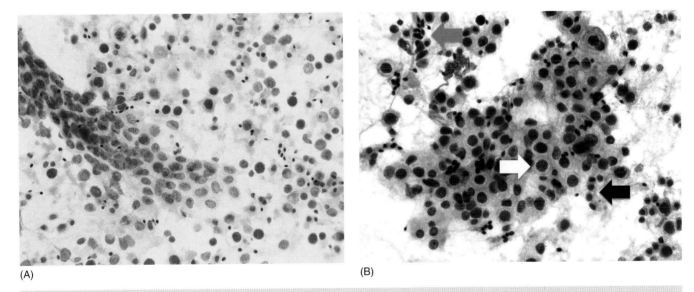

(A)

(B)

FIGURE 7.15 Normal testis. (A) This TP contains a sheet of mesothelial cells from the tunica and germ cells that demonstrate complete spermatogenesis (Pap-stained TP, medium power). (B) TP showing numerous spermatocytes (white arrow), spermatids (black arrow), and mature spermatozoa (grey arrow) (Pap-stained TP, medium power). TP, touch preparation.

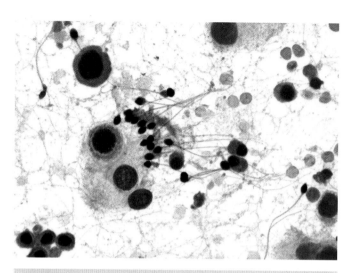

FIGURE 7.16 Normal testis. TP showing spermatocytes and sperm with elongated tails (Pap-stained TP, high power). TP, touch preparation.

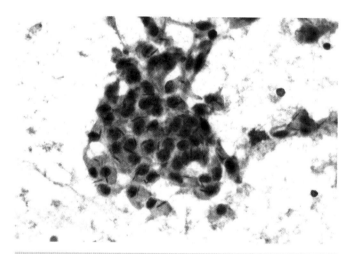

FIGURE 7.17 Normal Sertoli cells. This TP shows a homogenous population of Leydig cells. These cells have poorly delineated cell borders and a vesicular, oval nucleus, with smooth contours and a distinct, large nucleolus. Note the intracytoplasmic needle-shaped crystalloids of Charcot–Böttcher (Pap-stained TP, high power). TP, touch preparation.

BENIGN AND MALIGNANT LESIONS

Touch imprint cytology is most frequently used in the assessment of neoplasms of the genitourinary tract. Touch preps are rarely used in the assessment of benign diseases of the genitourinary tract, and therefore fewer of these entities are covered in this chapter.

Kidney

Percutaneous FNA and core biopsy with touch preparation are less invasive than open biopsy and often used to diagnose renal lesions. Imaging studies today are incidentally detecting an increasing number of small renal masses (≤4 cm). Indications for performing renal tumor biopsy have been further expanded by the development of conservative and minimally invasive treatments for low-risk RCC, and the discovery of novel targeted treatments for metastatic disease. Many review articles suggest that FNA and core biopsy are complimentary procedures, and that combined they increase the diagnostic accuracy of renal lesions (6,7). However, some studies have shown that compared to FNA alone, core biopsy, and touch prep has higher accuracy and diagnostic yield in the diagnosis of renal lesions (8). Perhaps this is because core biopsy permits more specific histologic classification and grading. Preoperative biopsy has limited ability to identify non–clear-cell histological subtype, Fuhrman grade, or sarcomatoid features of renal tumors (9).

Nonneoplastic Entities

Nonneoplastic entities that mimic malignancy and hence may be encountered with touch preparations of the kidney include infectious conditions such as pyelonephritis, including xanthogranulomatous pyelonephritis, and a renal abscess. Xanthogranulomatous pyelonephritis is a diffuse destructive inflammatory process, often ending in a nonfunctional kidney. The etiology is chronic infection often associated with *Escherichia coli* and *Proteus mirabilis*. The key findings include foamy histiocytes, neutrophils, plasma cells, and multinucleated giant cells. Occasionally, associated reactive renal tubular cells may be seen.

Renal Cell Epithelial Neoplasms

Renal epithelial tumors include benign neoplasms such as oncocytomas and malignant tumors such as clear cell, chromophobe, or papillary tumors. These tumors may present with variable growth patterns including nested, solid, papillary, or cystic growth. Their cytoplasmic and nuclear features are variable and there may be significant overlap in the cytomorphological appearance with granular to clear cytoplasm, as well as round uniform nuclei to nuclei that are of higher grade with large prominent nucleoli. Touch imprint cytology is often used to evaluate image-guided core needle biopsies of renal lesions onsite and to determine adequacy and appropriately triage samples. There are several entities on touch preps that present with diagnostic challenges. These include the recognition of normal kidney elements, identifying well-differentiated kidney tumors, distinguishing oncocytomas from other granular cell RCCs (Table 7.1) (10,11), as well as recognizing the multiple variants of urothelial carcinoma that may have cytomorphological overlap with entities such as collecting duct carcinoma or PRCC. A discussion of urothelial tumors that may be encountered in the kidney is dealt with in the subsequent section on urothelial tumors.

Oncocytoma

Renal oncocytoma is a rare, benign renal epithelial tumor composed of large cells with abundant granular eosinophilic mitochondria-rich cytoplasm (Figure 7.18A and 7.18B) thought to arise from intercalated cells of the collecting duct. Touch imprint cytology shows cells with low nuclear to cytoplasmic ratios, as well as round and uniform nuclei (Figure 7.19). Occasionally, on touch preparations, delicate fibrovascular septae may be seen. The differential diagnosis includes normal proximal tubules, chromophobe renal cell carcinoma (CHRCC), and clear cell carcinoma, eosinophilic variant. Ancillary testing may be helpful including the use of immunohistochemistry.

TABLE 7.1 Cytomorphology of Granular (Eosinophilic) Renal Cell Tumors

Cytomorphology	Oncocytic Tumor	Clear Cell Carcinoma	Papillary Renal Cell Carcinoma
Papillary pattern	No	No	Yes
Tubular pattern	No	No	Yes
Sheets with transgressing vessels	Sometimes	Yes	No
Cell shape	Polygonal	Polygonal	Cuboidal–columnar
Cell size	Medium-large	Medium-large	Medium
Nucleus location	Eccentric	Eccentric	One pole
High-grade nuclei	Sometimes	Sometimes	Sometimes
Abundant cytoplasm	Sometimes	Sometimes	No
Cytoplasmic vacuoles	No	Yes	No
Granular cytoplasm	Yes	Sometimes	Only type 1

Source: Adapted from Ref. (12). Lin X. Cytomorphology of clear cell papillary renal cell carcinoma. *Cancer Cytopathol*. 2016;125:48-54.

These tumors are typically negative for vimentin, show patchy staining with CK7 (Figure 7.20) and strong staining with parvalbumin (Figure 7.21). Molecular testing is not routinely used in the diagnosis of oncocytomas. The most common genetic abnormality is the loss of chromosome 1 and Y, which is also present in CHRCCs.

Metanephric Adenoma

Metanephric adenoma is a rare, benign neoplasm of epithelial cells. Due to its resemblance to some renal cell neoplasms such as papillary adenoma or PRCC, it becomes a diagnostic challenge to correctly identify on touch preparations. Imprints are usually very cellular. The tumor cells are uniform and have hyperchromatic nuclei. The neoplastic cells have an unusually scant amount of cytoplasm. The cells tend to form clusters or small tubules. The background has minimal or no necrosis. There may be psammoma bodies, infrequent mitotic figures, or apoptotic bodies. The differential diagnosis includes normal renal tubules, solid variant of PRCC, and Wilms tumor. Metanephric adenoma tumor cells are positive for WT-1 and CD57, but are negative for CK7.

Clear Cell Renal Cell Carcinoma

Conventional clear cell renal cell carcinoma (CCRCC) is the most common renal malignancy, comprising approximately 70% of all renal tumors. The hallmark of these tumors is the presence of neoplastic epithelial cells that have clear cytoplasm with a characteristic presence of delicate and arborizing small vessels. CCRCC is associated with the dominantly inherited familial disease syndrome known as von Hippel–Lindau (VHL) disease. The latter involves a germline mutation of the *VHL* gene at chromosome 3p25. Individuals that are affected are susceptible to cystic tumors of multiple organ systems, including their kidneys, pancreas, and genital tract.

These tumors can have a variable microscopic architecture growth pattern including alveolar, microcystic, tubular, or nested. They have a delicate network of vessels surrounding tumor cell nests (Figure 7.22). The cells have clear cytoplasm with a distinct cell membrane (Figure 7.23). Cells with more granular (eosinophilic) cytoplasm are seen in higher grade carcinomas. In touch preparations, tumor cells tend to be cohesive and have abundant cytoplasm with vacuoles and/or granules (Figure 7.24).

Occasional tumors may display hyaline globules within the cytoplasm. The nuclear features are variable, but in general lower grade tumors tend to have round or more oval nuclei with less prominent nucleoli (Figure 7.25). The nucleoli are more conspicuous in higher grade nuclei correlating well with the Fuhrman nuclear grading system (Figure 7.26). The International Society of Urological Pathology (ISUP) grading system is a new modification of the Fuhrman nuclear grading system (Table 7.2).

The differential diagnosis of CCRCC includes other renal tumors such as translocation tumors or other subtypes of RCC with clear cell areas including PRCC, clear cell PRCC, or even CHRCC. The nuclei of metastatic CCRCC may show a high degree of cytological atypia (Figure 7.27), but most often the cytoplasm in these metastases retains characteristic clear cell morphology. Immunohistochemistry is a very useful adjunct tool for confirming the diagnosis of CCRCC. These tumors typically express vimentin, epithelial membrane antigen (EMA), CD10, and PAX-8. PAX-8 is a useful pan-renal cell marker with strong nuclear staining (Figure 7.28), whereas carbonic anhydrase IX (CAIX) with strong, diffuse, membranous staining is a more specific CCRCC marker.

Chromophobe Renal Cell Carcinoma

CHRCC represents approximately 4% to 5% of all adult renal tumors. Their cell of origin is considered to be intercalated cells of the collecting duct. These tumors tend to have a low malignant potential. They occur predominantly in adults with only rare cases described in the pediatric population. Touch preparations may be cellular with clusters of cells showing a mosaic-like pattern of small and large cells (Figure 7.29). The key findings in imprint cytology preparations are the presence of polygonal cells with granular, eosinophilic cytoplasm, and well-defined cytoplasmic boundaries. These cells are usually more voluminous than those typically seen in CCRCC. The prominent cytoplasmic clearing or halo seen around the nucleus in tumor cells within core biopsy or resection specimens may not be evident in cytology samples. Such clear cytoplasmic spaces resembling perinuclear halos seem to be best appreciated in cells with abundant dense cytoplasm (13). The tumor cells have nuclei that are round, and occasionally binucleated (Figure 7.30). Nuclei can also have intranuclear inclusions (Figure 7.31). The differential diagnosis of

TABLE 7.2   The International Society of Urological Pathology Grading System for Renal Cell Carcinoma

Grade 1	Inconspicuous or absent nucleoli at ×400 magnification
Grade 2	Nucleoli distinctly visible at ×400 but inconspicuous at ×100 magnification
Grade 3	Nucleoli distinctly visible at ×100 magnification
Grade 4	Presence of rhabdoid or sarcomatoid differentiation; presence of tumor giant cells or cells showing extreme nuclear pleomorphism with clumping

CHRCC includes oncocytoma and eosinophilic variant of CCRCC. Ancillary testing may be helpful. These tumors are most often strongly and diffusely positive for Hale colloidal iron stain and membranous CK7 staining.

Papillary Renal Cell Carcinoma

PRCC is a distinct variant of RCC that represents 10% to 15% of all adult renal cell carcinomas. They have a slight male predominance. Although they have a sporadic occurrence, there are occasional tumors that are associated with familial renal cell carcinoma syndromes such as hereditary PRCC syndrome. In addition, PRCC tends to be frequently associated with end-stage kidney disease. These tumors are usually well-circumscribed, have a distinct fibrous capsule, are friable and hemorrhagic, and have a cystic appearance. Their architecture is predominantly papillary or tubulopapillary (Figure 7.32). The presence of papillae with true fibrovascular cores is very helpful to diagnose these tumors. There are two subtypes of PRCC: type 1 and type 2 (Figure 7.33). Type 1 is more common than type 2, usually has lower grade nuclear features, and generally has a better prognosis.

Touch preparations from both PRCC type 1 and type 2 may show characteristic features such as papillary clusters with fibrovascular cores surrounded by cuboidal-appearing tumor cells with abundant lightly granular cytoplasm (Figure 7.34). There are often detached cells present in the background (Figure 7.35). The nuclear features of PRCC are variable depending on the subtype. In general, tumor cells have round to oval nuclei with moderate to marked pleomorphism. In some cases, nuclear grooves may be visible. The ISUP nuclear grading system is now widely used for grading of PRCC (Table 7.1). Other features that may be seen in both type 1 and type 2 PRCC include hemosiderin pigment, foamy macrophages, and psammoma bodies.

Although there is an overlap in the cytomorphological appearance of type 1 and type 2 PRCC, there are some distinct features. Type 1 PRCC demonstrates a single layer of cells arranged around papillary cores. Their nuclei are generally small with minimal to mild nuclear pleomorphism and fairly inconspicuous nucleoli. Papillae are also shorter and more blunted. Type 2 PRCC tumor cells are larger with eosinophilic cytoplasm and they appear pseudostratified. Their nuclei are much larger, more pleomorphic, and have more prominent nucleoli (Figure 7.36).

The differential diagnosis of PRCC includes tumors within the kidney that may have a papillary appearance or architecture such as papillary adenomas, clear cell PRCC, translocation RCC, collecting duct carcinoma, mucinous and tubular spindle cell carcinoma, and acquired cystic disease-associated RCC. A combination of clinical presentation, distinct cytomorphology, and ancillary testing will help in correctly classifying these lesions. More challenging is the evaluation of a metastatic tumor with a papillary appearance on touch preparations with nondistinct cytomorphological features such as large cells with a granular appearance and significant nuclear atypia including prominent nucleoli (Figure 7.37). To enable accurate subtyping, pan-RCC markers such as PAX-8 will be helpful. To further subtype these tumors, a panel of immunohistochemical markers can be utilized. PRCC tumor cells strongly express CK7 (Figure 7.38) and alpha-methylacyl-CoA racemase (AMACR). Other positive markers for PRCC include CD10, EMA, and RCC. Although there is significant overlap, PRCC type 1 tumors tend to express CK7 and vimentin more often, whereas type 2 PRCC tends to express CK20 and E-cadherin more frequently. Molecular testing including the use of fluorescence in-situ hybridization (FISH) may be helpful in confirming the presence of the characteristic trisomy of chromosomes 7 and 17 in difficult PRCC cases.

Sarcomatoid and Rhabdoid Renal Cell Carcinoma

Sarcomatoid RCC (SRCC) is defined in the World Health Organization (WHO) classification of renal tumors as any RCC histological type with foci of malignant high-grade spindle cells. The proportion of the sarcomatoid component varies from being minimal to almost entirely sarcomatoid. A sarcomatoid component may be seen in any RCC subtype, but is most commonly encountered in CCRCC (70%–80%), CHRCC (4%–8%), and PRCC (4%–8%). Touch preparations of SRCC may reveal sheets of spindle cells with marked pleomorphism. The spindle cell morphology is highly variable with occasional cases showing prominent myxoid background. Rarely, there may be chrondosarcomatous or osteosarcomatous differentiation. The histological tumor type of origin may be present, such as a distinct clear cell component if the tumor is arising from a CCRCC or a papillary architecture if arising from PRCC. The differential diagnosis of SRCC includes sarcomas such as leiomyosarcoma or angiomyolipoma (smooth muscle predominant variant) (Figure 7.39A and 7.39B).

Rhabdoid RCC (RRCC) is currently considered to be any histological subtype of RCC containing high-grade malignant cells with prominent rhabdoid morphology (Figure 7.40). Rhabdoid morphology may be seen in up to 5% to 8% of all RCCs and is mostly commonly seen in CCRCC. Touch preparations from cases of RRCC characteristically show large highly pleomorphic cells with abundant globule-like cytoplasm with a rhabdoid appearance (Figure 7.41). Their nuclei are large, irregular, and usually have an eccentric appearance. Nucleoli may be prominent. Most often, the rhabdoid component shows the coexistence of the RCC subtype from which the rhabdoid component originates. The differential diagnosis of RRCC includes sarcomas such as rhabdomyosarcoma. For both SRCC and RRCC, ancillary testing to establish the associated RCC subtype is helpful, including the use of immunohistochemistry (IHC) and molecular testing.

Hematolymphoid Neoplasms

Lymphomas are occasionally encountered in the kidney as the initial presentation either as primary, secondary, or posttransplant lymphomas. The subtypes of lymphoma commonly encountered in the kidney include diffuse large B cell lymphoma (Figure 7.42A and 7.42B), mucosa-associated lymphoid tissue (MALT) lymphoma, or follicular lymphoma. Other entities that may be seen include plasmacytoma/myeloma and myeloid sarcoma. Risk factors for renal lymphoma include acquired immunodeficiency syndrome (AIDS) or the posttransplant setting (Figure 7.43). Primary renal lymphomas are rare and more frequently these tumors are associated with secondary involvement. Touch preparations are useful to rapidly evaluate a renal mass and appropriately triage material for a suspected lymphoma (e.g., flow cytometry). Touch preps typically demonstrate a predominance of abnormal lymphoid cells. Cytopathology in this setting plays a critical role, as it can prevent the patient from unnecessary nephrectomy.

Metastatic Tumors to the Kidney

Metastases to the kidney are rare and if they present as a single mass, they may mimic a primary renal tumor clinically, on imaging, and are also a pitfall in cytology. Such cases are particularly challenging if the initial presentation of metastatic disease is in the kidney. Tumors that are most frequently metastatic to the kidney include lung, breast, head and neck, and colon carcinoma. Metastatic tumors to the kidney can be multiple as well as bilateral. The touch imprint appearance of metastatic carcinoma may mimic renal cell carcinoma (Figure 7.44) or a high-grade poorly differentiated urothelial carcinoma (Figure 7.45). Ancillary testing using immunohistochemistry is often necessary to confirm the diagnosis.

Renal Pelvis, Ureter, Urinary Bladder, and Urethra

Urothelial Lesions

Urothelial carcinoma is the most common histologic type of carcinoma involving the urinary tract. These carcinomas account for greater than 90% of all cancers involving the urinary tract. They arise most commonly in the urinary bladder, but can also occur in the renal pelvis, ureters, and urethra. Urothelial lesions can be flat or papillary. They include benign (inverted and exophytic) papillomas, tumors of uncertain malignant potential papillary urothelial neoplasm of low malignant potential (PUN-LMP), and malignant tumors. Papillary and flat urothelial carcinomas include urothelial carcinoma in situ (CIS) and multiple variants of urothelial carcinoma such as small cell carcinoma, squamous cell carcinoma, and adenocarcinoma (Table 7.3). Urothelial carcinomas are composed of irregular infiltrating nests of tumor cells, with possibly glandular or squamous differentiation. Nuclear features include pleomorphism (Figure 7.46), elongated to round nuclei, irregular nuclear outlines and grooves, and irregular chromatin distribution with one to many nucleoli.

The most important cytological criteria for the diagnosis of urothelial neoplasms in touch imprint preparations include increased nuclear size, increased nuclear-to-cytoplasmic ratio, nuclear pleomorphism, hyperchromasia, nuclear eccentricity, and nuclear membrane irregularity, as well as cytoplasmic homogeneity. Low-grade papillary urothelial neoplasms display minimal architectural disorder, and exhibit lower grade nuclear cytologic atypia. Low-grade lesions lack distinguishable nuclear pleomorphism and tumor cells have no nucleoli or mitoses. In contrast, high-grade urothelial tumors tend to have a much more disorderly appearance with prominent

TABLE 7.3   The 2016 WHO Classification of Urothelial Tumors of the Urinary Tract

Noninvasive Urothelial Lesions
Urothelial papilloma
Inverted urothelial papilloma
Urothelial proliferation of uncertain malignant potential
Urothelial dysplasia
Papillary urothelial neoplasm of low malignant potential
Urothelial carcinoma in situ
Noninvasive papillary urothelial carcinoma, low grade
Noninvasive papillary urothelial carcinoma, high grade
Infiltrating Urothelial Carcinoma
Nested, including large nested variant
Microcystic variant
Micropapillary variant
Lymphoepithelioma-like variant
Plasmacytoid/signet ring cell/diffuse variant
Sarcomatoid variant
Giant cell variant
Poorly differentiated variant
Lipid-rich variant
Clear cell variant

WHO, World Health Organization.

architectural (e.g., crowding and overlapping) and cytological (e.g., clumped chromatin, irregular nuclear outlines, prominent nucleoli, and mitoses) abnormalities (Figures 7.47 and 7.48). These tumors are usually cellular with discohesive cells (Figure 7.49). High-grade tumors can sometimes demonstrate focal squamous differentiation with keratinization. The distinction of an in situ component from an invasive carcinoma is not usually possible with touch preparations, unless the architecture is preserved. Helpful immunomarkers for urothelial carcinoma include positive staining with CK7, CK20, high molecular weight cytokeratin (34ßE12+), p63, uroplakin, and GATA3 (Figure 7.50).

Squamous Cell Lesions of the Urothelial Tract

A number of benign and malignant squamous lesions may be encountered in the urinary tract, particularly in the urinary bladder (Table 7.4). It is important that pathologists are aware of these lesions, as they may be encountered in cytology samples.

Small Cell Carcinoma of the Urothelial Tract

Small cell carcinoma of the urothelial tract is a rare form of urothelial carcinoma for which standard therapy is not available. Although small cell carcinoma can occur anywhere in the urothelial tract, most cases have been described in the urinary bladder. The clinical presentation of small cell urothelial carcinoma is indistinguishable from conventional urothelial carcinoma, with most patients presenting with hematuria and dysuria. The diagnosis of small cell urothelial carcinoma is made primarily on the basis of cytomorphology. These tumors contain small to medium-sized round cells with hyperchromatic nuclei and are often associated with marked necrosis and mitoses (Figure 7.51). At higher magnification, small uniform cells with minimal cytoplasm and nuclear molding are characteristic. Their nuclei contain evenly dispersed powdery ("salt and pepper") chromatin. Nucleoli are inconspicuous. They often coexist with other forms of in situ or invasive carcinoma. Neuroendocrine differentiation is not required. These tumors are largely indistinguishable from small cell carcinoma arising from other sites (14).

Metastatic or Secondary Tumors Involving the Urinary Tract

Metastatic or secondary tumors to the urinary tract are rare. It may be difficult to distinguish primary urothelial carcinomas reliably from metastases. These tumors may involve the urinary tract via direct extension as well as metastasis. There may be significant overlap of their cytomorphology and immunoprofile. For example, squamous cell carcinoma originating in the cervix and extending into the bladder may be difficult to separate from a primary urothelial carcinoma with squamous differentiation. In such cases, a history of a known prior cancer and radiological findings may be necessary to confirm tumor origin.

Prostate

Touch imprint preparation of prostate glands is infrequently performed, but may be undertaken in certain settings. Touch preparation has been previously studied in the evaluation of prostatic capsule involvement by prostate cancer (1). Transrectal core needle biopsies have been shown to significantly improve the detection of prostate carcinoma (15). In problematic cases, touch preparation of these prostate core biopsies has helped improve their diagnostic yield (2). Touch imprints from fresh prostate needle biopsy specimens are also a reliable source of material for molecular testing (16). However, cytologists are more likely to encounter prostate cancer in touch preparations when dealing with metastatic disease. Touch imprint cytology was previously proven to be useful in detecting metastatic prostate cancer in pelvic lymph nodes, helping to overcome certain deficits of frozen section such as the presence of micrometastases or handling fatty lymph nodes that are difficult to process (17).

Benign Prostate Conditions

There are several benign conditions that may mimic prostate adenocarcinoma such as atrophy, hyperplasia, adenosis, mucinous metaplasia, squamous metaplasia, granulomatous prostatitis, nephrogenic metaplasia, and radiation atypia. However, these entities are extremely difficult to diagnose in imprint preparations. Most of these conditions usually have bland-appearing epithelial cells or exhibit only minimal

TABLE 7.4 Squamous Cell Lesions of the Urinary Tract

Squamous metaplasia
   Nonkeratinizing
   Keratinizing
Condyloma acuminatum
Squamous papilloma
Urothelial carcinoma with squamous differentiation
Verrucous carcinoma
Squamous cell carcinoma

cytological atypia. Architectural findings are typically necessary, to determine if there is an infiltrative appearance. Other infrequent benign cytologic findings and possible pitfalls that may be encountered are the presence of transitional cells, ganglion cells, Cowper's glands (with foamy mucinous glands), and seminal vesicles (18,19).

Prostate Adenocarcinoma

Prostatic adenocarcinoma is the most common solid tumor in men in the United States. Up to 95% of prostate cancer cases are acinar, whereas up to 5% can be ductal subtype. The majority of tumors arise in the peripheral zone of the prostate gland. Key diagnostic criteria of prostatic carcinoma are based on a constellation of findings that include an assessment of architectural, luminal, cytoplasmic, and nuclear features (Figure 7.52). Table 7.5 highlights several diagnostic features that may be diagnostically helpful on touch preparations. At low magnification, the presence of microacini (without basal cells) within cell clusters is useful. At higher magnification, the presence of large nuclei with prominent nucleoli (especially if >3 μm) is a helpful feature (Figure 7.53). Mitotic figures are rare, except in high-grade tumors. Prostatic intraepithelial neoplasia (PIN) cannot be differentiated from invasive carcinoma in cytological preparations alone (20). Prostate cancer is graded using the Gleason score, which is a measurement of how aggressive the tumor is based on architectural patterns. There are several variants of prostatic adenocarcinoma such as the foamy, atrophic, ductal, mucinous (colloid), intraductal, lymphoepithelioma-like, signet ring, and pseudo-hyperplastic variants. The differential diagnosis commonly includes poorly differentiated urothelial carcinoma. Clinical history, serum prostate specific antigen (PSA), and the use of immunohistochemistry can help in separating these two malignancies.

Prostate carcinoma is known to metastasize widely to bone, lung, lymph nodes, and other sites. Metastatic prostate carcinoma tends to demonstrate similar architectural (e.g., acinar arrangement) (Figure 7.54) and cytological (e.g., glandular cells with prominent nucleoli) features (Figure 7.55). Touch preparations of metastatic lesions may also show loose clusters, sheets, or single pleomorphic cells

with no appreciable acini. Certain metastatic prostate carcinoma cases can present with small cell or neuroendocrine features. The cytomorphological features overlap with small cell carcinoma of nonprostatic origin (21). These features include cells with minimal cytoplasm, nuclear molding, hyperchromasia, fine dusty chromatin, inconspicuous nucleoli, nuclear crush artifact, and karyorrhexis (Figure 7.56). Immunohistochemistry may be helpful. Prostate specific markers include androgen receptor, PSA, prostate specific acid phosphatase (PSAP), and NKX3.1. However, it is important to be aware that some of these markers may be negative in hormone-treated metastatic prostate carcinoma (22). Hence, it is also critical to perform a diagnostic workup including serum PSA to identify the primary source for the patient's metastasis, particularly if the patient has multiple lesions.

TESTIS

Nonneoplastic Lesions

As alluded to earlier, touch preparations of testicular core needle biopsies are often employed during the evaluation of male infertility, looking for complete spermatogenesis (4,5,23,24). Azoospermia may be caused by primary or secondary testicular failure. Primary testicular failure can be due to failure of spermatogenesis within the testes, including maturation arrest, partial or complete absence of germ cells, or Sertoli-cell-only syndrome. Other causes of infertility, where sperm are likely to be encountered in touch preparations, include ejaculatory dysfunction or ductal obstruction. Nonneoplastic lesions that may be encountered in biopsy samples include sperm granuloma, infections, nonspecific granulomatous orchitis, Leydig cell hyperplasia, infarction, and testicular involvement in systemic diseases (e.g., vasculitis, amyloidosis).

Testicular Neoplasms

Neoplasms of the testis can be classified into germ cell tumors, sex cord-stromal tumors, hematopoietic tumors (e.g., lymphoma, plasmacytoma, leukemia), miscellaneous tumors (e.g., mesothelioma, rete testis carcinoma, tumors

TABLE 7.5 Key Diagnostic Features of Prostatic Adenocarcinoma

- Amphophilic cytoplasm
- Nuclear enlargement
- Hyperchromasia
- Enlarged nucleoli
- Absent basal cells
- Luminal secretions
- Luminal (acidic/blue) mucus
- Luminal crystalloids
- Mitotic figures

of ovarian-type epithelium), and metastases. Germ cell tumors may arise in the testis or from multiple midline extragonadal sites. Table 7.6 lists the WHO classification of germ cell tumors of the testis. Only commonly encountered germ cell tumors are discussed in this section. Table 7.7 compares the key cytological features of some of these germ cell tumors. A variety of paratesticular tumors may also be encountered such as adenomatoid tumor, papillary cystadenoma of the epididymis, sarcomas including desmoplastic small round cell tumor, and melanotic neuroectodermal tumor. Touch imprint cytology of primary testicular neoplasms may be seen during their intraoperative assessment (25), or encountered with rapid onsite evaluation of metastatic disease.

Seminoma

Classic seminoma accounts for almost half of testicular germ cell tumors. Spermatocytic seminoma is more rare. Touch imprints from a case of typical seminoma are cellular (Figure 7.57) and show a predominantly dispersed cell population of large cells with scant to moderately abundant vacuolated cytoplasm. Spermatocytic seminoma has cells of three sizes: germ cells with large, medium, and small nuclei. Tumor cell nuclei are round, slightly irregular, demonstrate finely granular chromatin, and may have one or more central prominent nucleoli (26). Variable numbers of lymphocytes, plasma cells, and epithelioid histiocytes may be present. A "tigroid" background, when present, is very distinctive (27). Brisk mitotic activity is often present. Immunohistochemistry may be helpful such as the use of placental alkaline phosphatase (PLAP), OCT3/4, and CKIT.

Embryonal Carcinoma

Embryonal carcinomas are mostly seen in young patients. Many of them present with metastatic disease at the time of diagnosis. Even though pure embryonal carcinomas are rare, this tumor is one of the most common components of a mixed germ cell tumor and therefore will be commonly encountered. Their growth pattern may be solid, glandular, or papillary. Touch imprints may show single cells and/or syncytial aggregates of cells with indistinct cytoplasm, large nuclei, and prominent nucleoli (Figure 7.58). Cell groups may have a microglandular pattern (28). CD30, OCT3/4, SALL4, and SOX2 are good immunomarkers for embryonal carcinoma.

Yolk Sac Tumor

Yolk sac tumor is a rare testicular tumor that primarily affects children and young adults. These tumors can have many microscopic patterns such as reticular (lace-like), papillary, cord-like, endodermal sinus (with many Schiller–Duval bodies), hepatoid, macrocystic, macrocystic, myxomatous, as well as a solid and sarcomatoid pattern. Touch imprints may show a wide spectrum of cytomorphology based on these growth patterns. Samples are usually cellular. Tumor cells have bubbly cytoplasm and nuclei with a pleomorphic chromatin pattern, ranging from fine to coarse. Their nucleoli range from being small to prominent and pleomorphic. Extracellular hyaline material may be seen. Immunohistochemistry may be helpful in confirming the diagnosis including the use of glypican-3 and alpha-fetoprotein (AFP).

TABLE 7.6 The 2016 WHO Classification of Germ Cell Tumors of the Testis

Noninvasive Germ Cell Neoplasia
  Germ cell neoplasia in situ
  Specific forms of intratubular germ cell neoplasia
Tumors of a Single Histological Type (Pure Forms)
  Seminoma
  Seminoma with syncytiotrophoblast cells
  Nonseminomatous germ cell tumors
  Embryonal carcinoma
  Yolk sac tumor, postpubertal-type
  Trophoblastic Tumors
      Choriocarcinoma
      Nonchoriocarcinomatous trophoblastic tumors
      Placental site trophoblastic tumor
      Epithelioid trophoblastic tumor
      Cystic trophoblastic tumor
  Teratoma, postpubertal-type
  Teratoma with somatic-type malignancy
Nonseminomatous Germ Cell Tumors of More Than One Histological Type
  Mixed germ cell tumors
Germ Cell Tumors of Unknown Type
  Regressed germ cell tumors

WHO, World Health Organization.

TABLE 7.7 Morphologic Features of Germ Cell Neoplasms

	Classic Seminoma	Embryonal Carcinoma	Yolk Sac Tumor
Tumor growth	Usually diffuse	Papillary, solid	Variable
Chromatin pattern	Usually fine	Coarse	Fine
Nucleolus size	Large	Large	Small
Mitotic activity	Frequent	Brisk	Rare
Cell borders	Distinct	Indistinct	Variable
Cytoplasm	Clear	Dark, amphophilic	Variable
Lymphocytes	Present	Variable	Variable
Granulomas	Present	Absent	Absent

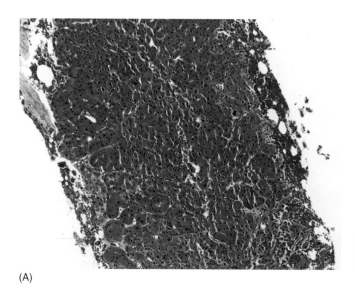

(A)

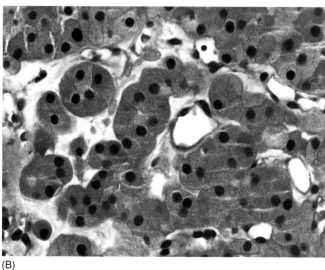

(B)

FIGURE 7.18 Oncocytoma. These tumors are composed of solid nests of tumor cells. The cells have abundant granular eosinophilic cytoplasm with round uniform nuclei. ((A) H&E-stained core biopsy, low power; (B) H&E-stained core biopsy, high power.) H&E, hematoxylin and eosin.

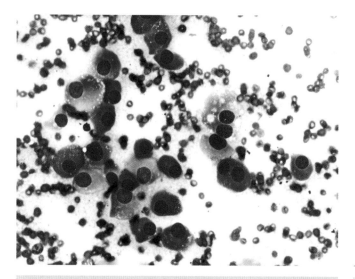

FIGURE 7.19 Oncocytoma. TP showing several single cells with abundant dense to granular cytoplasm and well defined cell borders. As in this case, occasional binucleate cells may be encountered. Nuclei are round and have inconspicuous nucleoli. The background is notably clean without necrosis (DQ-stained TP, medium power). DQ, Diff-Quik; TP, touch preparation.

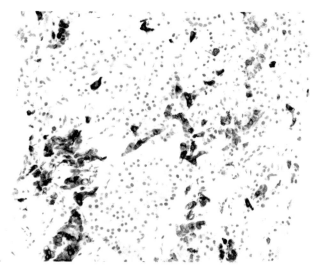

FIGURE 7.20 Oncocytoma. Tumor cells demonstrate patchy CK7 immunoreactivity (CK7 stain, medium power).

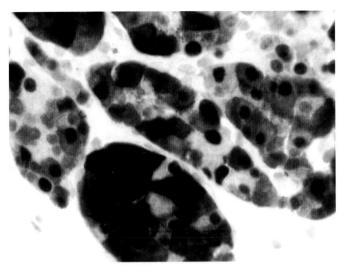

FIGURE 7.21 Oncocytoma. Strong parvalbumin positive staining is shown in tumor cells (Parvalbumin stain, high power).

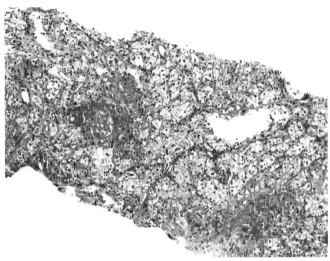

FIGURE 7.22 Renal cell carcinoma, clear cell type. Core biopsy with solid nests of clear tumor cells separated by a prominent delicate vascular network (H&E-stained core biopsy, low power). H&E, hematoxylin and eosin.

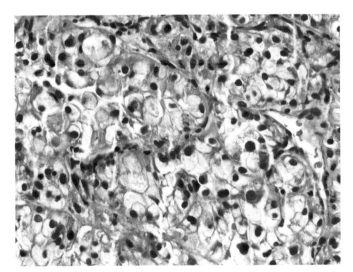

FIGURE 7.23 Renal cell carcinoma, clear cell type. Tumor cells have characteristic clear cytoplasm (H&E-stained core biopsy, medium power). H&E, hematoxylin and eosin.

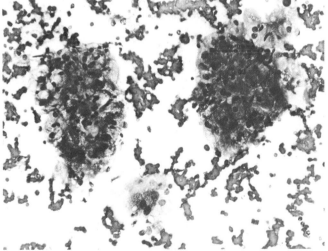

FIGURE 7.24 Renal cell carcinoma, clear cell type. TP showing cohesive groups of tumor cells. The tumor cells have abundant vacuolated cytoplasm (DQ-stained TP, medium power). DQ, Diff-Quik; TP, touch preparation.

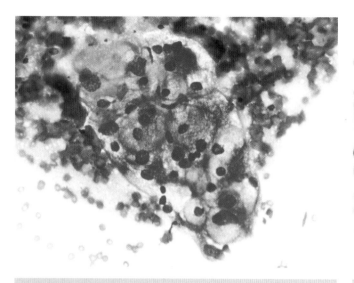

FIGURE 7.25 Renal cell carcinoma, clear cell type. Low-grade carcinoma with tumor cells showing finely granular chromatin and absent to small nucleoli (DQ-stained TP, high power). DQ, Diff-Quik; TP, touch preparation.

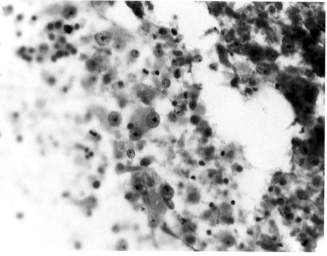

FIGURE 7.26 Renal cell carcinoma, clear cell type. High-grade carcinoma with tumor cells showing nuclear pleomorphism and macronucleoli (Pap-stained TP, high power). TP, touch preparation.

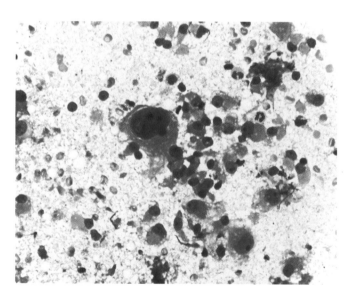

FIGURE 7.27 Metastatic renal cell carcinoma, clear cell type. These dyshesive tumor cells have high-grade features including marked nuclear pleomorphism and macronucleoli. Cells with fragile cytoplasm disrupt easily leaving behind several stripped naked nuclei (DQ-stained TP, high power). DQ, Diff-Quik; TP, touch preparation.

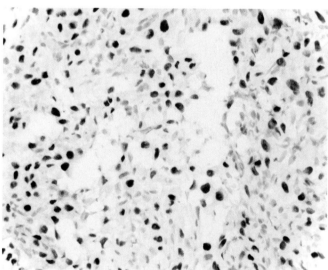

FIGURE 7.28 Renal cell carcinoma, clear cell type. Tumor cell nuclei are PAX-8 positive (PAX-8-stained, medium magnification).

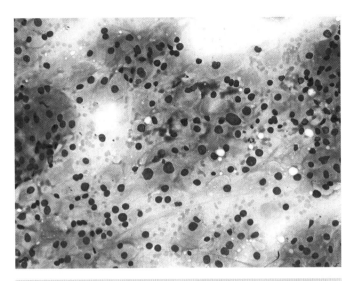

FIGURE 7.29 Renal cell carcinoma, chromophobe type. This TP shows polygonal tumor cells with abundant pale cytoplasm and nuclear pleomorphism (DQ-stained TP, medium power). DQ, Diff-Quik; TP, touch preparation.

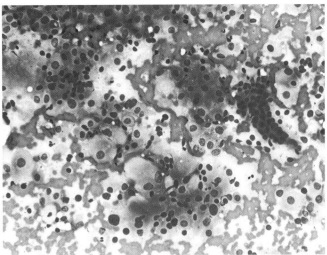

FIGURE 7.30 Metastatic renal cell carcinoma, chromophobe type, involving the liver. Tumor cells have abundant cytoplasm relative to the bile duct cell group seen in the right field of the image. Note the presence of binucleated tumor cells (DQ-stained TP, medium power). DQ, Diff-Quik; TP, touch preparation.

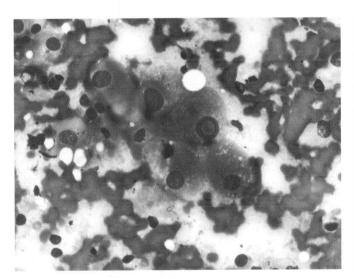

FIGURE 7.31 Renal cell carcinoma, chromophobe type. Note the prominent intranuclear cytoplasmic inclusion, which is a common finding in this subtype of renal cell carcinoma (DQ-stained TP, high power). DQ, Diff-Quik; TP, touch preparation.

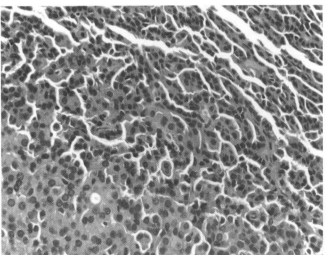

FIGURE 7.32 Renal cell carcinoma, papillary type. Tumor showing tightly packed tubulopapillary structures (H&E-stained core biopsy, low power). H&E, hematoxylin and eosin.

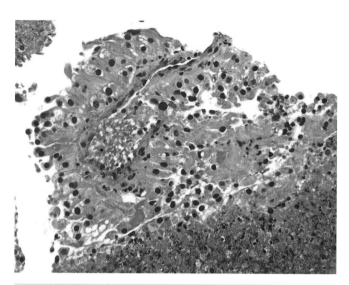

FIGURE 7.33 Renal cell carcinoma, papillary type 2. This tumor papilla is lined by cells with abundant eosinophilic cytoplasm and pseudostratified nuclei (H&E-stained core biopsy, medium power). H&E, hematoxylin and eosin.

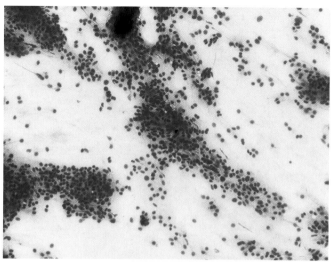

FIGURE 7.34 Renal cell carcinoma, papillary type. Imprint preparation showing papillary clusters with fibrovascular cores (DQ-stained specimen, low power). DQ, Diff-Quik.

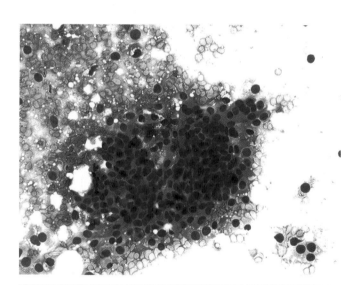

FIGURE 7.35 Renal cell carcinoma, papillary type. TP showing a cluster of uniform tumor cells with minimal cytoplasm and similar detached cells in the background (DQ-stained TP, medium power). DQ, Diff-Quik; TP, touch preparation.

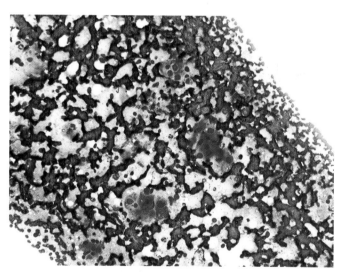

FIGURE 7.36 Renal cell carcinoma, papillary type 2. TP showing epithelial tumor cells with abundant cytoplasm and pleomorphic nuclei (DQ-stained TP, medium power). DQ, Diff-Quik; TP, touch preparation.

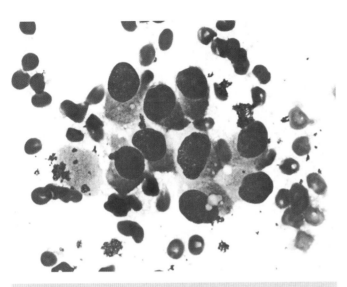

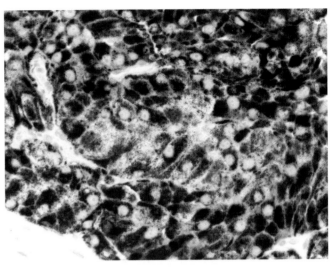

FIGURE 7.37 Metastatic renal cell carcinoma, papillary type 2. These tumor cells have high-grade nuclear features (DQ-stained TP, high power). DQ, Diff-Quik; TP, touch preparation.

FIGURE 7.38 Renal cell carcinoma, papillary type. Tumor cells show CK7 immunoreactivity. CK7 expression is more common in type 1 tumors (CK7 stain, medium power).

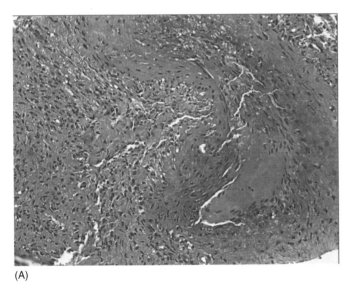

(A)

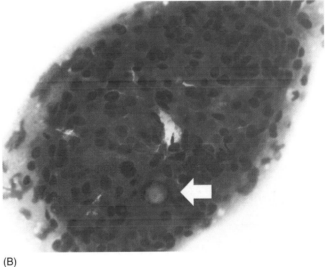

(B)

FIGURE 7.39 Angiomyolipoma. The smooth muscle component of this benign neoplasm with an abnormal thick-walled blood vessel is shown. The adipose tissue component is not represented in this image. A touch preparation shows a cohesive group of polygonal cells with granular cytoplasm admixed with a scant adipocyte (arrow). ((A) H&E-stained core biopsy, low power; (B) DQ-stained TP, high power.) DQ, Diff-Quik; H&E, hematoxylin and eosin; TP, touch preparation.

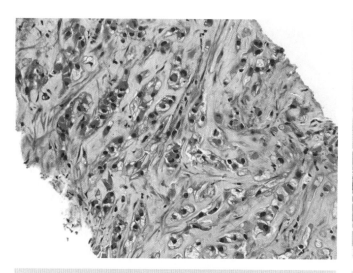

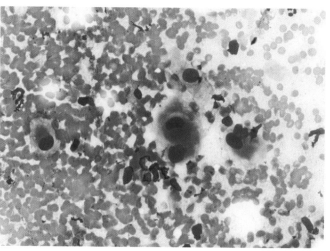

FIGURE 7.40   Renal cell carcinoma with prominent rhabdoid differentiation. Core biopsy showing rhabdoid tumor cells in a myxoid stroma. Many of the polygonal cells have abundant eosinophilic cytoplasm with a globular intracytoplasmic inclusion (H&E-stained core biopsy, medium power). H&E, hematoxylin and eosin.

FIGURE 7.41   Renal cell carcinoma with prominent rhabdoid differentiation. Touch preparation showing isolated tumor cells with rhaboid features and large, atypical nuclei (DQ-stained TP, high power). DQ, Diff-Quik; TP, touch preparation.

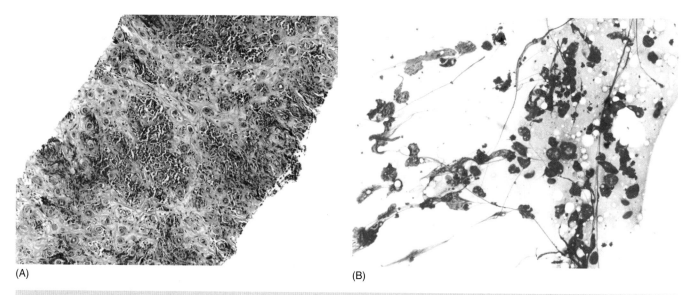

(A)   (B)

FIGURE 7.42   Diffuse large B-cell Non-Hodgkin lymphoma (DLBCL). Core biopsy showing atypical lymphocytes infiltrating atrophic renal parenchyma. The TP of this core shows dyshesive lymphocytes with atypical irregular nuclei. The cytoplasm from these fragile cells was easily disrupted, leaving behind scattered background lymphoglandualr bodies. ((A) H&E-stained core biopsy, low power; (B) DQ-stained TP, high power.) DQ, Diff-Quik; H&E, hematoxylin and eosin; TP, touch preparation.

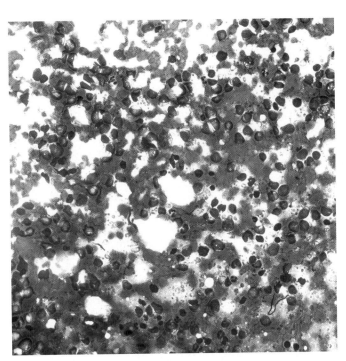

FIGURE 7.43 Posttransplant lymphoproliferative disorder (PTLD). The TP in this case shows a polymorphous population of atypical lymphoid cells. Note the prominent lymphoglandular bodies (DQ-stained TP, medium power). DQ, Diff-Quik; TP, touch preparation.

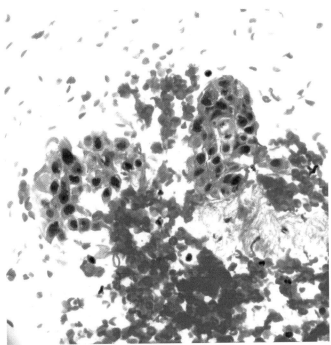

FIGURE 7.44 Metastatic lung non-small cell carcinoma involving the kidney. These clusters of tumor cells with moderate cytoplasm and atypical nuclei with macronucleoli resemble renal cell carcinoma (H&E-stained imprint, high power). H&E, hematoxylin and eosin.

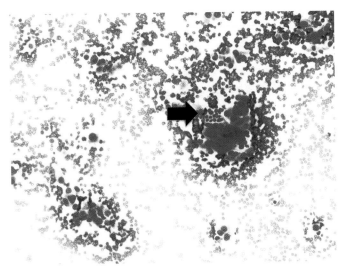

FIGURE 7.45 Metastatic lung non-small cell carcinoma involving the kidney. These clusters and single tumor cells resemble urothelial cell carcinoma. Note the much smaller entrapped benign distal tubule cells present in the middle of the image (arrow) (DQ-stained TP, medium power). DQ, Diff-Quik; TP, touch preparation.

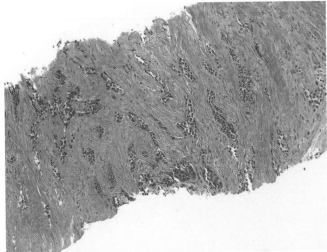

FIGURE 7.46 Invasive high-grade urothelial carcinoma. Core biopsy showing infiltrating irregular nests of tumor cells (H&E-stained core biopsy, low power). H&E, hematoxylin and eosin.

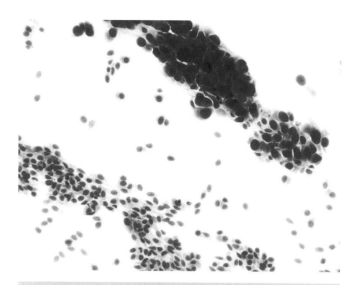

FIGURE 7.47 High-grade urothelial carcinoma. TP showing a cluster of malignant urothelial cells at the top of the image, with background normal urothelium (DQ-stained TP, medium power). DQ, Diff-Quik; TP, touch preparation.

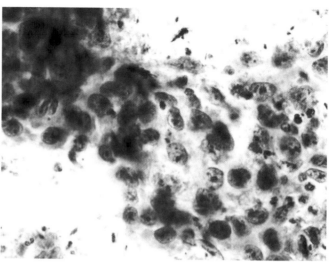

FIGURE 7.48 High-grade urothelial carcinoma. TP showing urothelial tumor cells with marked pleomorphism. The tumor cells have enlarged hyperchromatic nuclei, coarse chromatin, an increased N:C ratio, and prominent nucleoli (Pap-stained TP, high power). N:C, nuclear:cytoplasmic; TP, touch preparation.

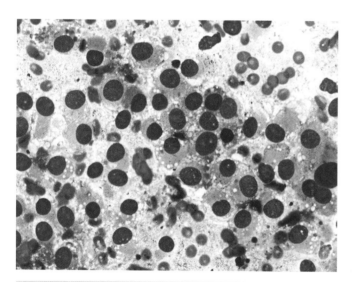

FIGURE 7.49 High-grade urothelial carcinoma. Cellular TP showing numeorus dyshesive tumor cells with intracy-toplasmic vacuoles (DQ-stained TP, high power). DQ, Diff-Quik; TP, touch preparation.

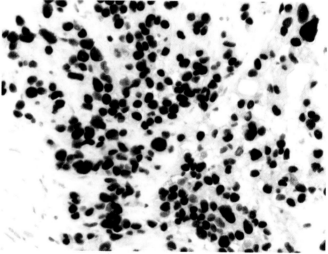

FIGURE 7.50 High-grade urothelial carcinoma. GATA3 positive tumor cells (GATA3 stain, medium power).

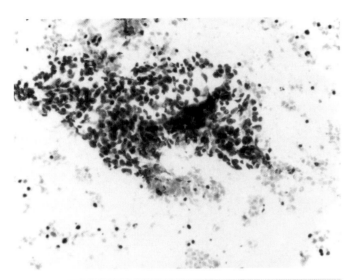

FIGURE 7.51 Small cell carcinoma of the urinary bladder. These carcinoma cells have minimal cytoplasm, stippled chromatin, and are associated with extensive cellular necrosis (Pap-stained TP, medium power). TP, touch preparation.

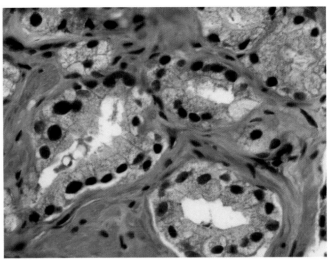

FIGURE 7.52 Prostatic adenocarcinoma. These small infiltrating prostate glands have pale amphophilic cytoplasm, basally lined enlarged nuclei, and prominent nucleoli (H&E-stained core biopsy, high power). H&E, hematoxylin and eosin.

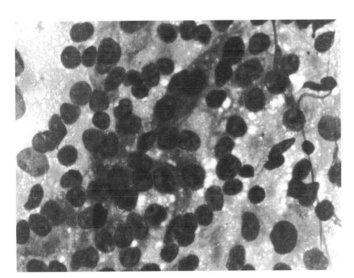

FIGURE 7.53 Prostatic adenocarcinoma. This imprint preparation shows a vague microacinar cell arrangment. Tumor cells have pleomorphic nuclei with prominent nucleoli (DQ-stained TP, high power). DQ, Diff-Quik; TP, touch preparation.

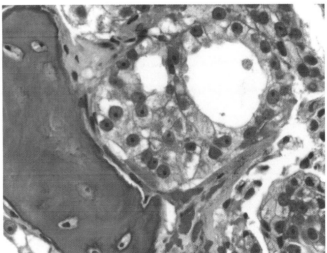

FIGURE 7.54 Metastatic prostatic adenocarcinoma involving bone. Note the microacinar growth pattern and tumor cells with macronucleoli, both features characteristic of prostatic carcinoma (H&E-stained core biopsy, high power). H&E, hematoxylin and eosin.

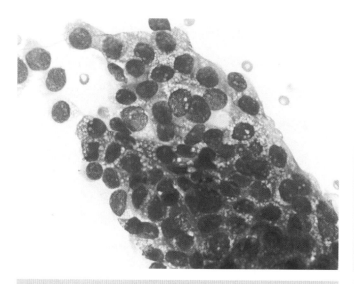

FIGURE 7.55 Metastatic prostatic adenocarcinoma. Sheet of overlapping tumor cells with vacuolated cytoplasm, pleomorphic nuclei, and prominent nucleoli (DQ-stained TP, high power). DQ, Diff-Quik; TP, touch preparation.

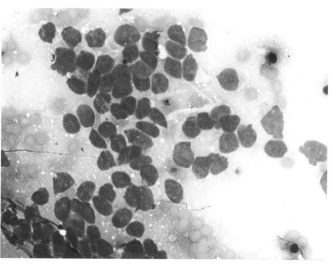

FIGURE 7.56 Metastatic prostatic adenocarcinoma with small cell features. These tumor cells have minimal cytoplasm, show focal nuclear molding, have powdery chromatin, and inconspicuous nucleoli. Note the scant background karyorrhectic debris (DQ-stained TP, high power). DQ, Diff-Quik; TP, touch preparation.

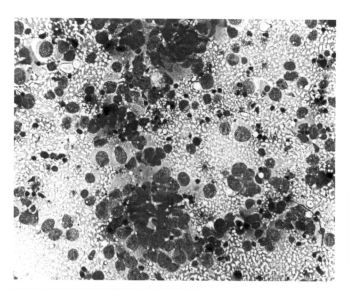

FIGURE 7.57 Seminoma. TP showing discohesive tumor cells with round nuclei and small scattered lymphocytes. Many cells have been stripped of their fragile glycogenated cytoplasm causing a tigroid background (DQ-stained TP, high power). DQ, Diff-Quik; TP, touch preparation.

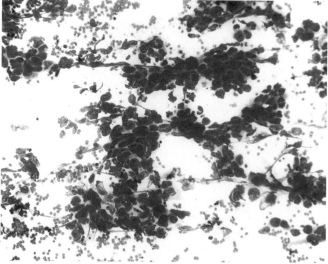

FIGURE 7.58 Embryonal carcinoma. TP showing clusters of poorly differentiated malignant cells with scant cytoplasm (DQ-stained TP, high power). DQ, Diff-Quik; TP, touch preparation.

TUMORS OF THE PENIS

Except for condyloma acuminata (genital warts), benign-tumors of the penis are uncommon. Condylomas are associated with low-risk Human Papilloma Virus types (6 or 11). The majority of malignant tumors originate from squamous epithelium (squamous cell carcinoma). The most common type of carcinoma is keratinizing squamous cell carcinoma (Figure 7.59). These cancers are graded from well to poorly differentiated according to nuclear atypia. Occasionally, penile squamous cell carcinoma may present with metastatic foci in regional or distant sites. Other types of penile carcinomas include basaloid, condylomatous, verrucous, papillary, and sarcomatoid carcinoma. Occasionally, urothelial carcinoma may be encountered. Less frequent tumors originate from soft tissue (sarcomas) or lymphoid tissue (lymphoma). Metastases from other primary tumor sites may also occur, but are rare (29).

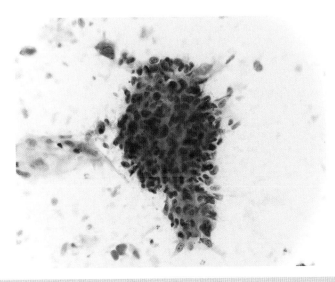

FIGURE 7.59 Penile squamous cell carcinoma. TP showing a group of poorly differentiated carcinoma cells (Pap-stained TP, high power). TP, touch preparation.

REFERENCES

1. Brannigan RE, Shin E, Rademaker A, et al. The usefulness of touch preparation cytological evaluation and prostatic capsule involvement in prediction of prostate cancer recurrence. *J Urol.* 1998;160:1741-1747.

2. Mannweiler S, Pummer K, Auprich M, et al. Diagnostic yield of touch imprint cytology of prostate core needle biopsies. *Pathol Oncol Res.* 2009;15:97-101.

3. Ibarrola de Andrés C, Castellano Megías VM, Perez Barrios A, et al. Seminal vesicle epithelium as a potential pitfall in the cytodiagnosis of presacral masses. A report of two cases. *Acta Cytol.* 2000;44:399-402.

4. Yildiz-Aktas IZ, Monaco SE, Khalbuss WE, et al. Testicular touch preparation cytology in the evaluation of male infertility. *Cytojournal.* 2011;8:24.

5. Kim ED, Greer JA, Abrams J, et al. Testicular touch preparation cytology. *J Urol.* 1996;156:1412-1414.

6. Parks GE, Perkins LA, Zagoria RJ, et al. Benefits of a combined approach to sampling of renal neoplasms as demonstrated in a series of 351 cases. *Am J Surg Pathol.* 2011;35:827-835.

7. Volpe A, Finelli A, Gill IS, et al. Rationale for percutaneous biopsy and histologic characterisation of renal tumours. *Eur Urol.* 2012;62:491-504.

8. Scanga LR, Maygarden SJ. Utility of fine-needle aspiration and core biopsy with touch preparation in the diagnosis of renal lesions. *Cancer Cytopathol.* 2014;122:182-190.

9. Abel EJ, Carrasco A, Culp SH, et al. Limitations of preoperative biopsy in patients with metastatic renal cell carcinoma: comparison to surgical pathology in 405 cases. *BJU Int.* 2012;110:1742-1746.

10. Liu J, Fanning CV. Can renal oncocytomas be distinguished from renal cell carcinoma on fine-needle aspiration specimens? A study of conventional smears in conjunction with ancillary studies. *Cancer.* 2001;93:390-397.

11. Strojan Fležar M, Gutnik H, Jeruc J, et al. Typing of renal tumors by morphological and immunocytochemical evaluation of fine needle aspirates. *Virchows Arch.* 2011;459:607-614.

12. Lin X. Cytomorphology of clear cell papillary renal cell carcinoma. *Cancer.* 2017;125:48-54.

13. Tejerina E, González-Peramato P, Jiménez-Heffernan JA, et al. Cytological features of chromophobe renal cell carcinoma, classic type. A report of nine cases. *Cytopathology.* 2009;20:44-49.

14. Shin HJ, Caraway NP. Fine-needle aspiration biopsy of metastatic small cell carcinoma from extrapulmonary sites. *Diagn Cytopathol.* 1998;19:177-181.

15. Ukimura O, Coleman JA, de la Taille A, et al. Contemporary role of systematic prostate biopsies: indications, techniques, and implications for patient care. *Eur Urol.* 2013;63:214-230.

16. Chieco P1, Bertaccini A, Giovannini C, et al.. Telomerase activity in touch-imprint cell preparations from fresh prostate needle biopsy specimens. *Eur Urol.* 2001;40:666-672.

17. Gentry JF. Pelvic lymph node metastases in prostatic carcinoma. The value of touch imprint cytology. *Am J Surg Pathol.* 1986;10:718-727.

18. Greenebaum E. Megakaryocytes and ganglion cells mimicking cancer in fine needle aspiration of the prostate. *Acta Cytol.* 1988;32:504-508.

19. Pérez-Guillermo M1, Acosta-Ortega J, García-Solano J. Pitfalls and infrequent findings in fine-needle aspiration of the prostate gland. *Diagn Cytopathol.* 2005;33:126-137.

20. Valdman A, Jonmarker S, Ekman P, et al. Cytological features of prostatic intraepithelial neoplasia. *Diagn Cytopathol.* 2006;34:317-322.

21. Parwani AV, Ali SZ. Prostatic adenocarcinoma metastases mimicking small cell carcinoma on fine needle aspiration. *Diagn Cytopathol.* 2002;27:75-79.

22. Mai KT, Roustan Delatour NL, Assiri A, et al. Secondary prostatic adenocarcinoma: a cytopathological study of 50 cases. *Diagn Cytopathol.* 2007;35:91-95.

23. Lin WW, Abrams J, Lipschultz LI, et al. Image analysis assessment of testicular touch preparation cytologies effectively quantifies human spermatogenesis. *J Urol.* 1998;160:1334-1336.

24. Kahraman S, Yakin K, Samli M, et al. A comparative study of three techniques for the analysis of sperm recovery: touch-print cytology, wet preparation, and testicular histopathology. *J Assist Reprod Genet.* 2001;18:357-363.

25. Hooda RS, Hoda SA, Reuter VE. Intraoperative touch-imprint cytology of germ cell neoplasms. *Diagn Cytopathol.* 1996;14: 393-394.

26. Fleury-Feith J, Bellot-Besnard J. Criteria for aspiration cytology for the diagnosis of seminoma. *Diagn Cytopathol.* 1989;5:392-395.

27. Caraway NP, Fanning CV, Amato RJ, et al. Fine-needle aspiration cytology of seminoma: a review of 16 cases. *Diagn Cytopathol.* 1995;12:327-333.

28. Khan L, Verma S, Singh P, et al. Testicular embryonal carcinoma presenting as chest wall subcutaneous mass. *J Cytol.* 2009;26: 39-40.

29. Skoog L, Collins BT, Tani E, et al. Fine needle aspiration cytology of penile tumors. *Acta Cytol.* 1998;42:1336-1340.

CHAPTER 8

Pancreatobiliary, Liver, and Gastrointestinal Tract

Reetesh K. Pai

INTRODUCTION

Touch imprint cytology can be a helpful ancillary study when evaluating small biopsies of pancreatic tumors, gastric neoplasms, and primary or metastatic lesions of the liver. Furthermore, touch preparations can be prepared during intraoperative evaluation of gastrointestinal lesions or tumors that undergo resection. Initial assessment of a tumor by touch preparation can help assess for adequacy of the tissue sample and can allow for appropriate triage of patient samples for ancillary immunohistochemical and molecular studies.

NORMAL

Pancreas

Touch imprints of normal pancreas predominantly yield pancreatic acinar parenchyma (Figure 8.1) and a minor component of ductal epithelium (Figure 8.2). Intact pancreatic lobules are very cellular and contain intermixed pancreatic ducts closely associated with clusters of acinar cells, imparting a cluster of grapes appearance. The cellularity of intact pancreatic lobules can be alarming and care must be taken to not misinterpret these cellular lobules as representing a neoplasm, particularly an acinar cell carcinoma or neuroendocrine tumor.

Gastrointestinal

Normal small intestinal mucosa is easily recognized at low power magnification by the regularly dispersed goblet cells within sheets of glandular epithelium (Figure 8.3). Touch imprints of normal gastric mucosa will typically yield surface foveolar epithelium (Figure 8.4); oxyntic glandular epithelial cells including parietal and chief cells, are not commonly seen. Gastric foveolar epithelium is characterized by a small apical mucin cap present in the superficial one-third of the epithelial cell. The mucin cap does not distort the nucleus. The apical mucin cap is a helpful feature when distinguishing neoplastic mucinous epithelium derived from the pancreas from normal gastric mucosa. In neoplastic mucinous epithelium derived from the pancreas, the cytoplasmic mucin typically displaces and distorts the nucleus and fills the entire cytoplasm of the cell. Normal colon is characterized by honeycomb sheets of glandular cells with abundant cytoplasmic mucin that typically fills the entire cytoplasm.

Liver

Normal liver is predominantly composed of large polygonal hepatocytes arranged in thin trabeculae. Binucleation, prominent nucleoli, and intranuclear inclusions can be seen and should not be mistaken for neoplasia. Bile duct epithelium is also commonly present and resembles pancreatic ductal epithelium.

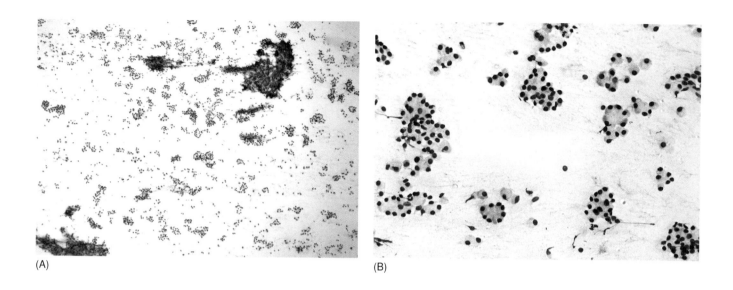

(A)   (B)

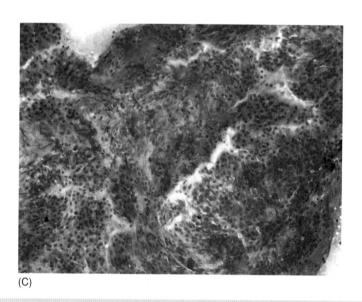

(C)

FIGURE 8.1   Normal pancreas. Benign pancreatic parenchyma consists predominantly of acinar cells, which will predominate in TP of pancreatic tissue. (A) This TP demonstrates intact acinar units arranged in cohesive grape-like clusters easily visualized at low power magnification (DQ-stained TP, low power). (B) The acinar units of normal pancreas are composed of cells with uniform round nuclei and abundant granular cytoplasm. The acinar units are delicate and single dispersed acinar cells are commonly seen (DQ-stained TP, high power). (C) Intact pancreatic lobules contain clusters of acinar units intimately associated with benign ductal epithelium. Intact pancreatic lobules are highly cellular and care must be taken to not over-interpret these cellular aggregates as neoplastic (DQ-stained TP, high power). DQ, Diff-Quik; TP, touch preparation.

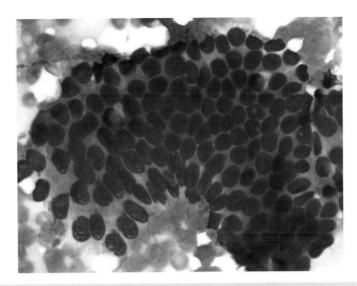

FIGURE 8.2 Benign pancreatic duct. Normal ductal epithelium is less frequently seen in TPs of pancreatic tissue. As shown in this TP ductal cells are arranged in flat organized sheets without nuclear overlap or anisonucleosis (DQ-stained TP, high power). DQ, Diff-Quik; TP, touch preparation.

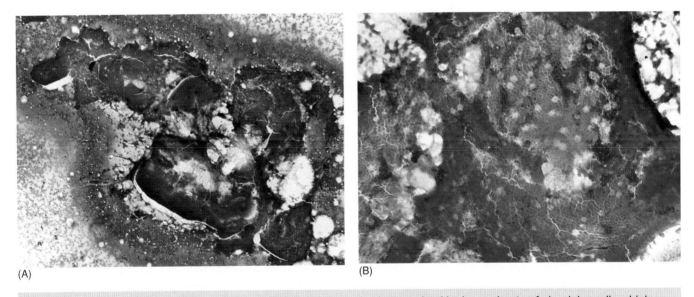

(A)

(B)

FIGURE 8.3 Normal small intestinal mucosa. (A) The mucosa is characterized by large sheets of glandular cells which can have a villous architectural arrangement with associated regularly dispersed goblet cells containing cytoplasmic mucin. The regularly dispersed goblet cells appear as clear "holes" within the glandular sheets making it relatively easy to identify small intestinal mucosal epithelium at low power magnification (DQ-stained TP, low power). (B) Higher magnification of small intestinal mucosa demonstrating sheets of glandular epithelium with dispersed goblet cells (DQ-stained TP, high power). DQ, Diff-Quik; TP, touch preparation.

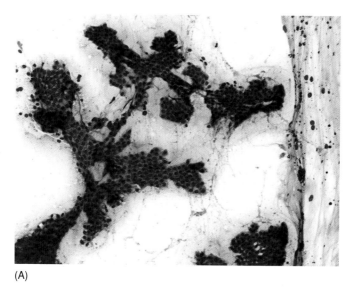

(A)

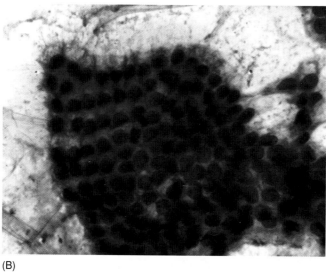

(B)

FIGURE 8.4   Normal gastric mucosa. (A) TP of normal gastric mucosa showing surface gastric foveolar epithelium, which is arranged in flat sheets of glandular epithelium that are typically smaller in size than small intestinal epithelium (DQ-stained TP, low power). (B) Normal gastric foveolar epithelium contains characteristic apical mucin caps within the superficial one-third of the cytoplasm. This apical mucin does not distort the nuclei within the cells (DQ-stained TP, high power). DQ, Diff-Quik; TP, touch preparation.

BENIGN ENTITIES

Touch imprint cytology is infrequently used in the assessment of benign diseases of the pancreas, liver, and gastrointestinal tract. Benign mass lesions can be seen in these organs and if biopsied touch preparations may need to be performed onsite to help determine their etiology and to exclude a malignancy.

Pancreatobiliary Tract

Benign entities in the pancreatobiliary tract include acute and chronic pancreatitis, and autoimmune IgG4-related sclerosing pancreatitis. Benign cystic lesions, such as a pseudocyst, low-grade mucinous neoplasms, and serous cystadenoma, are typically not sampled by core biopsy, but rather are aspirated or sampled with a larger needle to acquire small tissue fragments (e.g., procore or sharkcore). Acute pancreatitis can show granular debris mixed with acute inflammatory cells and reactive ductal cells, whereas chronic pancreatitis usually shows very scant cellularity as a result of fibrosis in the pancreas. The presence of plasma cells and fragments of spindle cells with a patternless pattern should raise suspicion for autoimmune IgG4-related sclerosing pancreatitis. Immunostaining with CD138 can confirm the presence of plasma cells, and additional immunostains for IgG and IgG4 could be done. The findings should also be correlated with serum IgG4 levels.

Solid pseudopapillary neoplasm of the pancreas predominantly occurs in young women in the second and third decades of life. These tumors are composed of cytologically bland cells with oval nuclei and fine chromatin that are characteristically associated with branching capillaries (Figure 8.5). Necrosis is often present but should not be interpreted as representing an aggressive neoplasm. Ancillary immunohistochemical studies are necessary to confirm the diagnosis. These tumors demonstrate nuclear beta-catenin expression and lymphoid enhancing factor-1 (LEF-1) expression (1). Importantly, solid pseudopapillary neoplasms can be positive for synaptophysin, a potential pitfall that could lead to a misdiagnosis of neuroendocrine tumor. Chromogranin is typically negative in solid pseudopapillary neoplasm.

Gastrointestinal Tract

The most common benign neoplasms sampled by core needle biopsy are submucosal mass lesions of the stomach, in order to evaluate for a leiomyoma, schwannoma or neurogenic tumor, and gastrointestinal tumors (see malignant section). Leiomyomas appear as spindle cells with plump, spindled cigar-shaped nuclei, and some eosinophilic cytoplasmic extensions. In contrast, neurogenic tumors typically have longer, comma-shaped nuclei and more of a myxoid-type background. An important clue can be variable cellularity with nuclear palisading of cells in cellular areas.

Liver

Most tumors of the liver that are biopsied are malignant tumors, given that small needle biopsies can be challenging in benign liver lesions. However, occasional bile duct adenomas with bland-appearing glandular arrangements of bile duct cells in a clean background could be seen.

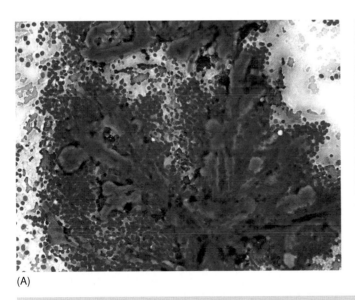

(A)

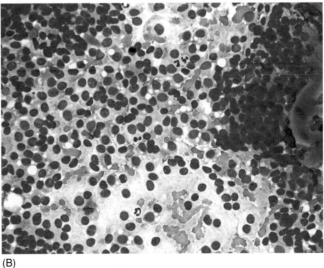

(B)

FIGURE 8.5 Solid pseudopapillary neoplasm of the pancreas. (A) This touch imprint is hypercellular with neoplastic cells arranged in characteristic branching fragments with prominent central capillaries associated with perivascular amorphous myxoid substance (DQ-stained TP, low power). (B) The individual tumor cells display oval nuclei and fine chromatin, which may be misinterpreted as a neuroendocrine tumor (DQ-stained TP, high power). DQ, Diff-Quik; TP, touch preparation.

MALIGNANT ENTITIES

Pancreatobiliary Tract

The most useful criteria for ductal adenocarcinoma of the pancreas (Figure 8.6) include the following: (a) anisonucleosis defined as 4:1 nuclear size variation within a cell group, (b) nuclear membrane irregularities, (c) nuclear overlapping and architectural disarray (i.e., loss of the normal "honeycomb" architecture of ductal epithelial cells), and (d) nuclear enlargement (2). The most specific cytomorphologic feature is anisonucleosis (4:1 nuclear size variation) and this feature should be present before a diagnosis of ductal adenocarcinoma is rendered. Other features such as chromatin clearing, macronucleoli, increased mitoses, and nuclear hyperchromasia are not particularly helpful as they are frequently absent in well-differentiated ductal adenocarcinoma. Increasingly, surgical resections are performed for pancreatic cysts, most commonly intraductal papillary mucinous neoplasm (IPMN), which is a precursor to pancreatic ductal adenocarcinoma. Direct smears of cyst fluid from resected pancreatic IPMN will yield thick extracellular mucin that is colloid-like in appearance and may contain histiocytes (Figure 8.7). Notably, not all neoplastic mucinous cysts of the pancreas will have thick mucin and in up to one-third of IPMN cases the cyst fluid will be thin and watery. In IPMNs with low-grade dysplasia, little to no neoplastic mucinous epithelium may be present in the cyst fluid, and if present, the cells are typically arranged in small tight epithelial clusters. Cyst fluid from an IPMN with intermediate to high-grade dysplasia is more cellular and papillary groups of neoplastic epithelium are more often observed. Cyst fluid chemistry and molecular analysis has become a very useful ancillary diagnostic study. Neoplastic mucinous cysts have elevated carcinoembryonic antigen (CEA) and cyst fluid from an IPMN often harbors KRAS and/or GNAS mutations (3).

Solid cellular epithelioid neoplasms of the pancreas that have overlapping cytomorphologic features include neuroendocrine tumors, acinar cell carcinoma, and solid pseudopapillary neoplasm (Table 8.1). Neuroendocrine tumors of the pancreas are very vascular and touch imprints can be very bloody. The cytomorphologic features of neuroendocrine tumors can be quite variable. Most tumors demonstrate plasmacytoid morphology with metachromatic cytoplasmic granules; however, other morphologic findings, including spindled morphology, can be observed (Figure 8.8). Neuroendocrine tumors can also display marked nuclear pleomorphism raising concern for an aggressive high-grade carcinoma. However, in the absence of increased mitotic activity, necrosis, and elevated Ki67 labeling by immunohistochemistry, marked nuclear pleomorphism should not be considered indicative of a high-grade neuroendocrine tumor. In cases that appear aggressive or present in a metastatic setting, a Ki67 immunostain may be performed to help determine grade (e.g., grade 1 Ki67 <3%, grade 2 Ki67 3%–20%, grade 3 Ki67 >20%).

Acinar cell carcinoma of the pancreas is rare, accounting for 1% to 2% of all pancreatic neoplasms. These tumors are very cellular and touch imprints will yield abundant cellular material for evaluation. The cells are arranged in sheets and acini, and are very delicate resulting in numerous stripped nuclei with prominent nucleoli seen in the background of cytologic preparations (Figure 8.9). Large central nuclei with prominent nucleoli are a characteristic feature of acinar cell carcinoma. Acinar cell carcinomas will demonstrate positive staining for trypsin and chymotrypsin by immunohistochemistry. Pancreatoblastoma will also be positive for trypsin and chymotrypsin and is very difficult to distinguish from acinar cell carcinoma using cytomorphologic features. Squamoid nests are a characteristic feature of pancreatoblastoma, but may be very focal within the tumor.

Gastrointestinal Tract, Including Presentation as Metastatic Disease

Approximately 20% to 25% of patients with colorectal carcinoma present with metastasis. The most common site of distant metastasis is the liver, but peritoneal metastasis accounts for 4% to 8% of patients who present with metastases. The different subtypes of colorectal carcinomas have different patterns of distant metastatic spread,

TABLE 8.1 Cytomorphologic Features of Solid Cellular Epithelioid Neoplasms of the Pancreas

Tumor Type	Group Morphology	Cytoplasm	Nuclei	Nucleoli
Neuroendocrine tumor	Single cells with occasional rosettes, plasmacytoid morphology	Granular cytoplasm with metachromatic granules or punched out vacuoles	Eccentric nuclei with "salt and pepper" chromatin	Usually absent or rare
Acinar cell carcinoma	Acini, sheets, stripped naked nuclei	Abundant granular cytoplasm	Round nuclei with coarse chromatin, smooth membranes	Prominent
Solid pseudopapillary neoplasm	Loose aggregates associated with branching capillaries	Scant cytoplasm	Oval, fine chromatin, nuclear grooves common	Absent

which can affect the type of biopsies performed (4). Conventional colorectal carcinoma with gland formation and dirty necrosis more often metastasizes to the liver. In contrast, mucinous colorectal carcinoma with or without signet ring cell differentiation more often metastasizes to the peritoneum. The cytomorphologic features of conventional colorectal carcinoma include crowded clusters of glandular cells with high nuclear:cytoplasmic ratios, elongated nuclei with irregular nuclear membranes, and palisading of nuclei. There is often a background of necrosis (Figure 8.10). Mucinous colorectal adenocarcinoma lacks a background of necrosis and instead shows areas associated with copious extracellular mucin (Figure 8.11). The tumor cells may also display intracytoplasmic mucin and signet ring cell morphology may be observed.

Ancillary diagnostic immunohistochemistry can help establish colorectal origin in cases with an unknown primary site. The most common multimarker immunohistochemical panel used to establish colorectal origin is CK7, CK20, and CDX2. Conventional colorectal carcinoma is typically CK20-positive, CDX2-positive, and CK7-negative. However, the immunoprofile in colorectal carcinoma is affected by the molecular phenotype. Tumors with high-level microsatellite instability will frequently lack CDX2 and CK20 staining. In addition, tumors with BRAF mutation will often lack CDX2 staining and exhibit positive CK7 expression (5). Knowledge of these staining patterns and their molecular associations is important to prevent the erroneous assumption that origin from other sites is more likely than colorectal origin.

Touch imprints of gastric and esophageal intestinal-type adenocarcinoma are typically very cellular and resemble adenocarcinomas seen elsewhere in the gastrointestinal tract (Figure 8.12). Diffuse-type gastric adenocarcinoma can be subtle as the cells may have bland nuclei and dispersed singly in cytologic preparations with only occasional clusters (Figure 8.13). Cytoplasmic mucin is seen in signet ring cells. Immunohistochemical stains for cytokeratin are helpful in establishing the diagnosis of adenocarcinoma. When metastatic, evaluation of gastric and esophageal adenocarcinoma

for HER2 by either immunohistochemistry or fluorescence in-situ hybridization (FISH) should be performed.

Neuroendocrine tumors of the gastrointestinal tract resemble those seen in the pancreas. Most neuroendocrine tumors of the gastrointestinal tract are well-differentiated, encompassing low- and intermediate-grade tumors. The small intestine is the most common site for gastrointestinal neuroendocrine tumors. They account for nearly half of all small intestinal tumors. The ileum is the most common site involved in the small intestine and if metastatic to the liver, may produce a carcinoid syndrome. Duodenal tumors may produce Zollinger-Ellison syndrome due to gastrin production. Touch preparations of neuroendocrine tumors will demonstrate uniform tumor cells arranged in small clusters and dispersed singly. Single tumor cells often have plasmacytoid morphology with metachromatic cytoplasmic granules. The tumor cells are very delicate, which may result in numerous bare nuclei (Figure 8.14). Care must be taken not to misinterpret bare nuclei as evidence of a lymphoproliferative disorder.

Gastrointestinal stromal tumor (GIST) is the most common mesenchymal tumor in the gastrointestinal tract. GISTs are most commonly found in the stomach and small intestine, but can be seen anywhere in the gastrointestinal tract. Given its mural location, fine needle aspiration biopsy is typically required to establish the diagnosis of GIST. If performed, touch preparations of core biopsies will demonstrate a spindle cell neoplasm with bland blunt-ended nuclei (Figure 8.15). Other spindle cell neoplasms in the gastrointestinal tract include leiomyoma, which is most frequently identified in the esophagus/esophagogastric junction, and schwannoma, which can occur in the stomach. Some GISTs, particularly those that arise in the stomach, may exhibit an epithelioid morphology and should not be misinterpreted as carcinoma. Formalin-fixed paraffin-embedded tissue for ancillary immunohistochemical studies is essential to confirm the diagnosis of GIST. C-kit (CD117) and DOG-1 ("discovered on GIST-1") are both typically positive in GIST.

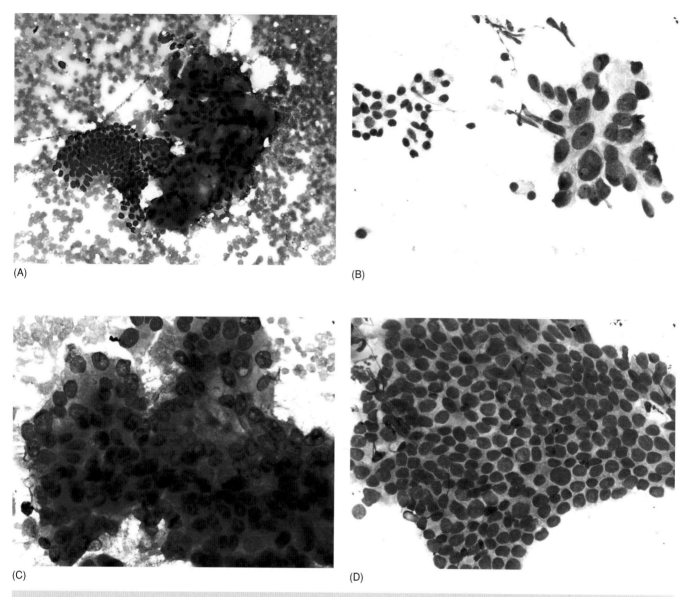

FIGURE 8.6 Pancreatic ductal adenocarcinoma. (A) Compared with normal ductal epithelium (left side of image), pancreatic adenocarcinoma (right side of image) is characterized by enlarged nuclei, nuclear membrane irregularities, architectural disarray, and anisonucleosis (DQ-stained TP, medium power). (B) Similarly, adenocarcinoma (right side of image) is easily distinguished from normal acinar cells (left side of image) (DQ-stained TP, high power). (C) Ductal adenocarcinoma typically displays architectural disarray and loss of the normal organized arrangement of normal ductal epithelium (DQ-stained TP, high power). (D) Anisonucleosis, defined as 4:1 nuclear size variation within a cell group, is typically observed in ductal adenocarcinoma regardless of the degree of differentiation (DQ-stained TP, high power). DQ, Diff-Quik; TP, touch preparation.

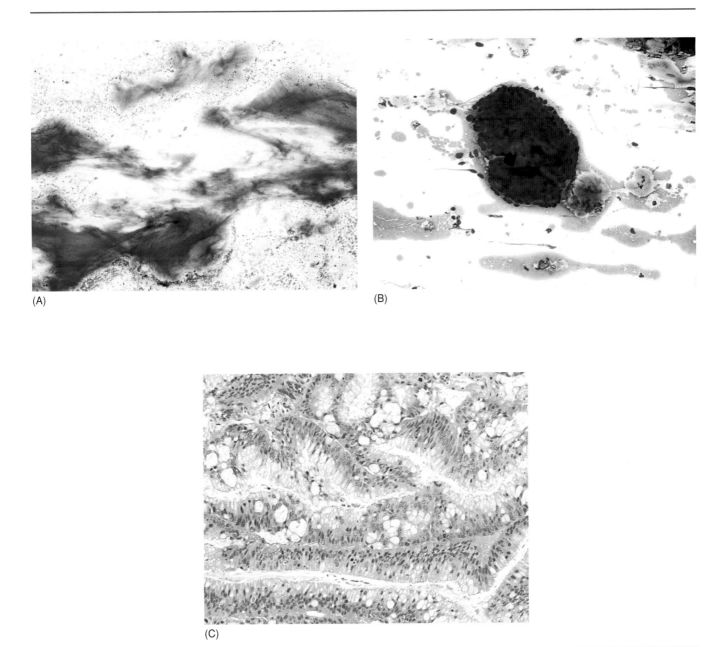

(A)

(B)

(C)

FIGURE 8.7 IPMN. (A) This specimen from a cystic lesion in the head of the pancreas demonstrates the characteristic thick mucin of a neoplastic mucinous cyst (DQ-stained TP, low power). (B) Papillary clusters of neoplastic epithelium are present, indicative of an IPMN (DQ-stained TP, high power). (C) The surgical resection specimen demonstrates an IPMN with high-grade dysplasia (H&E-stained, medium power). DQ, Diff-Quik; H&E, hematoxylin and eosin; IPMN, intraductal papillary mucinous neoplasm; TP, touch preparation.

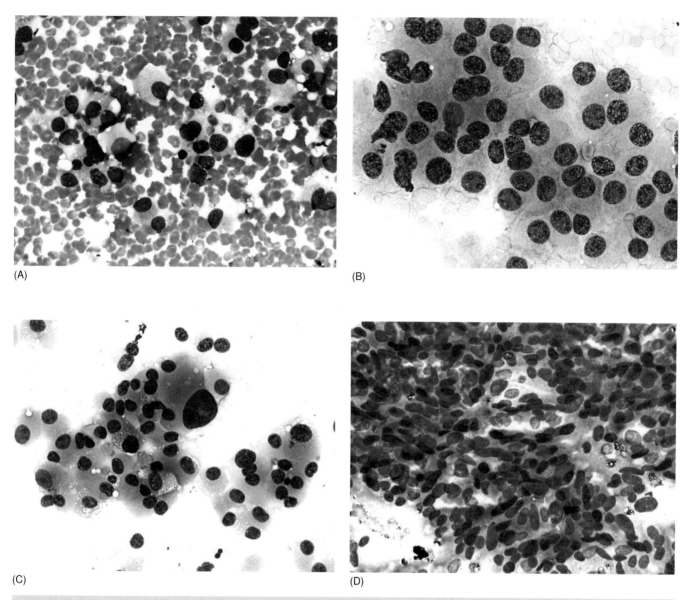

(A)

(B)

(C)

(D)

FIGURE 8.8 Pancreatic endocrine tumor. (A) TP showing the plasmacytoid appearance of tumor cells with characteristic metachromatic granules within the cytoplasm (DQ-stained TP, high power). (B) Neuroendocrine tumor cells display granular chromatin imparting a "salt and pepper" appearance (DQ-stained TP, high power). (C) Neuroendocrine tumors such as this can exhibit marked nuclear pleomorphism and prominent nucleoli (DQ-stained TP, high power). (D) Neuroendocrine tumor with a spindled cytomorphology raising diagnostic concern for a spindle cell soft tissue neoplasm (DQ-stained TP, high power). DQ, Diff-Quik; TP, touch preparation.

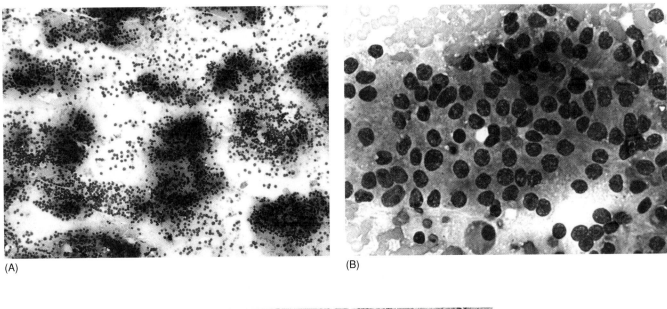

(A)

(B)

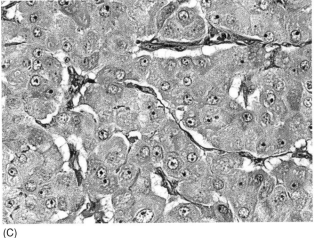

(C)

FIGURE 8.9 Acinar cell carcinoma of the pancreas. (A) This touch imprint is hypercellular with neoplastic cells arranged in irregular acini, sheets, and trabecula. Note the numerous stripped round nuclei (DQ-stained TP, low power). (B) These tumor cells have prominent nucleoli with granular cytoplasm (DQ-stained TP, high power). (C) The surgical resection specimen correlates with the touch imprints and demonstrates tumor cells with prominent nucleoli and granular eosinophilic cytoplasm (H&E-stained, high power). DQ, Diff-Quik; H&E, hematoxylin and eosin; TP, touch preparation.

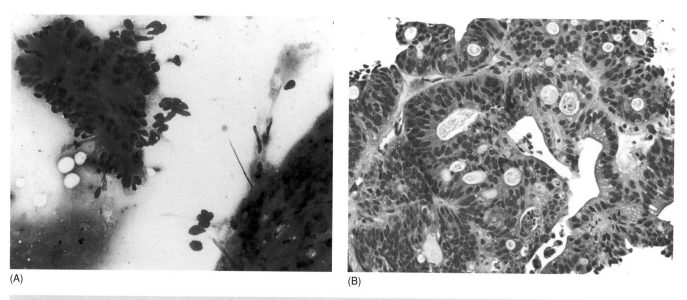

FIGURE 8.10 Metastatic colorectal adenocarcinoma to the liver, conventional type. (A) The TP is characterized by malignant glandular epithelium with elongated palisading nuclei typical of colorectal origin (DQ-stained TP, high power). (B) Corresponding core biopsy demonstrating infiltrating glands typical of colorectal adenocarcinoma associated with dirty necrosis (H&E-stained, medium power). DQ, Diff-Quik; H&E, hematoxylin and eosin; TP, touch preparation.

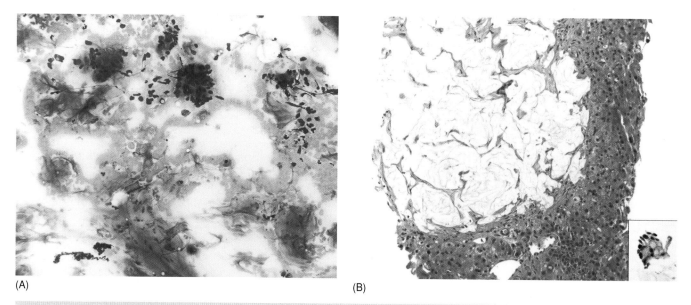

FIGURE 8.11 Metastatic colorectal adenocarcinoma with mucinous features to the liver. (A) Imprint demonstrating copious extracellular mucin associated with neoplastic glandular epithelium (DQ-stained TP, low power). (B) The core biopsy demonstrates copious extracellular mucin with rare clusters of neoplastic mucinous epithelium (inset, bottom right). (H&E-stained, medium power; Inset: DQ-stained TP, high power). DQ, Diff-Quik; H&E, hematoxylin and eosin; TP, touch preparation.

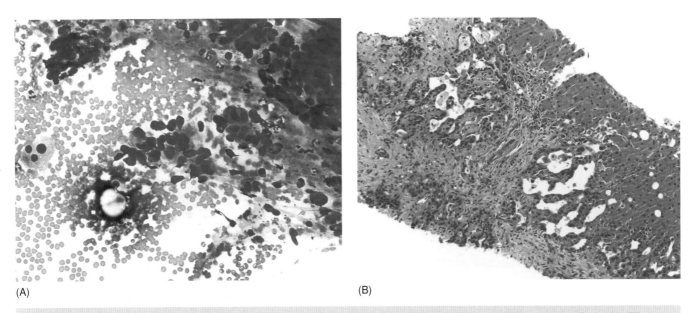

(A)

(B)

FIGURE 8.12 Esophagogastric adenocarcinoma, intestinal type, metastatic to the liver. (A) The tumor cells in this TP show cytomorphologic features that resemble adenocarcinomas seen elsewhere in the gastrointestinal tract (DQ-stained TP, high power). The clinical history and endoscopic evaluation of the esophagus and stomach are essential to determining primary site of origin as there is no characteristic or specific immunohistochemical staining profile for adenocarcinomas of the upper gastrointestinal tract. (B) The corresponding core biopsy demonstrates infiltrating adenocarcinoma (H&E-stained, low power). DQ, Diff-Quik; H&E, hematoxylin and eosin; TP, touch preparation.

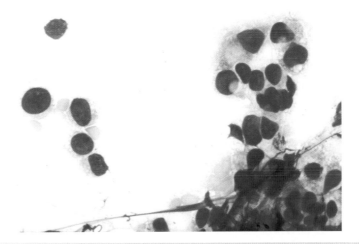

FIGURE 8.13 Gastric adenocarcinoma, signet ring cell/diffuse type, metastatic to a celiac lymph node. Dyshesive tumor cells are shown with vacuolated cytoplasm. Diffuse-type gastric adenocarcinoma can be subtle as the cells may have bland nuclei. Material for ancillary studies, including cytokeratin immunohistochemistry and mucin histochemical stains, can be helpful to establish the diagnosis (DQ-stained TP, high power). DQ, Diff-Quik; TP, touch preparation.

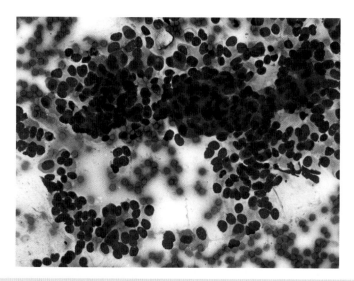

FIGURE 8.14 Duodenal neuroendocrine tumor. This TP shows uniform tumor cells arranged in clusters and dispersed singly. Some of the dyshesive tumor cells demonstrate a plasmacytoid morphology characteristic of neuroendocrine tumor. Stripped naked nuclei are also present; however, intact tumor cells demonstrate ample cytoplasm allowing for distinction from a lymphoproliferative disorder (DQ-stained TP, high power). DQ, Diff-Quik; TP, touch preparation.

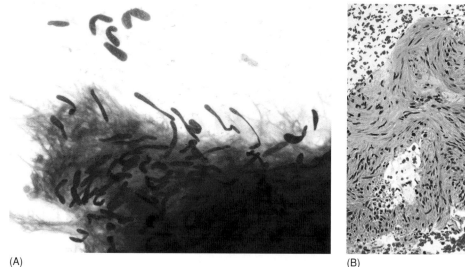

(A)

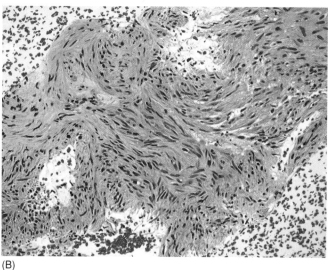

(B)

FIGURE 8.15 GIST. (A) TP showing bland spindle cells with indistinct cell borders associated with wispy cytoplasm (DQ-stained TP, high power). (B) Corresponding histopathology showing a spindle cell neoplasm (H&E-stained, medium power). DQ, Diff-Quik; GIST, gastrointestinal stromal tumor; H&E, hematoxylin and eosin; TP, touch preparation.

PRIMARY TUMORS OF THE LIVER

Touch imprints of hepatocellular carcinoma are typically very cellular and composed of neoplastic hepatocytes arranged in thickened hepatic trabeculae that are lined by spindle-shaped endothelial cells. The thickened trabecular arrangement of the cells allows for distinction of hepatocellular carcinoma from benign hepatic parenchyma (Figure 8.16). Other helpful features of hepatocellular carcinoma are increased nuclear:cytoplasmic ratios, granular cytoplasm, intranuclear inclusions, and large nuclei with prominent nucleoli. Poorly differentiated hepatocellular carcinoma may be difficult to distinguish from adenocarcinoma. The tumor cells in poorly differentiated hepatocellular carcinoma have marked nuclear pleomorphism and less abundant cytoplasm. Ancillary diagnostic immunohistochemistry can help distinguish hepatocellular carcinoma from adenocarcinoma. Markers of hepatic differentiation include HepPar-1, arginase-1, and glypican-3 (6).

Intrahepatic cholangiocarcinoma has two distinct morphologic subtypes, bile duct and cholangiolar, that correlate with different underlying molecular alterations (7). The bile duct type of intrahepatic cholangiocarcinoma morphologically resembles pancreatic ductal adenocarcinoma (Figure 8.17) and metastasis from the pancreas must be clinically excluded. The cholangiolar type of intrahepatic cholangiocarcinoma is composed of monotonous tumor cells with scant cytoplasm. Cholangiolar type cholangiocarcinoma is not as common as the bile duct type of intrahepatic cholangiocarcinomas. The cholangiolar type cholangiocarcinoma may lack significant cytologic nuclear atypia making diagnosis difficult based on cytomorphologic features. Core biopsy and cell block sections showing infiltration help to establish the diagnosis. Molecular alterations correlate with morphologic subtypes: *KRAS* is frequently mutated in bile duct type cholangiocarcinoma while *IDH1* is frequently mutated in cholangiolar type intrahepatic cholangiocarcinoma.

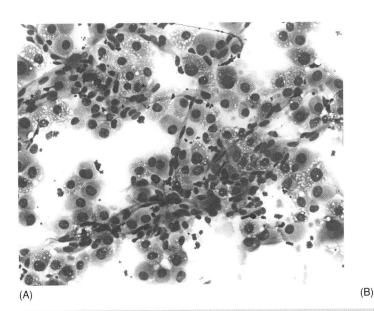
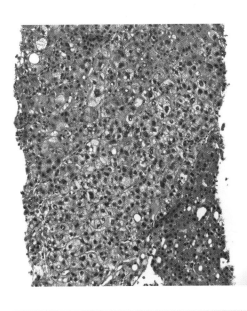

(A)

(B)

FIGURE 8.16 Hepatocellular carcinoma. (A) This imprint is very cellular and composed of neoplastic hepatocytes admixed with endothelial-lined vessels (DQ-stained TP, high power). (B) Core needle biopsy demonstrating thickened hepatic trabeculae (H&E-stained, low power). Ancillary staining of core biopsies with reticulin and CD34 can help to demonstrate abnormal trabecular architecture. DQ, Diff-Quik; H&E, hematoxylin and eosin; TP, touch preparation.

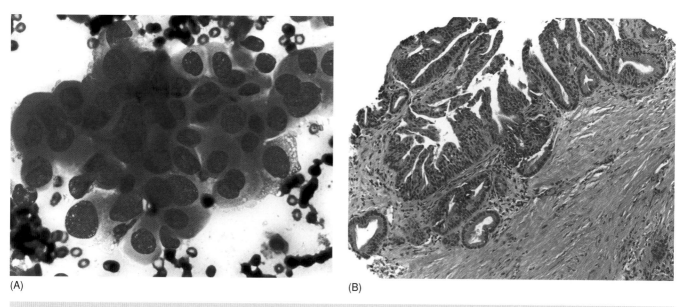

(A)   (B)

FIGURE 8.17 Cholangiocarcinoma, bile duct type. (A) This TP demonstrates cytomorphologic features indistinguishable from pancreatic ductal adenocarcinoma (DQ-stained TP, high power). (B) The core biopsy also demonstrates infiltrating adenocarcinoma morphologically similar to pancreatic ductal adenocarcinoma (H&E-stained, low power). DQ, Diff-Quik; H&E, hematoxylin and eosin; TP, touch preparation.

REFERENCES

1. Singhi AD, Lilo M, Hruban RH, et al. Overexpression of lymphoid enhancer-binding factor 1 (LEF1) in solid-pseudopapillary neoplasms of the pancreas. *Mod Pathol.* 2014;27:1355-1363.

2. Cohen MB, Egerter DP, Holly EA, et al. Pancreatic adenocarcinoma: regression analysis to identify improved cytologic criteria. *Diagn Cytopathol.* 1991;7:341-345.

3. Singhi AD, Nikiforova MN, Fasanella KE, et al. Preoperative GNAS and KRAS testing in the diagnosis of pancreatic mucinous cysts. *Clin Cancer Res.* 2014;20:4381-4389.

4. Hugen N, van de Velde CJ, de Wilt JH, Nagtegaal ID. Metastatic pattern in colorectal cancer is strongly influenced by histological subtype. *Ann Oncol.* 2014;25:651-657.

5. Landau MS, Kuan SF, Chiosea S, Pai RK. BRAF-mutated microsatellite stable colorectal carcinoma: an aggressive adenocarcinoma with reduced CDX2 and increased cytokeratin 7 immunohistochemical expression. *Hum Pathol.* 2014;45:1704-1712.

6. Fujiwara M, Kwok S, Yano H, Pai RK. Arginase-1 is a more sensitive marker of hepatic differentiation than HepPar-1 and glypican-3 in fine-needle aspiration biopsies. *Cancer Cytopathol.* 2012;120:230-237.

7. Liau JY, Tsai JH, Yuan RH, et al. Morphological subclassification of intrahepatic cholangiocarcinoma: etiological, clinicopathological, and molecular features. *Mod Pathol.* 2014;27:1163-1173.

CHAPTER 9

Head and Neck

Juan Xing and Deborah J. Chute

INTRODUCTION

Touch imprint cytology is an important diagnostic modality in the intraoperative diagnosis and rapid onsite evaluation of head and neck pathology. Compared to permanent histology sections, the concordance between touch imprint cytology and histology for the diagnosis of head and neck tumors is 90%. The sensitivity and specificity of touch imprint cytology in detecting head and neck malignancy are 88% and 92%, respectively (1). Touch imprint cytology is more sensitive than frozen section examination in the intraoperative diagnosis of thyroid lesions, especially in follicular variant of papillary thyroid carcinoma (86% vs. 29% sensitivity) (2). In certain scenarios, touch imprint cytology may be the only feasible diagnostic method to provide rapid assessment for calcified thyroid nodules, which can be seen in papillary thyroid carcinoma. For salivary gland tumors, especially the biphasic neoplasms, DQ-stained touch imprint cytology is one of the best ancillary studies to highlight chondromyxoid stroma. Intraoperative frozen section examination to confirm the presence of parathyroid tissue is common practice in surgical pathology. Studies have shown that parathyroid touch imprint cytology can rapidly and accurately identify the presence or absence of parathyroid tissue, which improves the efficacy of intraoperative diagnosis (3). Overall, touch imprint cytology is a rapid, cost effective, and reliable tool for initial evaluation of head and neck lesions for diagnosis, adequacy assessment, and specimen triage for ancillary studies.

NORMAL

Touch imprints of normal thyroid show predominantly watery colloid with a small amount of normal follicular cells (Figure 9.1). In comparison to aspirate smears, where the follicles may rupture resulting in irregularly shaped clusters arranged in two-dimensional sheets, the findings in touch preparations may show more intact follicles and three-dimensional clusters.

The normal parathyroid gland consists of three cell types interspersed by adipose tissue. The chief cells are small polygonal cells with central round nuclei. The oncocytic cells are slightly larger than chief cells with abundant granular cytoplasm and appear similar to oncocytic cells found in other organs. The water-clear cells are less frequently seen and have well-defined cell borders and abundant clear cytoplasm, which may mimic clear cell neoplasms of other organ systems such as clear cell renal cell carcinoma. The tissues submitted that may be mistaken for possible parathyroid gland during parathyroid exploration includes lymph node, thyroid tissue, and adipose tissue (typically brown fat). Lymph node and thyroid tissue can be rapidly and reliably identified by touch imprints highlighting lymphoglandular bodies and colloid, respectively.

Normal salivary gland tissue predominantly consists of acinar cells with a minor component of ductal epithelial cells and fibroadipose tissue. This can appear as clusters of grapes with acini appearing as aggregates of cells with a moderate amount of granular or vacuolated cytoplasm, clustered around a larger duct or blood vessel. Acinar cells can be serous with cytoplasmic granularity, mucinous with vacuolated cytoplasm, or mixed depending on the type of salivary gland being evaluated.

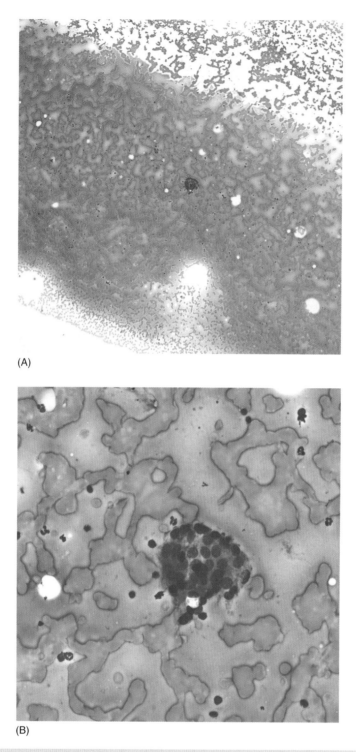

(A)

(B)

FIGURE 9.1 Normal thyroid gland. (A) Scant follicular cells are present in a background of abundant watery colloid (DQ-stained TP, low power). (B) The follicular cells are small, uniform, and evenly spaced (DQ-stained TP, high power). DQ, Diff-Quik; TP, touch preparation.

BENIGN ENTITIES

Thyroid Gland

Common benign entities in the thyroid gland include benign colloid nodules, chronic lymphocytic thyroiditis, and follicular/Hürthle cell adenoma. As with fine needle aspiration, touch imprint cytology cannot reliably differentiate follicular lesions, such as cellular/dominant adenomatoid nodule, follicular/Hürthle cell adenoma, or follicular/Hürthle cell carcinoma. However, if aspirates are nondiagnostic or bloody, a core needle biopsy (CNB) may provide an alternate way to evaluate the etiology of a thyroid nodule (e.g., benign vs. neoplastic). Benign colloid nodules show similar cytomorphology as seen in the normal thyroid gland including abundant colloid and a small to moderate amount of benign follicular cells. In addition, Hürthle cell metaplasia, nonspecific inflammatory cells, macrophages, and cyst lining cells can also be seen (Figure 9.2). Chronic lymphocytic thyroiditis demonstrates follicular/Hürthle cells in a background of polymorphous lymphocytes with a variable amount of colloid and typically increased plasma cells (Figure 9.3). Follicular/Hürthle cell neoplasms/lesions are hypercellular with predominantly a microfollicular or trabecular pattern. The cells are uniform and monotonous. There is increased cellularity compared to the amount of colloid present (Figure 9.4). In addition, it is important to recognize the nuclear features of follicular/Hürthle cell neoplasms/lesions, which include centrally located nucleoli within a round nucleus, as opposed to papillary thyroid carcinoma, which typically has oval nuclei with peripherally placed nucleoli and prominent grooves.

Parathyroid Gland

Common benign entities seen in the parathyroid gland include parathyroid hyperplasia and parathyroid adenoma. Imprints of involved glands show small groups of cells with small, hyperchromatic nuclei in an acinar or microfollicular arrangement with a clean background. Touch imprint cytology cannot reliably distinguish these two entities because the main diagnostic criterion is the presence or absence of a capsule. However, some cytological features such as the presence of a single cell population and cellular monotony are seen more commonly in adenoma. Since an adenoma is a monoclonal proliferation, molecular tests can be helpful in differentiating parathyroid adenoma from hyperplasia. Some molecular alterations seen in parathyroid adenoma include cyclin D1 translocations (8%) or overexpression (20%–40%), adenomatous polyposis coli (APC) expression, and somatic mutations of MEN1, which can be seen in about 25% to 40% of patients (4).

Salivary Gland

Touch imprint cytology is not frequently used to evaluate reactive and infectious entities of the salivary gland; however, it is a great diagnostic method used to facilitate the diagnosis of benign salivary gland neoplasms. A benign lesion that could cause a mass lesion in the salivary gland is chronic sclerosing sialadenitis, and if this is biopsied, the touch preparation findings will be scant (given the abundant fibrosis present) with limited chronic inflammatory cells. Pleomorphic adenoma is the most common benign salivary gland tumor in both children and adults. It can occur in any salivary gland, but arises most commonly in the parotid gland. Touch imprints demonstrate epithelial cells, myoepithelial cells, and chondromyxoid matrix (Figure 9.5). The proportion of the cellular components is variable from tumor to tumor. Tumors with a predominantly cellular component are known as cellular pleomorphic adenoma. Even in the same tumor, the cellular and matrix proportions may vary. The common differential diagnosis includes basal cell adenoma, myoepithelial tumors (e.g., epithelial myoepithelial carcinoma), and adenoid cystic carcinoma. Warthin tumor (papillary cystadenoma lymphomatosum) is a biphasic tumor composed of oncocytic cells with a dense polymorphous lymphoid background (Figure 9.6). It is the second most common salivary gland tumor and often occurs bilaterally in older male smokers. The differential diagnosis includes oncocytoma, lymph node metastasis, and the oncocytic variant of mucoepidermoid carcinoma. Oncocytoma is a rare benign salivary gland neoplasm. It affects the parotid gland in 80% to 90% of cases. Touch imprints show polygonal cells in sheets, papillary fragments, acinar-like structure, or singly. There is no lymphoid background, but stripped nuclei may be seen (Figure 9.7). The differential diagnosis includes Warthin tumor, the oncocytic variant of mucoepidermoid carcinoma, and a dominant nodule within oncocytic hyperplasia. Basal cell adenoma is another rare benign salivary gland epithelial neoplasm that occurs mainly in the parotid gland. It consists of a proliferation of small basaloid cells with peripheral palisading seen around cell sheets (Figure 9.8). The differential diagnosis includes basal cell adenocarcinoma, adenoid cystic carcinoma (solid variant), myoepithelial tumors, metastatic basaloid squamous cell carcinoma, and other benign entities such as cellular pleomorphic adenoma.

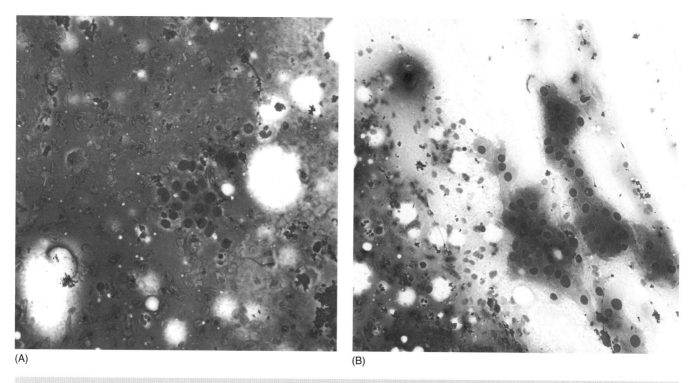

(A)   (B)

FIGURE 9.2 Benign colloid nodule. (A) Benign follicular cells with scant pigment-laden histiocytes are shown in a background of watery colloid (DQ-stained TP, high power). (B) Hürthle cell metaplasia is shown in a benign colloid nodule (DQ-stained TP, high power). DQ, Diff-Quik; TP, touch preparation.

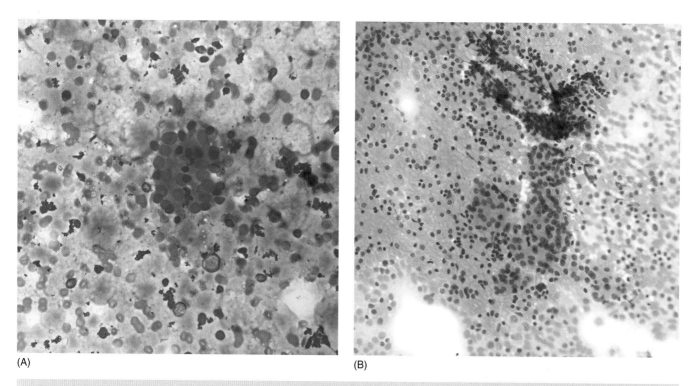

(A)   (B)

FIGURE 9.3 Chronic lymphocytic thyroiditis. (A) A group of benign follicular cells is shown in a background of mixed scattered polymorphous lymphocytes and watery colloid. Note that a few of the small lymphocytes infiltrate the oncocytic follicular cell clusters (DQ-stained TP, high power). (B) Groups of benign Hürthle cells are shown in a background of abundant lymphoid cells. A lymphoid tangle is present, caused by the fact that the small lymphocytes crush easily on TP (H&E-stained, medium power). DQ, Diff-Quik; H&E, hematoxylin and eosin; TP, touch preparation.

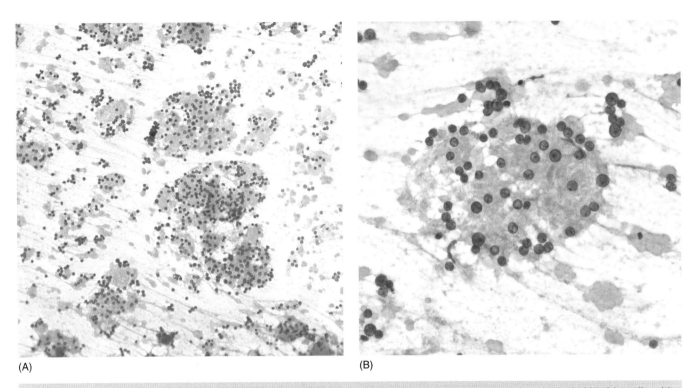

(A)

(B)

FIGURE 9.4 Hürthle cell adenoma. (A) Hürthle cell adenoma consists of numerous groups of exclusively Hürthle cells with no colloid (H&E-stained, low power). (B) The Hürthle cells are large polygonal cells with abundant granular cytoplasm, centrally located nuclei, and prominent central nucleoli (H&E-stained, high power). H&E, hematoxylin and eosin.

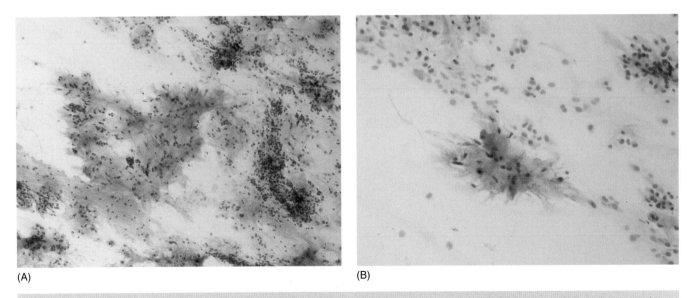

(A)

(B)

FIGURE 9.5 Pleomorphic adenoma. (A) Epithelial cells, myoepithelial cells, and chondromyxoid matrix are all present in this touch preparation. The epithelial cells are small, uniform, cohesive, and usually form a flat sheet or honeycomb pattern (H&E-stained, low power). (B) Myoepithelial cells can have a variable appearance including spindled, epithelioid, clear cell, and plasmacytoid shaped cells. They are commonly found individually, embedded in chondromyxoid matrix or in small loose clusters (H&E-stained, medium power). (*continued*)

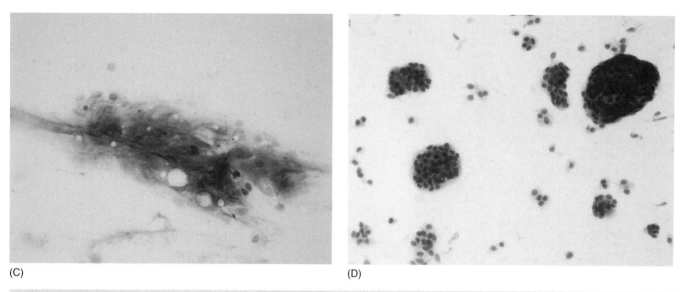

(C)   (D)

FIGURE 9.5 (*continued*) (C) Chondromyxoid matrix is best appreciated with DQ-staining that shows the characteristic fibrillary magenta colored stroma with embedded myoepithelial cells (DQ-stained TP, high power). (D) Cellular pleomorphic adenoma shows predominantly epithelial cells with minimal matrix (DQ-stained TP, high power). DQ, Diff-Quik; H&E, hematoxylin and eosin; TP, touch preparation.

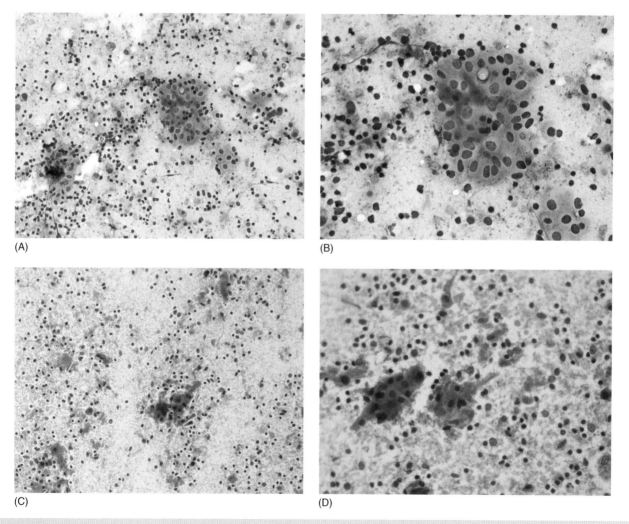

(A)   (B)

(C)   (D)

FIGURE 9.6 Warthin tumor. Flat sheet of oncocytic cells with bland centrally located nuclei and abundant cytoplasm are shown in a background of lymphoid cells and granular debris. ((A) and (B) DQ-stained TP, medium and high power; (C) and (D) H&E-stained, medium and high power.) DQ, Diff-Quik; H&E, hematoxylin and eosin; TP, touch preparation.

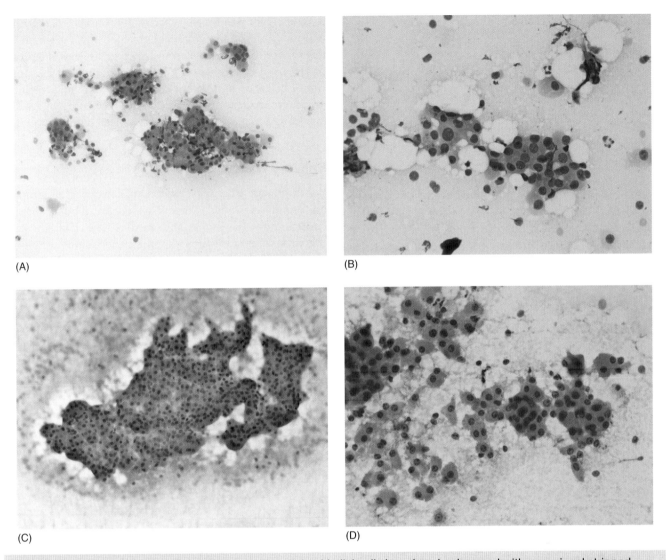

(A)

(B)

(C)

(D)

FIGURE 9.7 Oncocytoma. These TPs show polygonal epithelial cells in a clean background with occasional stripped dispersed nuclei. The oncocytic cells demonstrate abundant granular cytoplasm, round nuclei, and prominent central nucleoli. ((A) and (B) DQ-stained TP, medium and high power; (C) and (D) H&E-stained, medium and high power.) DQ, Diff-Quik; H&E, hematoxylin and eosin; TP, touch preparation.

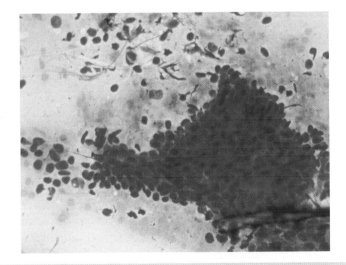

FIGURE 9.8 Basal cell adenoma. A syncytial fragment of small basaloid cells is seen. The cells exhibit scant cytoplasm and round to oval nuclei. The nuclei show peripheral palisading around the fragment (DQ-stained TP, high power). DQ, Diff-Quik; TP, touch preparation.

MALIGNANT ENTITIES

Thyroid Gland

Thyroid neoplasms account for about 1% of all cancers. Touch imprint cytology cannot reliably differentiate between follicular patterned lesions, such as a cellular/predominant adenomatoid nodule, follicular/Hürthle cell adenoma, or follicular/Hürthle cell carcinoma. However, touch imprint cytology is more sensitive than frozen section examination in intraoperative evaluation of other thyroid lesions, especially the follicular variant of papillary thyroid carcinoma (2). Papillary thyroid carcinoma represents about 85% of all malignant thyroid neoplasms. It is characterized by distinctive nuclear features including intranuclear cytoplasmic inclusions, nuclear contour irregularity, and grooves, peripherally located small nucleoli that hug the nuclear membrane, pale nuclear chromatin, enlarged cells with nuclear overlapping and crowding, and variable growth patterns (Figure 9.9). Although immunohistochemistry is rarely necessary in the diagnosis of papillary thyroid carcinoma, well-differentiated lung adenocarcinoma with a papillary growth pattern can show similar nuclear features and in such cases immunohistochemical stains can be very helpful. A panel consisting of galectin-3, HBME-1, fibronectin 1, CK19, and CITED1 shows good sensitivity and specificity for diagnosing papillary thyroid carcinoma (5,6). Medullary thyroid carcinoma is derived from parafollicular cells (C cells) and accounts for about 5% to 8% of thyroid malignancies with 80% being sporadic and 20% inherited. Touch imprint cytology is similar to fine needle aspiration and can show a variety of different patterns. In general, the imprints are cellular with cells arranged singly or in small loosely cohesive clusters. The cells can be round to oval, spindle shaped, plasmacytoid, and polygonal with moderate to abundant eosinophilic cytoplasm. The chromatin is finely stippled without a conspicuous nucleolus. Nuclear pleomorphism is often seen. The presence of amyloid in these tumors may be misinterpreted as colloid, but typically is more dense and will show apple green birefringence on polarization of a Congo Red stain (Figure 9.10). Anaplastic thyroid carcinoma accounts for 2% to 3% of all thyroid malignancies. Touch imprints are highly cellular with obvious malignant features, but not thyroid differentiation (Figure 9.11). Colloid is usually absent. Ancillary studies are necessary in these cases to render the correct diagnosis, as these tumors can mimic poorly differentiated metastatic carcinoma, squamous cell carcinoma, or even sarcoma.

Parathyroid Gland

Parathyroid carcinoma is a rare malignant neoplasm of the parathyroid gland. There is no single histological criterion, other than the presence of metastasis that is considered diagnostic for parathyroid carcinoma. Therefore, the value of touch imprint is limited in this setting. Furthermore, intraoperative frozen section in a patient with suspected parathyroid carcinoma should be discouraged, as it causes tumor cell seeding (7). The differential diagnosis includes parathyroid adenoma, thyroid follicular neoplasm, medullary carcinoma, and metastatic renal cell carcinoma.

Salivary Gland

For the past few decades, the field of salivary gland tumors has rapidly expanded. Currently there are about 13 benign entities and 23 malignant entities (8). Classification schemes, criteria for tumor grading and staging, immunohistochemical markers, and molecular profiles continue to evolve. In this section, only common entities likely to be encountered are covered. Mucoepidermoid carcinoma is the most common malignant salivary gland tumor seen in both adults and children, and occurs approximately equally in major and minor salivary glands. Touch imprints from these cancers show intermediate cells, mucin containing cells, and squamous cells in a background of mucinous material and debris (Figure 9.12). The differential diagnosis is broad and incudes anything that would mimic the mucinous component or the epidermoid component, or may have cystic changes. A small percentage of cases show *CRTC1-MAML2* fusion, which may be associated with a better outcome (9). Adenoid cystic carcinoma is the second most common carcinoma seen in adults and accounts for about 10% of all malignant salivary gland tumors. About 75% of these cases arise in minor glands and the remaining in major glands. It is a basaloid tumor consisting of epithelial cells, myoepithelial cells, and basement membrane material that resembles a pink "gumball" (Figure 9.13). *MYB-NFIB* fusion gene has been detected in some adenoid cystic carcinomas (ranging from 33% to 100%). Some studies show that this translocation is associated with a worse prognosis (9). Acinic cell carcinoma accounts for about 6% of all salivary gland tumors and 80% of them involve the parotid gland. It is the second most common malignant salivary gland tumor in children. The touch imprints are hypercellular with a clean background. The cells form tight clusters and have small bland peripherally located nuclei and abundant granular cytoplasm (Figure 9.14). The differential diagnosis includes mammary analog secretory carcinoma, which was previously thought to be a zymogen poor acinic cell carcinoma, in addition to oncocytic neoplasms.

Salivary duct carcinoma is an uncommon, high-grade primary salivary gland malignancy resembling an apocrine ductal carcinoma of the breast. The majority of these carcinomas affect major glands (85% occur in the parotid gland). It is also a common malignant element of carcinoma ex pleomorphic adenoma. The cells in these tumors are large and may demonstrate a range of cytologic atypia as well as apocrine-like eosinophilic cytoplasm (Figure 9.15). Interestingly, the immunoprofile of salivary duct carcinoma is similar to breast cancers. The tumor cells are positive for GCDFP-15, Her2, progesterone receptor, and occasionally estrogen receptor. About 90% of cases are also positive for androgen receptor, 58% for prostatic acid phosphatase, and 17% for prostatic specific antigen. Epithelial myoepithelial carcinoma is a rare entity and accounts for about 1% of salivary gland tumors. It usually involves the parotid gland, but may be seen in the other major and minor glands. Touch imprints are typically composed of cohesive clusters or sheets of ductal epithelial cells that are surrounded by individual or loosely cohesive clusters of myoepithelial cells (Figure 9.16). This tumor has been historically considered to represent a low-grade malignancy, but may perhaps be classified as an intermediate grade malignancy due to the relatively high risk of recurrence and metastasis. Basal cell adenocarcinoma is a rare salivary gland epithelial malignancy that accounts for 1% to 2% of salivary gland tumors. More than 90% of them occur in the parotid gland. It exhibits the same cytology and pattern as basal cell adenoma (Figure 9.17). The diagnosis is made due to the presence of an invasive and destructive growth pattern, neural and vascular invasion, lymph node metastasis, or rarely distant pulmonary metastasis. Most of these features can only be detected by histology. Basal cell adenocarcinoma is a low-grade malignancy with a good long-term prognosis.

Squamous Cell Carcinoma of the Head and Neck

Squamous cell carcinoma is the most common malignancy of the head and neck region. The most important risk factors are tobacco and alcohol abuse. High risk HPV infection accounts for about 70% to 80% of oropharyngeal squamous cell carcinoma in North America and Europe (10). The imprints from these carcinomas are often cellular with both syncytial fragments of large pleomorphic cells and singly dispersed cells with cytoplasmic tails. The cells show large nuclei, coarse chromatin, and dense waxy cytoplasm (Figure 9.18). If this diagnosis is suspected, a rapid Papanicolaou and H&E-stain can be helpful to highlight keratinization. Although the cytological diagnosis of head and neck squamous cell carcinoma is relatively straightforward, a few differential diagnoses to be kept in mind include radiation change, necrotizing sialometaplasia, papilloma, and variants of squamous cell carcinoma.

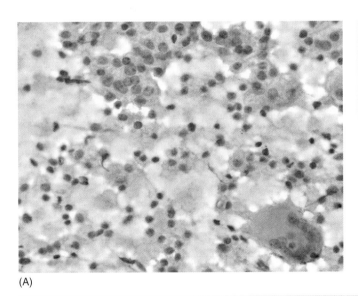

(A)

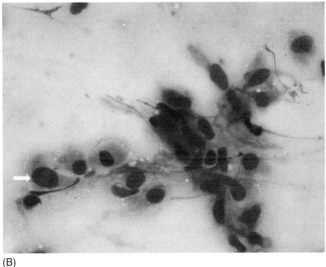

(B)

FIGURE 9.9 Papillary thyroid carcinoma. (A) A sheet of follicular cells is shown with pale powdery chromatin, many grooves, eccentrically located conspicuous nucleoli, and irregular nuclear contours. The right lower corner shows a multinucleated giant cell that is not specific, but is commonly seen in papillary thyroid carcinoma (H&E-stained, high power). (B) The follicular cells shown are overlapping and have enlarged, elongated nuclei, and nuclear irregularity. An intranuclear pseudoinclusion (arrow) is present (DQ-stained TP, high power). DQ, Diff-Quik; H&E, hematoxylin and eosin; TP, touch preparation.

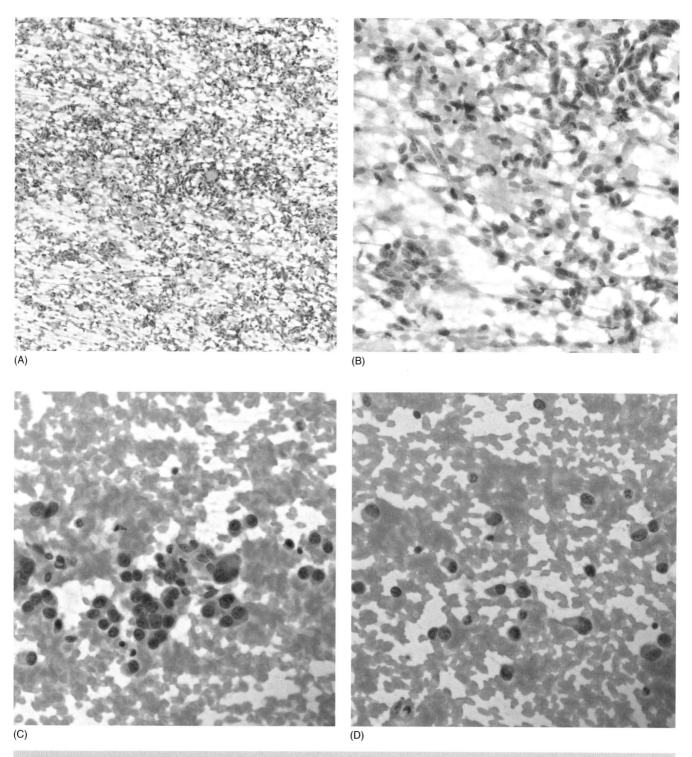

FIGURE 9.10 Medullary thyroid carcinoma. (A) Hypercellular imprint shows numerous single and loosely cohesive clusters of spindle cells. The eosinophilic clumps or spheres of amorphous materials are amyloid (H&E-stained, low power). (B) The cells are typically spindle shaped with stippled "salt and pepper" chromatin and lack nucleoli. In the center, there are homogeneous, amorphous eosinophilic clumps of amyloid, which can be misinterpreted as colloid (H&E-stained, high power). (C) Loosely cohesive clusters of cells are shown with round nuclei and stippled chromatin. Binucleated and multinucleated cells are seen (H&E-stained, high power). (D) This preparation shows individual plasmacytoid cells with stippled chromatin and abundant eosinophilic cytoplasm (H&E-stained, high power). H&E, hematoxylin and eosin.

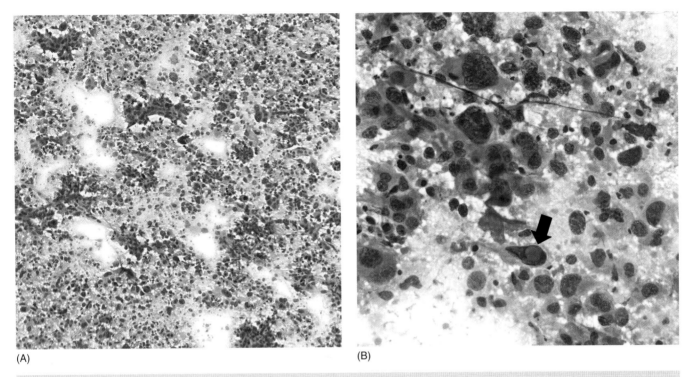

(A)   (B)

FIGURE 9.11 Anaplastic thyroid carcinoma. (A) Hypercellular imprint demonstrates single cells and clusters of large, highly pleomorphic cells (H&E-stained, low power). (B) Large bizarre cells are present with single or multiple nuclei and prominent nucleoli. Apoptosis and necrosis are also present. An intranuclear pseudoinclusion is present (arrow), which may indicate that the patient had a preexisting papillary thyroid carcinoma (H&E-stained, high power). H&E, hematoxylin and eosin.

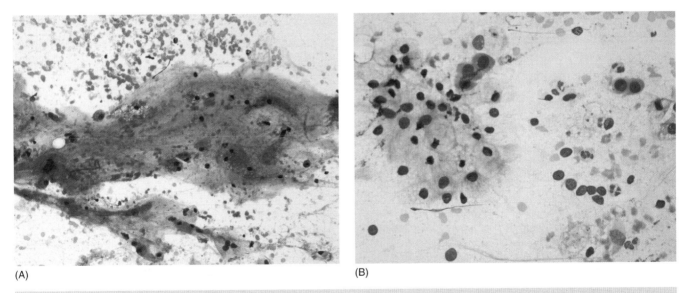

(A)   (B)

FIGURE 9.12 Mucoepidermoid carcinoma. (A) Scattered intermediate cells and muciphages are shown streaming within mucinous material (DQ-staining TP, medium power). (B) This imprint shows rare cells with abundant vacuolated cytoplasm, consistent with mucinous cells (DQ-stained TP, high power). (*continued*)

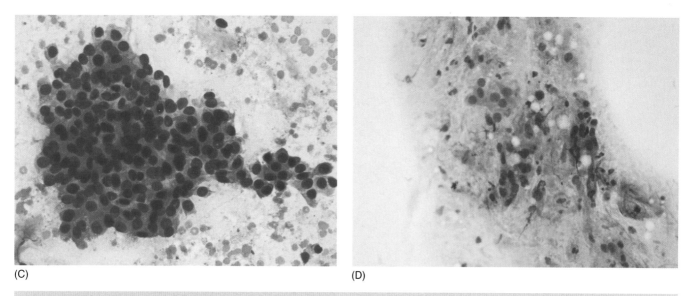

(C)   (D)

FIGURE 9.12 (*continued*) (C) This imprint demonstrates intermediate cells forming a cohesive cluster in a mucinous background (DQ-stained TP, high power). (D) Intermediate cells are shown with more cytological atypia; in this case the subsequent excision showed a high-grade mucoepidermoid carcinoma (H&E-stained, high power). DQ, Diff-Quik; H&E, hematoxylin and eosin; TP, touch preparation.

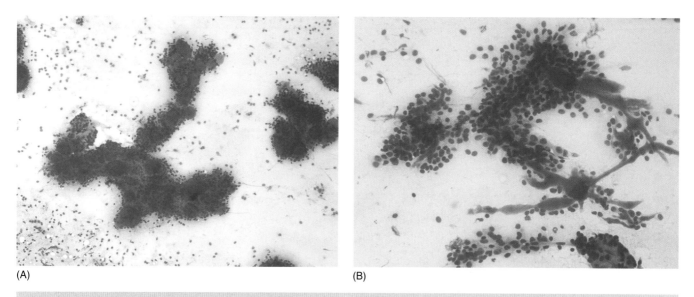

(A)   (B)

FIGURE 9.13 Adenoid cystic carcinoma. (A) Spherical hyaline globules are shown with a "gumball" appearance. These are associated with peripherally arranged basaloid cells that have small, monotonous hyperchromatic nuclei. The cells are not embedded within the globules, which is different from pleomorphic adenoma (DQ-stained TP, low power). (B) The hyaline material has a different shape, and is more dense than the fibrillary material seen in pleomorphic adenoma (DQ-stained TP, medium power). (*continued*)

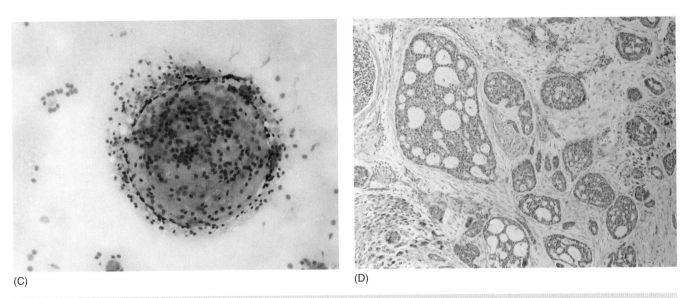

(C)

(D)

FIGURE 9.13 (*continued*) (C) Hyaline globules with associated cells resemble the corresponding histology section (H&E-stained, medium power). (D) Corresponding histology section shows characteristic cribriform pattern. The pseudo-cystic areas are filled with basophilic mucoid or hyaline, eosinophilic material, corresponding to the spehrical hyaline globules seen with cytology (H&E-stained, low power). DQ, Diff-Quik; H&E, hematoxylin and eosin; TP, touch preparation.

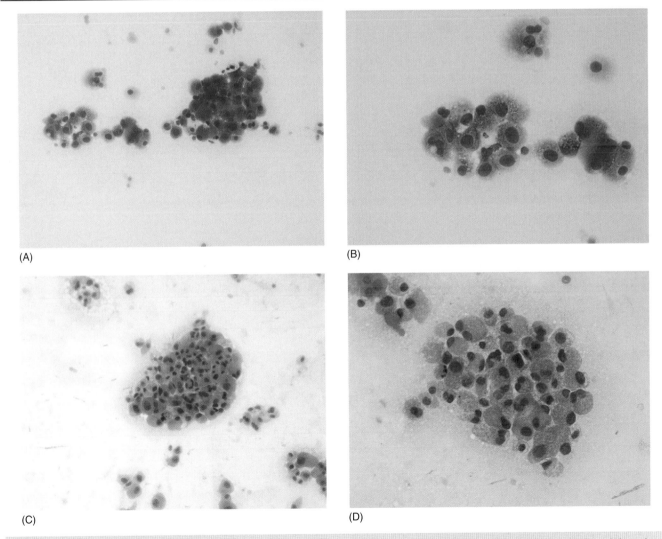

(A)

(B)

(C)

(D)

FIGURE 9.14 Acinic cell carcinoma. Tight clusters of cells are shown with small, bland, eccentrically located nuclei, and abundant granular cytoplasm with zymogen granules. ((A) and (B) DQ-stained TP, medium and high power; (C) and (D) H&E-stained, medium and high power.) DQ, Diff-Quik; H&E, hematoxylin and eosin; TP, touch preparation.

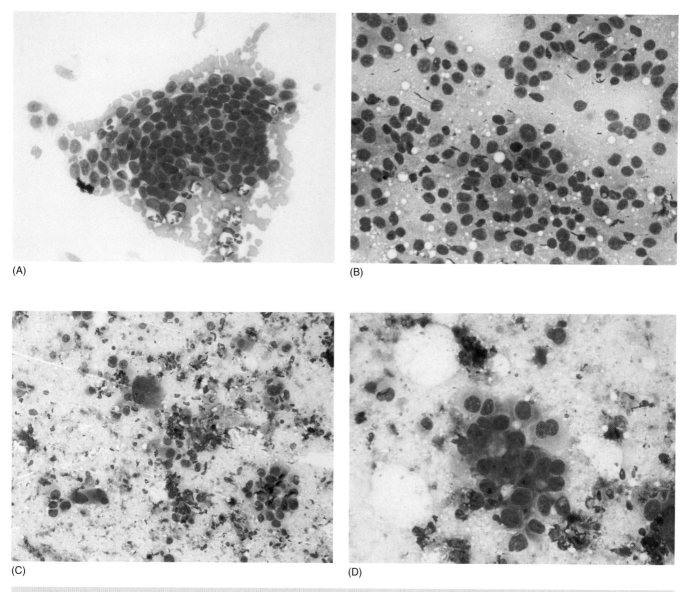

(A)

(B)

(C)

(D)

FIGURE 9.15   Salivary duct carcinoma. (A) Cohesive cluster of relatively uniform epithelial cells is shown. The cells have an increased nuclear-to-cytoplasmic ratio and several conspicuous nucleoli (DQ-stained TP, medium power). (B) Loosely cohesive and single atypical cells show nuclear pleomorphism, prominent nucleoli, and irregular nuclear contours (DQ-stained TP, high power). (C, D) These imprints demonstrate single and clustered malignant cells with background necrosis. Some cells show moderate amounts of apocrine-type cytoplasm (DQ-stained TP, medium and high power). DQ, Diff-Quik; TP, touch preparation.

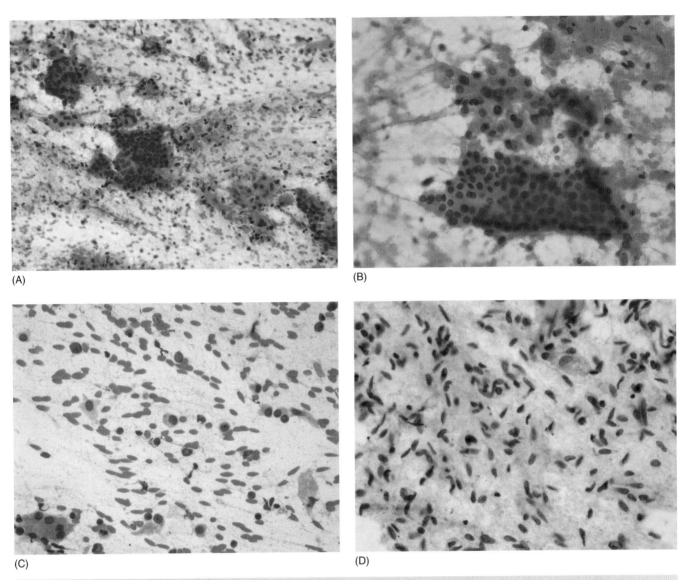

(A)

(B)

(C)

(D)

FIGURE 9.16 Epithelial-myoepithelial carcinoma. (A, B) Imprints show a two-cell population composed of sheets of epithelial cells and single or loosely cohesive clusters of myoepithelial cells that have moderate to abundant cytoplasm (H&E-stained, medium and high power). (C) Myoepithelial cells can present as different morphological types including basaloid cells, spindle cells, plasmacytoid cells and clear cells. This imprint shows scattered myoepithelial cells with a plasmacytoid appearance (H&E-stained, high power). (D) This imprint demonstrates many spindle-shaped myoepithelial cells. In contrast to epithelial-myoepithelial carcinoma, there is no second cell population (H&E-stained, high power). H&E, hematoxylin and eosin.

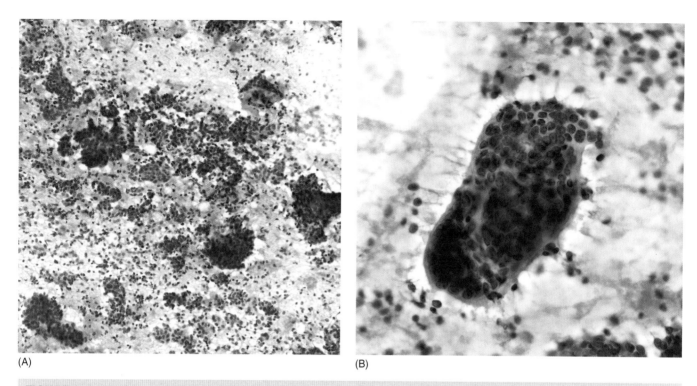

(A)   (B)

FIGURE 9.17 Basal cell adenocarcinoma. (A) Hypercellular imprint shows nests of cytologically bland basaloid cells (H&E-stained, low power). (B) This imprint demonstrates a membranous basal cell adenocarcinoma with an island of basaloid cells surrounded by a prominent hyalinized basement membrane (H&E-stained, high power). H&E, hematoxylin and eosin.

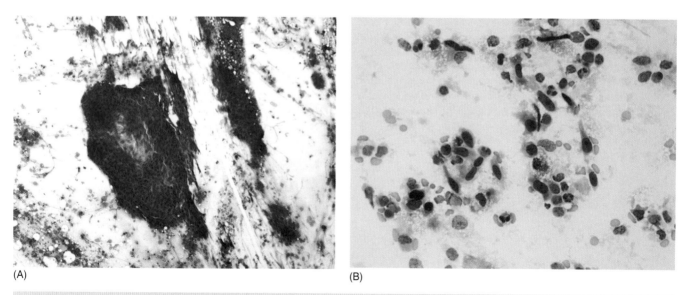

(A)   (B)

FIGURE 9.18 Squamous cell carcinoma. (A) The TP shows large syncytial fragments of pleomorphic squamous cells, which are often seen in non-keratinizing squamous cell carcinoma (DQ-stained TP, low power). (B) In this keratinizing squamous cell carcinoma, singly dispersed cells with large nuclei and dense cytoplasm are seen. Some cells show elongated cytoplasmic process, resembling "tadpole" cells (DQ-stained TP, high power). DQ, Diff-Quik; TP, touch preparation.

REFERENCES

1. Hussein MR, Rashad UM, Hassanein KA. Touch imprint cytologic preparations and the diagnosis of head and neck mass lesions. Ann Oncol. 2005;16(1):171-172.

2. Shen PU, Kuhel WI, Yang GC, Hoda SA. Intraoperative touch-imprint cytological diagnosis of follicular variant of papillary thyroid carcinoma. Diagn Cytopathol. 1997;17(1):80-83.

3. Geelhoed GW, Silverberg SG. Intraoperative imprints for the identification of parathyroid tissue. Surgery. 1984;96(6):1124-1131.

4. Thompson, LD. Benign Neoplasms of the Parathyroid Gland. Head and Neck Pathology. Philadelphia, PA: Elsevier Saunders; 2012:chap 26:651-652.

5. Prasad ML, Pellegata NS, Huang Y, et al. Galectin-3, fibronectin-1, CITED-1, HBME1 and cytokeratin-19 immunohistochemistry is useful for the differential diagnosis of thyroid tumors. Mod Pathol. 2005;18(1):48-57.

6. Abd-El Raouf SM, Ibrahim TR. Immunohistochemical expression of HBME-1 and galectin-3 in the differential diagnosis of follicular-derived thyroid nodules. Pathol Res Pract. 2014;210(12):971-978.

7. Thompson, LD. Malignant Neoplasms of the Parathyroid Gland. Head and Neck Pathology. Philadelphia, PA: Elsevier Saunders; 2012:chap 27:656.

8. Zarbo RJ. Salivary gland neoplasm: a review for the practicing pathologist. Mod Pathol. 2002;15(3):298-323.

9. Weinreb I. Translocation-associated salivary gland tumors: a review and update. *Adv Anat Pathol.* 2013;20(6):367-377.

10. Sturgis EM, Ang KK. The epidemic of HPV-associated oropharyngeal cancer is here: is it time to change our treatment paradigms? *J Nat Compr Canc Netw.* 2011;9(6):665.

CHAPTER 10

Bone and Soft Tissue

Liron Pantanowitz

INTRODUCTION

Touch and/or imprint cytology is very helpful when evaluating bone and soft tissue lesions. In one study, there was an accuracy of 82% when using imprint cytology to diagnose bone and joint lesions (1). In another study, the diagnostic accuracy of imprint cytology for bone core needle biopsies was 75% and for soft tissue core needle biopsies it was 86% (2). Percutaneous core needle biopsy is cost-effective and less invasive than an open biopsy (gold standard) in the workup of bone or soft tissue lesions (3). Core needle biopsy for the diagnosis of malignant musculoskeletal neoplasms also has high diagnostic and accuracy rates (4). Diagnostic yield, however, is often higher in lytic than in sclerotic bone lesions. A key limitation of fine-needle aspiration (FNA) of bone and soft tissue neoplasms, without an accompanying core biopsy, is the lack of tissue architecture. However, FNA performed concurrently with a core biopsy can increase diagnostic yield (5,6).

Rapid onsite evaluation (ROSE) of core biopsies for bone and soft tissue lesions has been shown to be helpful to assess adequacy, provide a preliminary diagnosis, (7) and properly triage specimens. In a study involving 354 CT-guided bone biopsies, investigators showed that these procedures accompanied by ROSE led to a lower percentage (6.5%) of unsatisfactory final diagnoses (8). Rapid assessment of a bone touch or imprint preparation is particularly valuable for clinicians when the final histopathologic diagnosis will be delayed because the specimen requires lengthy decalcification (9). A firm bone or sclerotic/ossified soft tissue lesion core biopsy can be easily rolled on a glass slide, allowing lesional cells to adhere to the surface (Figure 2.4).

A frozen section of musculoskeletal lesions may help confirm a diagnosis prior to definitive treatment. For example, orthopedic surgeons prefer to ascertain a diagnosis of a bone metastasis before they perform an intramedullary nailing for a pathologic fracture. An intraoperative consultation is also often requested to assess surgical margins. Intraoperative cytology is a valuable adjunct to frozen section that can enhance the diagnostic accuracy for bone and soft tissue lesions (10). Imprints performed for intraoperative evaluation of 118 musculoskeletal tumors in one study showed that the respective accuracy, sensitivity, specificity, and positive as well as negative predictive value were 96%, 94%, 100%, 100%, and 91% (11). In a related study of 52 patients who underwent a surgical procedure for a bone tumor, the diagnostic yield was 88% for imprints, 90% for frozen section, and 95% for final diagnoses based upon paraffin sections (12). Further details on the role of imprint cytology for intraoperative consultation of bone tumors is covered in Chapter 3 (section "Bone Tissue").

Diagnosing musculoskeletal lesions can be challenging because there are many different lesions. Trying to subtype all of these tumors with cytologic samples alone is diagnostically challenging, especially for low-grade malignant tumors or when there is cytomorphological overlap and notable heterogeneity of large tumors. On the contrary, touch imprint cytology is very reliable in diagnosing metastatic carcinoma and hematolymphoid malignancies involving musculoskeletal tissues (13). As in surgical pathology, an accurate evaluation of cytologic material for bone and soft tissue lesions requires close correlation with clinical and radiological findings.

BONE TISSUE

A wide variety of bone lesions can be encountered in practice including nonneoplastic entities (e.g., remodeling bone, osteonecrosis, infections) (Figure 10.1), benign and malignant primary bone tumors, as well as metastases. In this chapter, tumors of bone are classified according to the World Health Organization (WHO) (2013) (14).

Normal Bone and Cartilage

All bones have similar composition. Their cortex is composed of dense compact (cortical) bone (Figure 10.2). The medullary canal contains cancellous (trabecular or spongy) bone along with fatty and hematopoietic marrow (Figures 10.3 and 10.4). Both cortical and cancellous bone can be categorized into woven (haphazard arrangement) and lamellar (parallel) types. Woven bone is seen mostly during rapid bone growth and/or formation, including reactive conditions (e.g., fracture callus) or bone neo-plasms. Cartilage is comprised of chondrocytes embedded within avascular extracellular matrix. Hyaline cartilage is found mostly on articular surfaces.

Cytology samples may include any of the aforementioned normal bone elements. If present in increased amounts, they may be mistaken for malignancy. Osteoblasts typically line bone surfaces. They are called osteocytes when they are buried in bone matrix. They are more likely to be numerous and plump in woven bone. Osteoblasts have polarized nuclei, a conspicuous nucleolus, and a perinuclear halo. However, the halo or clearing in osteoblasts is usually more centrally located in the cytoplasm and not hugging the nucleus as closely as seen with plasma cells. In addition, the eccentrically located nucleus almost appears to protrude from one side of the cell. Morphologically, osteoblasts can have features that resemble plasma cells (Figure 10.5). Osteoclasts are multinucleated cells responsible for bone resorption. They have abundant cytoplasm and may have 4 to 20 nuclei (Figures 10.6 and 10.7).

Cartilage Tumors

Chondrogenic tumors may be benign (osteochondroma, chondroma, chondromyxoid fibroma, osteochondromyxoma, synovial chondromatosis, chondroblastoma) or malignant (chondrosarcoma). Chondromas are benign hyaline cartilage neoplasms that are often located within bone (enchondroma). They may be solitary or multiple. They are usually hypocellular and composed of sparse, bland chondrocytes that have minimal vacuolated cytoplasm and small, round nuclei. Cytology samples contain thick, metachromatic fragments of cartilage with scant small, round, uniform cells in lacunae (Figure 10.8) (15). Enchondromas in the hands and feet can be more cellular and often demonstrate more chondrocyte atypia. Chondromyxoid fibroma specimens are more cellular with spindle-shaped myofibroblastic cells and multinucleated giant cells and varying chondroid, myxoid, fibrous, and calcified extracellular matrix. Chondroblastoma usually occurs in male patients between 10 and 25 years of age, presenting as a painful lesion in the epiphyseal region of the long bones. Cytology samples contain variable amounts of single, discohesive mononuclear chondroblasts, as well as osteoclast-type giant cells and background matrix with characteristic "chicken wire" calcification (16). Chondroblasts are ovoid cells that have moderate amounts of cytoplasm and round nuclei with grooves, lobulation, and small nucleoli. They stain with S100 and SOX9, and sometimes cytokeratin.

Chondrosarcomas are malignant cartilage tumors. Most (85%) chondrosarcomas are primary, of conventional type, and they affect adults over the age of 50 years. Secondary chondrosarcoma may develop from an osteochondroma or enchondroma. Chondrosarcomas can be subclassified by location (intramedullary, juxtacortical, or peripheral) and

histology (conventional with hyaline and/or myxoid cartilage, mesenchymal, clear cell, or dedifferentiated). They can arise anywhere in the skeleton. The differential diagnosis includes chondroblastoma, chondroblastic osteosarcoma, and chondroid chordoma (17). Chondrosarcoma specimens are often cellular, display irregular cell arrangements in tumor fragments, and contain malignant chondrocytes characterized by having abundant cytoplasm and enlarged, pleomorphic, and hyperchromatic nuclei (Figure 10.9) (18). There may also be binucleation and mitoses present. The background shows cartilage matrix with myxoid changes and necrosis, but no osteoid as seen in chondroblastic osteosarcoma. Dedifferentiated chondrosarcoma may arise in 10% to 15% of cases, in which there is an abrupt transition from a low-grade cartilage tumor to a high-grade sarcoma (e.g., undifferentiated, leiomyosarcoma) or even osteosarcoma. A correct diagnosis requires recognition of both components. Hence, sampling error may be problematic (19). Clear cell chondrosarcoma variant is characterized by tumor cells with clear cytoplasm. These vacuolated plasmacytoid cells may mimic signet ring cell carcinoma (20). Mesenchymal chondrosarcomas have a bimorphic pattern including islands of well-differentiated hyaline cartilage admixed with poorly differentiated small round cells. Grading (graded I–III) may be difficult on cytology samples alone, but is an important predictor of local recurrence and metastasis.

Osteogenic Tumors

Benign osteogenic tumors (e.g., osteoma) are unlikely to yield cellular imprints because they have extensive bone mineralization and only few osteoblasts in these lesions. Osteoblastoma specimens with abundant woven bone are more likely to produce cellular touch preparations comprised of osteoblasts and occasional giant cells (Figure 10.10). Osteosarcomas are malignant bone tumors where the neoplastic cells produce osteoid. They may be primary or secondary (e.g., associated with Paget disease or radiation). They include a heterogenous group of tumors including conventional (primary intramedullary), telangiectatic (large vascular spaces), parosteal (low grade on bone surface), periosteal (intermediate grade on bone surface), and small cell osteosarcoma. They can be further categorized as osteoblastic (predominantly bone/osteoid), chondroblastic (mostly chondroid matrix), fibroblastic (with high-grade spindle cells), or osteosarcomas with another unusual feature (e.g., giant cell–rich osteosarcoma) (21–23). Imprint specimens may have variable cellularity with discohesive tumor cells and/or cell clusters (Figure 10.11). Tumor cells have marked nuclear atypia including hyperchromasia, irregular nuclear contours, prominent nucleoli, and atypical mitoses. The presence of neoplastic bone and osteoid matrix formation in close association with these malignant osteoblasts confirms the diagnosis (Figure 10.12), even in extraskeletal tumors (24,25). The differential diagnosis includes markedly reactive bone (e.g., callus), other sarcomas with bone formation (e.g., osteoblastic chondrosarcoma), and heterotopic ossification (e.g., myositis ossificans) in soft tissue locations (26).

Fibrous, Fibrohistiocytic, and Fibroosseous Tumors

Fibrogenic tumors of bone are rare and given their fibrotic nature are unlikely to produce cellular cytologic samples. This includes desmoplastic fibroma and fibrosarcoma of bone. The fibrohistiocytic tumors include nonossifying fibroma (NOF)/fibrous cortical defect (FCD), and benign fibrous histiocytoma (BFH) of bone. These two entities have the same histological features. NOF arises mainly in the long bone metaphysis of the lower extremities, whereas BFH tends to involve the nonmetaphyseal region of long bones or the pelvis. They contain a mixture of bland spindle-shaped cells, foamy macrophages, scattered osteoclast-type giant cells, and hemosiderin. Fibrous dysplasia is a common benign fibro-osseous bone neoplasm. Polyostotic disease is associated with McCune–Albright or Mazabraud syndromes. Fibrous dysplasia contains curvilinear woven bone that lacks osteoblastic rimming. Cytology samples may contain a mix of osteoblasts, osteoclasts, bland spindle cells, and foamy histiocytes (27). The differential diagnosis includes fracture callus, osteofibrous dysplasia, and osteosarcoma. Osteofibrous dysplasia is a benign lytic bone lesion of childhood that typically arises in the tibia or fibula. This fibro-osseous lesion is also comprised of trabeculae, but in these lesions they are rimmed by osteoblasts (Figure 10.13).

Small-Round-Cell Tumors

This group of tumors includes Ewing sarcoma/primitive neuroectodermal tumor (PNET) (Figure 10.14), small cell variant of osteosarcoma, hematopoietic tumors (e.g., lymphoma, plasma cell neoplasia), and metastatic nonmesenchymal malignancies with small cell features (e.g., small cell carcinoma, melanoma with small cell morphology). Immunostains and possibly other ancillary studies (e.g., flow cytometry, fluorescence in-situ hybridization [FISH]) may be required to confirm the diagnosis. Ewing sarcoma is discussed later (section "Small Round Cell Tumors"). Small cell osteosarcoma is characterized by small cells with round hyperchromatic nuclei and scant osteoid (28). Lymphomas of bone may be primary or secondary to systemic disease. Diffuse large B-cell lymphoma is the most common primary bone lymphoma. These lymphomas are composed of large atypical lymphoma cells that are associated with lymphoglandular bodies in the background (Figure 10.15). They are usually high grade, which is reflected by their increased mitotic activity and apoptosis/necrosis. Myeloma is the most common primary bone neoplasm, typically causing osteolytic lesions (Figures 10.16 and 10.17).

Giant Cell–Rich Tumors

Almost all bone lesions may contain giant cells. However, the differential for a bone tumor that is comprised of abundant giant cells includes giant cell tumor (GCT) of bone, brown tumor (of hyperparathyroidism), giant cell reparative granuloma, and giant cell-rich osteosarcoma (29). GCT of bone (osteoclastoma) is a benign but locally aggressive primary bone neoplasm that affects young adults between 20 and 40 years of age. Most of these tumors are lytic and arise in the epiphyseal-metaphyseal region of long tubular bones. They are locally aggressive and may rarely metastasize to the lungs and lymph nodes. GCT is characterized by a combination of ovoid mononuclear and osteoclast-like giant cells (Figure 10.18). Both of these cells exhibit similar bland nuclei (30). Giant cell–rich osteosarcoma by comparison contains malignant mononuclear and giant cells along with osteoid (Figure 10.19).

Miscellaneous Tumors

Chordoma

Chordomas are low-grade malignant bone tumors that arise from the clivus, sacrum, or coccyx. Elderly males are typically affected. The hallmark of these tumors is the presence of physaliphorous cells associated with chondromyxoid matrix (Figure 10.20) (31). Physaliphorous cells have abundant dense bubbly cytoplasm (Figure 10.21). Their nuclei are focally enlarged, pleomorphic, hyperchromatic, and may have nuclear inclusions, binucleation, and indentations that resemble lipoblasts. The differential diagnosis includes myxopapillary ependymoma, well-differentiated chondrosarcoma, extraskeletal myxoid chondrosarcoma (EMC), myoepithelial (mixed) tumors of soft tissue, and metastatic mucinous carcinoma (32). Immunostains typically show that the tumor cells are positive for cytokeratin, S100, epithelial membrane antigen (EMA), and brachyury (Figure 10.22) (33). Parachordoma is a rare soft tissue tumor that is believed to represent an extra-axial chordoma (Figure 10.23).

Adamantinoma

Adamantinoma of the long bones is a rare low-grade malignancy that presents largely as a lytic lesion in the mid shaft of the tibia. They are biphasic tumors composed of cytokeratin-positive epithelial (predominates in classic subtype) and osteofibrous (predominates in differentiated subtype) components (34). Variants include tumors with squamoid, basaloid, spindle, and tubular patterns. The differential diagnosis includes metastatic carcinoma.

Langerhans Cell Histiocytosis (Eosinophilic Granuloma)

Langerhans cell histiocytosis (LCH) is covered in Chapter 6 (section "Langerhans Cell Histiocytosis"). LCH is a neoplastic disease with a predilection for bone involvement in childhood. Langerhans tumor cells have moderate amount of cytoplasm, central ovoid nuclei with grooves, pale chromatin, and inconspicuous nucleoli (Figure 10.24). They are usually associated with abundant eosinophils (Figure 10.25) and sometimes Charcot–Leyden crystals (Figure 6.71), as well as multinucleated giant cells and lymphocytes (35). The differential diagnosis incudes osteomyelitis, fungal and parasitic infections, and Hodgkin lymphoma. Tumor cells are immunoreactive for S100, CD1a (Figure 10.26), CD68, and Langerin. *BRAF* p.V600E mutations are detected in many pediatric LCH lesions. BRAF V600E immunohistochemistry is available, but may not reliably stain all cases, especially in decalcified specimens.

Bone Metastases

Metastases are more common than primary bone tumors (36). The most common sites of origin include lung, breast, prostate, kidney, and thyroid carcinoma. Patients with metastatic carcinoma tend to be elderly, who may present with a pathologic fracture. In children, common metastatic lesions include neuroblastoma and rhabdomyosarcoma (RMS). Although any site may be involved, metastases have a predilection for bones containing red marrow. Unlike osteolytic lesions, osteoblastic metastases may not yield cellular touch preparations. Metastases generally resemble the primary tumor from which they originate. Hence, touch preparations of metastatic carcinoma tend to show clusters of malignant cells that are easy to recognize, often even at low magnification (Figures 3.7, 10.27–10.30). However, other tumors may be harder to recognize such as sarcomatoid renal cell carcinoma, which may resemble a primary bone sarcoma. Samples may also contain cellular features related to secondary changes including hemorrhage, reactive fibrosis, and osteoclast-like giant cells (Figure 10.31).

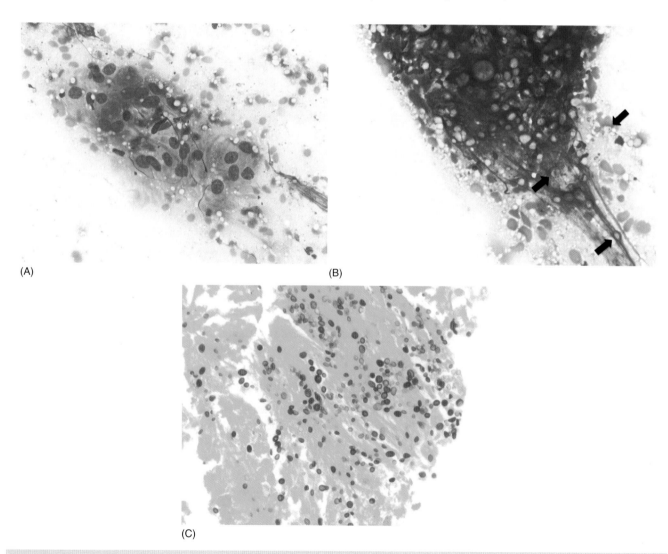

(A)

(B)

(C)

FIGURE 10.1 Bone cryptococcoma. (A) TP showing a nonnecrotizing granuloma. (B) Note the scattered encapsulated yeast (arrows). (C) Grocott's Methenamine Silver stain confirms the presence of pleomorphic Cryptococcus yeast. ((A) DQ-stained TP, medium power; (B) DQ-stained TP, high power; (C) GMS special stain, high power.) DQ, Diff-Quik; TP, touch preparation.

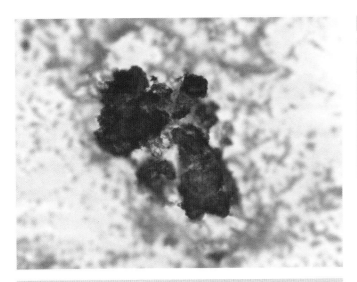

FIGURE 10.2 Benign cortical bone. Touch imprint showing a fragment of acellular dense compact bone (H&E-stained TP, low power). H&E, hematoxylin and eosin; TP, touch preparation.

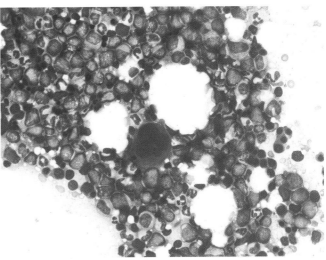

FIGURE 10.4 Normal bone marrow. TP showing trilineage bone marrow (DQ-stained TP, medium power). DQ, Diff-Quik; TP, touch preparation.

FIGURE 10.3 Normal bone marrow. TP of a bone core needle biopsy in which only normal marrow cells adhered to the glass slide. The large megakaryocytes may be mistaken for malignant cells (DQ-stained TP, low power). DQ, Diff-Quik; TP, touch preparation.

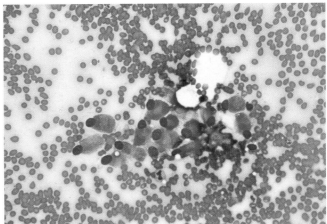

FIGURE 10.5 Benign osteoblasts. Osteoblasts are ovoid cells with abundant cytoplasm and a small polarized round nucleus. Unlike plasma cells their nucleus tends to protrude from the cell and the pale cytoplasmic "perinuclear hof" is separate from the nucleus (DQ-stained TP, medium power). DQ, Diff-Quik; TP, touch preparation.

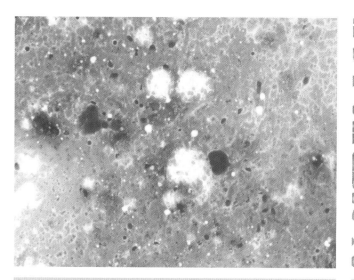

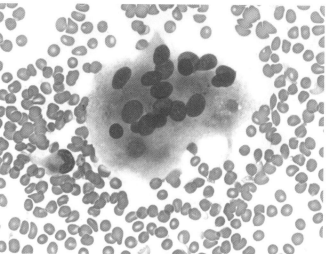

FIGURE 10.6 Benign osteoblasts and osteoclasts. This TP of a femoral head with AVN shows several small mononuclear osteoblasts and large multinucleated osteoclasts. Note the necrotic granular background (DQ-stained TP, low power). AVN, avascular necrosis; DQ, Diff-Quik; TP, touch preparation.

FIGURE 10.7 Benign osteoblast and osteoclast. TP comparing a mononuclear osteoblast (left) to a multinucleated osteoclast (right). Both cells have bland nuclei with fine chromatin and inconspicuous nucleoli (DQ-stained TP, high power). DQ, Diff-Quik; TP, touch preparation.

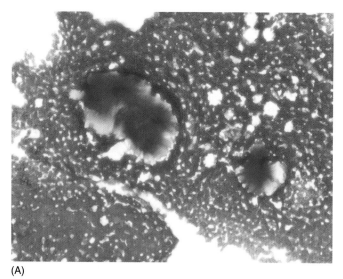

(A)

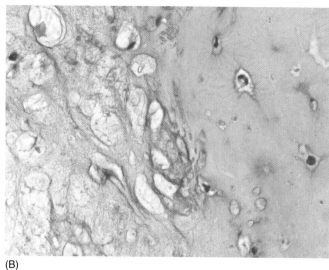

(B)

FIGURE 10.8 Enchondroma. (A) TP showing a hypocellular specimen with benign fragments of hyaline cartilage. (B) Benign cartilage showing focal degenerative change (left) and benign chondrocytes with pyknotic nuclei embedded within cartilage lacunae. ((A) DQ-stained TP, low power; (B) H&E-stained core biopsy, high power.) DQ, Diff-Quik; TP, touch preparation.

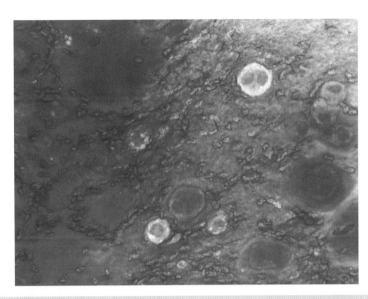

FIGURE 10.9 Primary chondrosarcoma, conventional type, grade 2. TP showing a moderately cellular specimen containing several atypical chondrocytes and abundant background chondroid matrix. Note the high N:C ratio and binucleation of these malignant cells (DQ-stained TP, medium power). DQ, Diff-Quik; N:C, nuclear:cytoplasmic; TP, touch preparation.

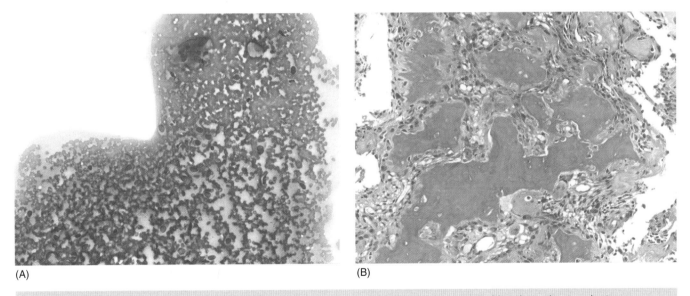

(A)

(B)

FIGURE 10.10 Osteoblastoma. (A) TP showing many osteoblasts and an occasional multinucleated osteoclast. (B) Corresponding core biopsy showing haphazard woven bone trabeculae rimmed by osteoblasts and scattered osteoclasts. ((A) DQ-stained TP, low power; (B) H&E-stained core biopsy, low power.) DQ, Diff-Quik; H&E, hematoxylin and eosin; TP, touch preparation.

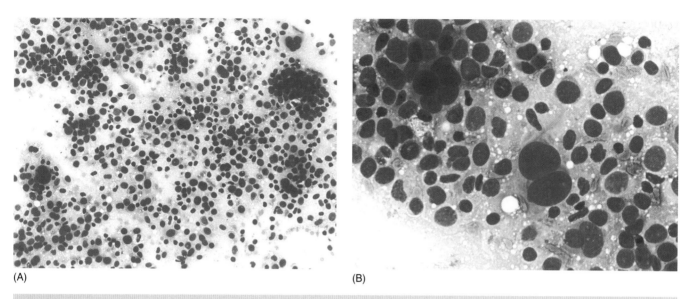

(A)   (B)

FIGURE 10.11   Osteoblastic osteosarcoma. (A) Hypercellular TP showing many discohesive large, round to ovoid osteo-blast-like tumor cells with scattered multinucleated tumor giant cells. (B) Tumor cells are highly pleomorphic and have high N:C ratios, round nuclei, and coarse chromatin. ((A) DQ-stained TP, low power; (B) DQ-stained TP, high power.) DQ, Diff-Quik; N:C, nuclear:cytoplasmic; TP, touch preparation.

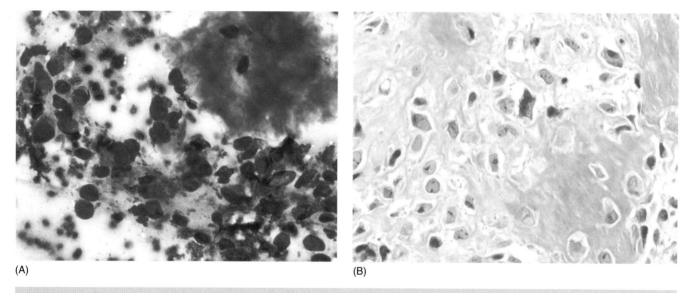

(A)   (B)

FIGURE 10.12   Osteoblastic osteosarcoma. (A) TP showing pleomorphic tumor cells with osteoid matrix. (B) Core biopsy showing malignant cells embedded within eosinophilic osteoid matrix. ((A) DQ-stained TP, high power; (B) H&E-stained core biopsy, high power.) DQ, Diff-Quik; H&E, hematoxylin and eosin; TP, touch preparation.

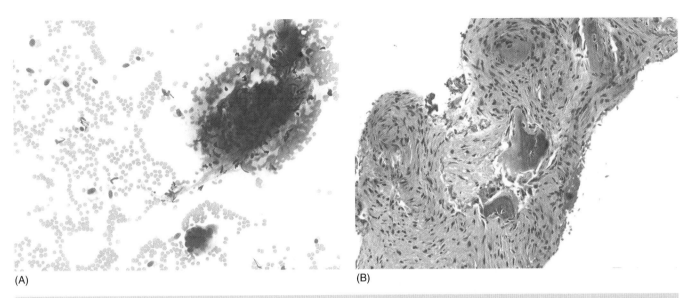

(A)

(B)

FIGURE 10.13 Osteofibrous dysplasia. (A) TP showing several single osteoblasts, a single multinucleated osteoclast, and fragment of dense fibrous stroma with spindle cells. (B) Core biopsy showing trabeculae of woven bone lined by osteoblasts and intervening collagenous stroma containing bland spindle cells. ((A) DQ-stained TP, low power; (B) H&E-stained core biopsy, low power.) DQ, Diff-Quik; H&E, hematoxylin and eosin; TP, touch preparation.

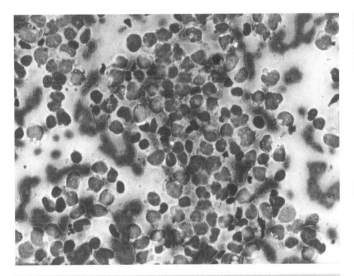

FIGURE 10.14 Ewing sarcoma involving bone. TP from the rib bone of a 25-year male showing a discohesive population of two cell types, including large light and small dark tumor cells (DQ-stained TP, medium power). DQ, Diff-Quik; TP, touch preparation.

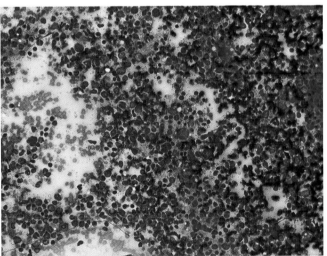

FIGURE 10.15 Primary diffuse large B-cell lymphoma of bone. Hypercellular TP showing an atypical population of large lymphocytes with associated lymphoglandular cytoplasmic bodies (DQ-stained TP, low power). DQ, Diff-Quik; TP, touch preparation.

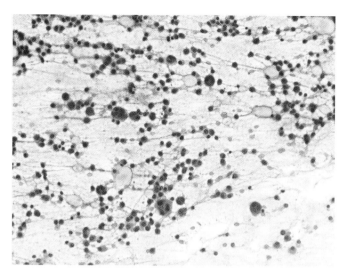

FIGURE 10.16 Plasmacytoma of bone. Intraoperative TP of a lumbar vertebral tumor showing many single plasma cells. The presence of binucleated and multinucleated cells is characteristic of a plasma cell neoplasm (H&E-stained TP, low power). H&E, hematoxylin and eosin; TP, touch preparation.

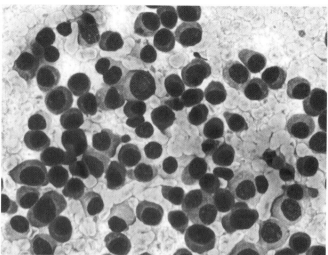

FIGURE 10.17 Plasmacytoma of bone. Plasma cells are discohesive and have moderate cytoplasm with a pale perinuclear hof abutting their eccentric, rounded nucleus (DQ-stained TP, high power). DQ, Diff-Quik; TP, touch preparation.

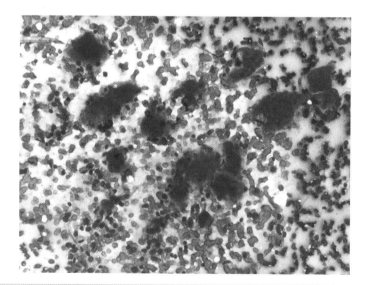

FIGURE 10.18 Giant cell tumor of bone. TP showing admixed mononuclear cells and numerous multinucleated osteoclast-like giant cells (DQ-stained TP, medium power). DQ, Diff-Quik; TP, touch preparation.

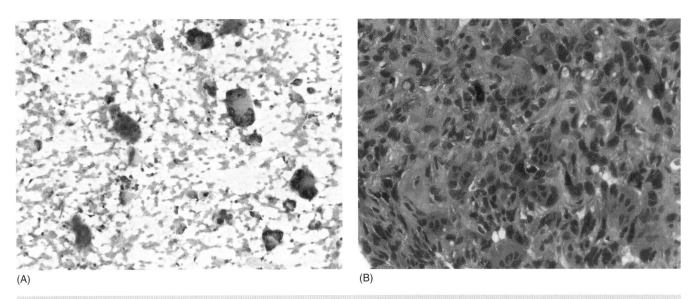

(A)

(B)

FIGURE 10.19 Giant cell-rich osteosarcoma. (A) Intraoperative TP showing malignant giant, multinucleated tumor cells with pleomorphic nuclei, and multinucleated osteoclast-like giant cells with uniform, benign round nuclei. (B) Malignant cells are shown with many scattered multinucleated osteoclast-like giant cells and osteoid. ((A) H&E-stained TP, low power; (B) H&E-stained core biopsy, medium power.) H&E, hematoxylin and eosin; TP, touch preparation.

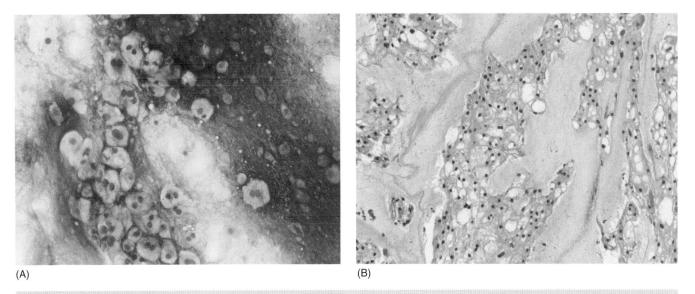

(A)

(B)

FIGURE 10.20 Chordoma. (A) TP showing chordoma tumor cells associated with abundant background myxoid matrix. Tumor cells have rounded nuclei and abundant bubbly cytoplasm. Binucleation is common. (B) Cords of tumor cells with clear to eosinophilic cytoplasm are shown set in a rich myxoid matrix. ((A) DQ-stained TP, low power; (B) H&E-stained core biopsy, low power.) DQ, Diff-Quik; H&E, hematoxylin and eosin; TP, touch preparation.

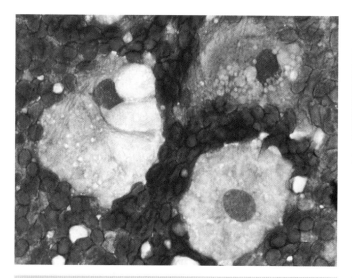

FIGURE 10.21 Chordoma. Physaliphorous tumor cells have abundant vacuolated "bubbly" cytoplasm. Note the prominent nucleoli in tumor cells and the indented nucleus in one of the cells (DQ-stained TP, oil magnification). DQ, Diff-Quik; TP, touch preparation.

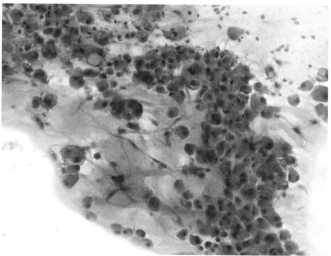

FIGURE 10.23 Parachordoma. TP of a chest wall mass showing epithelioid tumor cells that resemble chordoma cells present in a myxoid background (H&E-stained TP, low power). H&E, hematoxylin and eosin; TP, touch preparation.

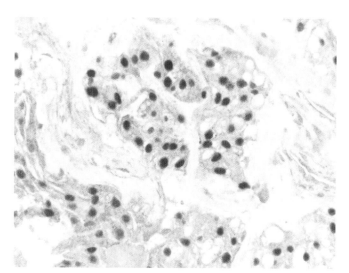

FIGURE 10.22 Chordoma. Tumor cells demonstrate nuclear immunoreactivity with brachyury (brachyury immunohistochemistry, medium power).

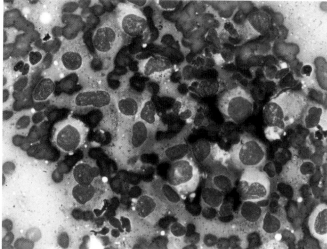

FIGURE 10.24 Langerhans cell histiocytosis of bone. Langerhans cells with moderate cytoplasm are shown with either ovoid or reniform nuclei. Some of the cells have longitudinal nuclear grooves (DQ-stained TP, high power). DQ, Diff-Quik; TP, touch preparation.

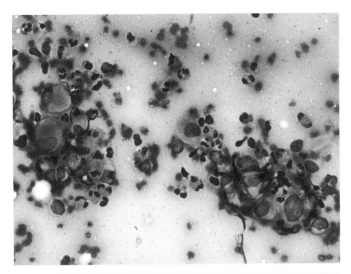

FIGURE 10.25 Langerhans cell histiocytosis of bone. Langerhans cells are shown associated with numerous eosinophils (DQ-stained TP, medium power). DQ, Diff-Quik; TP, touch preparation.

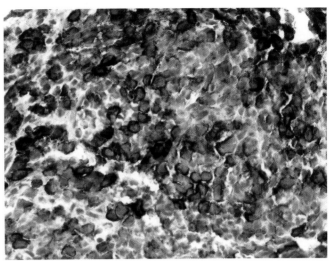

FIGURE 10.26 Langerhans cell histiocytosis of bone. Core biopsy with Langerhans cells that are CD1a positive (CD1a stain, medium power).

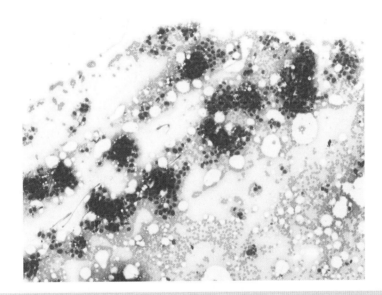

FIGURE 10.27 Metastatic breast carcinoma to bone. TP showing multiple clusters of carcinoma cells (DQ-stained TP, low power). DQ, Diff-Quik; TP, touch preparation.

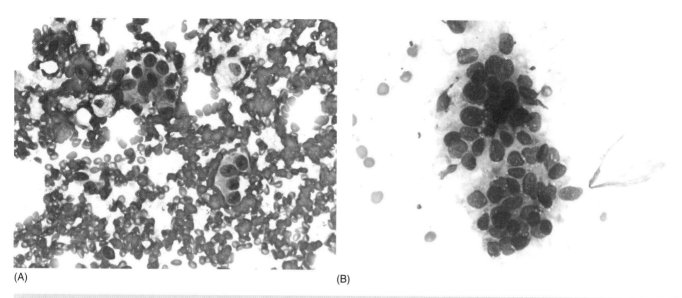

(A)   (B)

FIGURE 10.28 Metastatic lung carcinoma to bone. (A) TP of a vertebral core needle biopsy showing cohesive groups of metastatic lung adenocarcinoma. (B) TP showing metastatic basaloid squamous cell carcinoma. ((A) DQ-stained TP, medium power; (B) DQ-stained TP, high power.) DQ, Diff-Quik; TP, touch preparation.

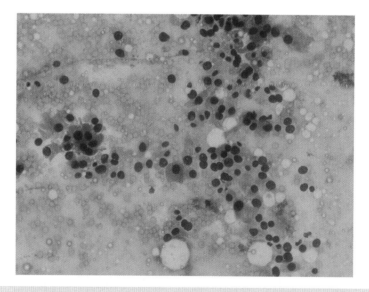

FIGURE 10.29 Metastatic lung adenocarcinoma to bone. TP with mostly discohesive tumor cells and only a focal cluster of carcinoma cells (DQ-stained TP, low power). DQ, Diff-Quik; TP, touch preparation.

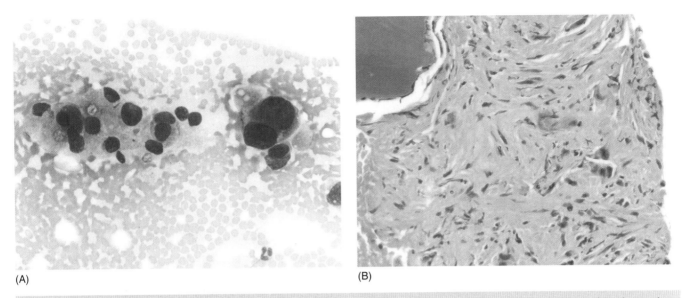

(A)

(B)

FIGURE 10.30 Metastatic lung adenocarcinoma to bone. (A) Pleomorphic tumor cells are shown with cytoplasmic mucin vacuoles indicative of their glandular origin. (B) Corresponding core biopsy showing scant intramedullary carcinoma cells associated with a dense desmoplastic stromal reaction. ((A) DQ-stained TP, medium power; (B) H&E-stained core biopsy, medium power.) DQ, Diff-Quik; H&E, hematoxylin and eosin; TP, touch preparation.

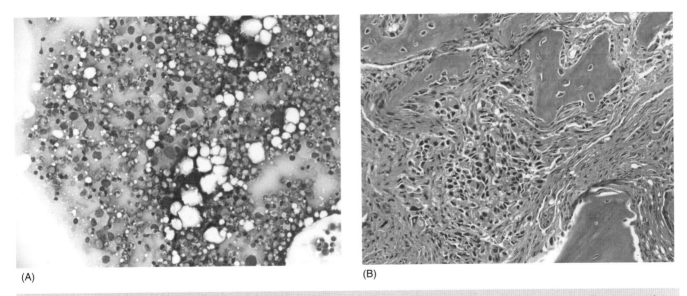

(A)

(B)

FIGURE 10.31 Metastatic urothelial carcinoma with bone remodeling. (A) TP showing scant large tumor cells scattered among abundant distracting normal hematopoietic marrow. (B) Core biopsy showing high-grade urothelial carcinoma associated with dense marrow fibrosis and remodeling of woven bone. ((A) DQ-stained TP, low power; (B) H&E-stained core biopsy, low power.) DQ, Diff-Quik; H&E, hematoxylin and eosin; TP, touch preparation.

SOFT TISSUE

The cytologic evaluation of soft tissue lesions involves pattern recognition of the background features and the predominant cell type present in the specimen (37). Based on this assessment soft tissue lesions can be categorized into one of the following categories: lipomatous lesion/tumor, spindle cell lesion/tumor, small round cell lesion/tumor, myxoid lesion/tumor, epithelioid lesion/tumor, giant cell lesion/tumor, and pleomorphic lesion/tumor.

Normal Soft Tissue

Soft tissue includes muscles (Figure 10.32) and tendons, fat, fibrous tissue, fascia, nerves, blood vessels, ligaments, and synovium. It is important to recognize these cellular elements in touch preparations. They are usually present due to contamination or in nondiagnostic specimens where the targeted lesion was missed during sampling. Many soft tissue tumors contain increased numbers of mast cells, which contain densely packed granules that may obscure the nucleus (Figure 10.33).

Lipomatous Tumors

There is a broad differential for fatty lesions ranging from benign nonneoplastic entities (e.g., fat necrosis (Figure 10.34), lipomatosis) to benign neoplasms (e.g., lipoma, hibernoma, lipoblastoma), and malignancies (e.g., liposarcoma). This also includes fat-containing variants of other tumors (e.g., solitary fibrous tumor (SFT)). Lipomas are the most common soft tissue neoplasms seen in adults. The cytomorphology of a lipoma is usually indistinguishable from benign vascularized, mature adipose tissue. Unlike FNA where adipocytes may get easily disrupted during aspiration, with imprints there are fewer acellular slides with only fat globules. Diagnosing variants of lipoma requires the presence of other mesenchymal elements, which may include spindle cells and/or floret-like cells (Figure 10.35) in spindle cell/pleomorphic lipoma, increased vessels with angiolipoma (Figure 10.36), or hematopoietic cells with myelolipoma. Hibernoma consists of brown fat and can be distinguished cytologically by finding mature adipocytes containing multiple fine vacuoles and granular cytoplasm.

Liposarcoma is the most common soft tissue sarcoma of adults. These fatty tumors usually contain lipoblasts, which are adipocytes with one or more cytoplasmic vacuoles and an atypical hyperchromatic nucleus that may be scalloped due to indentations caused by fat vacuoles (Figure 10.37). They need to be distinguished from mimics including foamy macrophages (e.g., fat necrosis, silicone granulomas) and pseudolipoblasts that may be seen in lipoma variants (e.g., chondroid lipoma), xanthomas, hibernoma, lipoblastoma, myxofibrosarcoma, epithelioid

hemangioendothelioma (with blister cells), sebaceous carcinoma (Figure 10.38), and signet ring cell carcinoma. There are several subtypes of liposarcoma (38). Well-differentiated liposarcoma or atypical lipomatous tumor (ALT) is a locally aggressive, but nonmetastasizing, lipogenic neoplasm. Touch preparations may show uniloculated adipocytes, rarely multivacuolated lipoblasts, and atypical stromal cells with pleomorphic and hyperchromatic nuclei (Figure 10.39). FISH to demonstrate *MDM2* amplification can help confirm the diagnosis (Figure 10.40). Dedifferentiated liposarcoma is characterized by a transition from an ALT to a nonlipogenic sarcoma of variable histology (e.g., pleomorphic sarcoma, leiomyosarcoma). Myxoid liposarcoma is composed of rare lipoblasts with background myxoid material (Figure 10.41). Finding thin branched ("chicken wire") blood vessels in these specimens can be helpful. A subset of these liposarcomas may show high-grade progression to a solid sheet of primitive tumor cells with round cell morphology (Figure 10.42). Myxoid/round cell liposarcomas typically show *FUS-DDIT3*, or less often *EWSR1-DDIT3*, rearrangements. Pleomorphic liposarcoma is a high-grade sarcoma that contains variable amounts of pleomorphic lipoblasts. The malignant cells in these tumors are usually discohesive and large, and demonstrate anaplastic features including bizarre nuclei.

Spindle Cell Lesions

This category of soft tissue lesions/neoplasms encompasses a very wide spectrum of benign and malignant conditions. Reactive lesions (pseudosarcomas) with spindle cells include granulomatous inflammation (Figure 10.43) and nodular fasciitis. Benign mesenchymal tumors with a predominant spindle cell pattern include leiomyoma, neurogenic tumors (neurofibroma, schwannoma), and fibromatosis. Malignancies with mostly spindle cells include sarcomas (e.g., fibrosarcoma, leiomyosarcoma, synovial sarcoma, gastrointestinal stromal tumor, malignant peripheral nerve sheath tumors (MPNST)), as well as nonmesenchymal tumors (e.g., spindle cell carcinoma, spindle cell melanoma). Extracranial meningiomas, which may infrequently be encountered as ectopic or metastatic tumors, can also have spindled cells. Their rarity and unique cytomorphology often pose a significant diagnostic dilemma. Although the majority of samples show tightly cohesive clusters of spindled cells, it is important that specimens are carefully inspected for characteristic whorls (Figure 10.44) (39). Meningeal cells may also have intranuclear inclusions and show nuclear grooves, and there may be psammoma bodies present. Meningiomas are immunoreactive for pancytokeratin and EMA.

Benign Spindle Cell Lesions

Nodular fasciitis is a common soft tissue tumor that may mimic sarcoma. These lesions usually present as a rapidly enlarging mass in adults and often occur on the forearm. Cytology samples often have mixed patterns (e.g., myxoid areas, regions with inflammatory cells) and variable cellularity (hypo- and hypercellular areas) (40). Samples contain mostly spindle-shaped fibroblasts (Figure 10.45) with bland nuclei, admixed with some polygonal myofibroblasts that may mimic ganglion cells, admixed with giant cells and inflammatory cells. Ubiquitin-specific protease 6 (*USP6*) FISH is a useful ancillary test for nodular fasciitis (41). Related fibroblastic/myofibroblastic mass-forming proliferations include proliferative fasciitis, proliferative myositis, myositis ossificans (Figure 10.46), and ischemic fasciitis. These entities all contain reactive spindled fibroblasts mixed with variable numbers of plump myofibroblasts, osteoclast-like giant cells, and scant lymphocytes.

Desmoid-type fibromatosis is a myofibroblastic proliferation of deep soft tissue, occurring most often on the trunk or proximal limbs. They may arise sporadically or associated with Gardner's syndrome or familial adenomatosis polyposis (FAP). Cytology specimens may be of variable cellularity and show short, bland, bipolar spindle cells (Figure 10.47), usually without significant atypia. There are often also numerous naked nuclei seen, along with collagenized or less often myxoid stroma. Tumor cell nuclei stain positively for beta-catenin.

Schwannoma (Figure 10.48) and neurofibroma (Figure 10.49) are both benign neurogenic tumors with overlapping features, and are thus often diagnosed simply as benign nerve sheath tumors. Most are sporadic, but they may occur in the setting of neurofibromatosis. Malignant transformation usually arises in patients with neurofibromatosis. Neurofibroma is more heterogeneous than schwannoma, being composed of Schwann cells as well as nerve axons, fibroblasts, and perineural cells. With touch preparations, lesional cells tend to form cohesive fragments of bland, spindled, comma, and bullet-shaped cells. Sometimes Verocay bodies may be seen. Tumor cells have wavy, irregular nuclei with pointed (fishhook) ends. Their chromatin is bland and nucleoli may not be noticeable. Ancient schwannoma is hard to recognize in cytology specimens alone, but may reveal focal marked nuclear pleomorphism (42). Cellular schwannoma is composed almost exclusively of Antoni A tissue. Specimens accordingly tend to be hypercellular and show closely packed spindled cells (Figure 10.50). The cells in cellular schwannoma are often more hyperchromatic, mitotically active, and associated with lymphoid aggregates. Immunostaining shows diffuse, strong S100 positivity in schwannoma and neurofibroma, as well as CD34 staining in neurofibromas.

Extrapleural SFT is a fibroblastic tumor that may be located superficially or in deep soft tissues. Although most SFTs are benign, they can behave aggressively. A diagnosis of SFT on cytology alone is challenging (43), because their prominent hemangiopericytic branching vascular pattern may not be appreciable. Touch preparations show predominantly spindle cells with only mild cytologic atypia. It is not uncommon to also find single cells and naked nuclei. Immunostains show that tumor cells are positive for CD34, STAT6, and CD99, and may stain variably with EMA and BCL2. Malignant SFT is rare, and may occur de novo or from a preexisting benign SFT. Malignant SFT specimens are usually hypercellular with noticeable nuclear atypia, increased mitoses, and necrosis (44).

Malignant Spindle Cell Lesions

In cytology specimens malignant spindle cell neoplasms are generally characterized by increased cellularity, marked nuclear atypia, increased mitoses including abnormal mitotic figures, the presence of necrosis, and an increased proliferation rate (high Ki67 index). Many sarcomas have spindle cell cytomorphology. This includes fibroblastic sarcomas such as low-grade fibromyxoid sarcoma (LGFMS), adult (Figure 10.51) and infantile fibrosarcoma, and myxofibrosarcoma.

Leiomyosarcoma may present as an extrauterine intraabdominal mass, deep soft tissue mass of extremities, or as a superficial (cutaneous) tumor. They may also involve the great vessels, especially the inferior vena cava. Cytology preparations contain tumor cell fascicles with spindle cells that may be deceptively bland (Figure 10.52) showing only mild nuclear atypia or limited mitotic activity. The cells have blunt-ended (cigar-shaped) nuclei, perinuclear vacuoles, occasional intranuclear vacuoles, and inconspicuous nucleoli (45). Some high-grade cases may have osteoclast-like multinucleated cells. Immunostains are positive for alpha-smooth muscle actin, desmin, calponin, and caldesmon. Retroperitoneal tumors in women may show ER positivity. In immunocompromised patients (e.g., AIDS or transplant recipients), they may be associated with Epstein–Barr virus (EBV) infection, and are accordingly positive for EBV-encoded small RNA (EBER) in situ hybridization (Figure 10.53).

Synovial sarcoma is a spindle-cell neoplasm that can be monophasic (spindle-cell component only) or biphasic (spindle and epithelial components). Poorly differentiated, synovial sarcoma is uncommon and shows more round cell morphology. Monophasic synovial sarcoma shows a monotonous population of single cells and/or clusters/sheets of short spindle cells. These cells have scant cytoplasm, elongated hyperchromatic nuclei with irregular nuclear borders, sometimes multiple nucleoli, and coarse chromatin (Figure 10.54). Synovial sarcoma stains positively for cytokeratin and EMA, BCL2, TLE-1, calponin, and CD99. FISH for the t(x;18)(p11;q11) translocation (*SS18-SSX* fusion transcript) is diagnostically helpful (46).

MPNSTs are typically deep-seated tumors. They may be associated with neurofibromatosis, radiation, or rarely arise from ganglioneuromas. They have a tendency to recur locally, and distant metastases occur frequently. MPNST is more cellular and displays greater cytological atypia than other neurogenic tumors (Figure 10.55). Cytology specimens may include spindle or epithelioid neoplastic cells as well as mitotic figures. Necrosis and metaplastic tissue (e.g., cartilage, bone, and muscle) may be seen.

Several vascular tumors may be composed predominantly of spindle cells. This includes Kaposi sarcoma, which consists of loosely cohesive clusters of bland spindled tumor cells and a bloody background (Figure 10.56) (47). Spindle cell angiosarcoma also yields similar spindle-shaped cells, but with more hyperchromatic and pleomorphic nuclei that have prominent nucleoli. Vasoformative features such as erythrophagocytosis, cytoplasmic vacuoles containing red blood cells, and intracellular eosinophilic inclusions may be seen in some cases (Figure 10.57) (48). Helpful immunostains to differentiate Kaposi sarcoma include vascular markers (CD31, CD34, FLI1, ERG), stains showing lymphatic differentiation (D2-40), and human herpesvirus-8 (HHV8) infection (LANA-1).

The differential diagnosis of a spindle cell malignancy includes spindle cell carcinoma (sarcomatoid carcinoma) and melanoma. Spindle cell carcinomas are high-grade malignancies that can be seen in many organs (e.g., lung, thyroid). Specimens from these spindle cell tumors tend to be highly cellular and may consist of single cells and/or clusters. Tumor cells are frequently pleomorphic, may have anaplastic features, and demonstrate necrosis. Pleomorphic tumor cells may show giant cell and bizarre cell morphology. Immunopositivity for epithelial cell markers is diagnostically helpful. Spindle cell melanoma may also mimic sarcoma (Figure 10.58). Binucleated and multinucleated cells may be identified, but melanin is usually absent or present in only rare cells. Immunostains show that tumor cells are positive for melanocytic markers S100, HMB45, MelanA, SOX10, tyrosinase, and MITF.

Small-Round-Cell Tumors

The differential diagnosis of soft tissue tumors with round cell morphology includes Ewing sarcoma/PNET, RMS, desmoplastic small-round-cell tumor (DSRCT), poorly differentiated sarcomas (e.g., synovial sarcoma, malignant SFT (Figure 10.59), round cell liposarcoma), cellular variant of EMC, small cell osteosarcoma (Figure 10.60), and nonmesenchymal malignancies (e.g., lymphoma (Figure 10.61), carcinoma (Figure 10.62), melanoma with small cell morphology, myeloid sarcoma, Wilms' tumor, hepatoblastoma, retinoblastoma). Rapidly growing pilomatricoma composed predominantly of basaloid cells can also mimic small round cell tumors (SRCTs) (Figure 10.63) (49).

This group of tumors accounts for the majority of childhood malignancies. Because of their morphologic similarities the SRCTs pose a differential diagnostic problem, particularly when they are poorly differentiated. Helpful cytomorphological clues include cytoplasmic vacuoles and a tigroid background due to glycogen in Ewing sarcoma, tadpole-shaped cells in embryonal RMS, sheets of undifferentiated small round cells surrounded by collagenous stroma in DSRCT, lymphoglandular bodies in non-Hodgkin lymphoma (NHL), paranuclear blue bodies in neuroendocrine tumors, eosinophilic fibrillar material, and Homer–Wright rosettes in neuroblastoma, acinar formation in hepatoblastoma, and blastema cells with tubular differentiation in nephroblastoma (50,51). FNA and/or core needle biopsies are reliable minimally invasive procedures for obtaining adequate numbers of dissociated, viable cells in order to perform diagnostic ancillary techniques such as flow cytometry, immunohistochemistry, FISH, and if necessary polymerase chain reaction (PCR).

RMS is a malignant tumor with muscle differentiation. Embryonal RMS (botryoid and spindle cell types) is the most common variant, which occurs in young children in their head and neck or urogenital region. Alveolar RMS occurs in older children, primarily on the extremities or in the paraspinal area. It has a poorer prognosis than embryonal RMS. Alveolar RMS is highly cellular and shows predominantly dissociated cells and naked nuclei. Tumor cells are round with a high nuclear to cytoplasmic ratio, have scant cytoplasm, and round hyperchromatic nuclei with finely granular chromatin and nucleoli (Figure 10.64). Mitotic figures are frequent. With embryonal RMS specimens more mature rhabdomyoblasts may be identified (52). Also, large tadpole-shaped tumor cells may be seen in embryonal RMS (53). Pleomorphic RMS occurs almost exclusively in adults and consists of bizarre polygonal, round and spindle cells. Embryonal and alveolar RMS cannot always be differentiated based on cytology alone. Therefore, FISH is often employed to detect the FKHR (or FOXO1) breakpoint on chromosome 13 or PCR to identify FKHR-PAX3/PAX7 fusion transcripts in alveolar RMS. By comparison, embryonal RMS has complex karyotypes. RMS tumor cells demonstrate positive immunostaining for desmin, myogenin (Figure 10.65), MyoD1, and myoglobin. There may also be occasional focal staining with actin, synaptophysin, chromogranin, cytokeratin, and CD99.

Ewing sarcoma/PNET is more common in bones than in soft tissues. They occur predominantly in children and young adults between the ages 5 and 25 years. Cytology preparations contain single small round tumor cells and sometimes even groups of small cells (Figure 10.66). There is usually a dual population of viable pale cells with cytoplasm and darker apoptotic cells. The presence of rosettes is an uncommon finding (Figure 10.67). Tumor cells have scant vacuolated cytoplasm, round nuclei that are hyperchromatic, and show only moderate pleomorphism (54,55). A tigroid background may be present in touch preparations (Figure 10.68), but is not as common as occurs with FNA. Tumor cells stain positive for Periodic acid–Schiff (PAS) (due to glycogen), CD99, and are rarely immunoreactive for cytokeratin, S100, and desmin. FISH using a break-apart probe for the *EWSR1* gene (at 22q12) is diagnostically helpful. Most (90%) tumors have t(11;22) with *EWSR1-FLI1* fusion and others (5%–10%) have t(21;22) with *EWSR1-ERG* fusion. Other rare translocations involving the *EWSR1* gene include t(2;22), t(7;22), and t(17;22).

DSRCT is a rare neoplasm with poor prognosis seen mainly in males in their third decade. It commonly arises in the retroperitoneum, omentum, and pelvis. Tumors are comprised of small round blue cells and abundant desmoplastic stroma. Occasionally, there may be focal epithelial differentiation characterized by rosettes and glandular structures. Cytology samples are relatively highly cellular and composed of cell groups and/or dissociated cells. Stromal fragments with acellular stroma may not be seen. Tumor cells have a high nuclear to cytoplasmic ratio, oval or round nuclei, moderate nuclear pleomorphism, and small nucleoli (56). Mitoses may be frequent. Immunoreactivity includes mixed epithelial (EMA), myogenic (desmin), and neural (S100) expression. Desmin shows characteristic dot-like and paranuclear staining. Tumor cells may also be positive for CD56, NSE, chromogranin, synaptophysin, CD99, and WT1. These tumors have a characteristic t(11;22) (p13;q12) translocation. However, unlike Ewing sarcoma the rearranged gene on chromosome 11 is *WT1* and not *FLI1*.

Myxoid Tumors

Myxoid tumors range from benign lesions to low- and high-grade myxoid sarcomas (57,58). The differential diagnosis of a hypocellular myxoid lesion/neoplasm includes a ganglion cyst and myxoma. Myxoma is a benign well-circumscribed soft tissue tumor of adults. They are often intramuscular and may be juxta-articular in location (e.g., often arise around the knee). Extraskeletal myxomas (heart, breast, skin) are part of the Carney complex. Cytology specimens contain rare bland fibroblasts and foamy macrophages with abundant background extracellular myxoid matrix (Figure 10.69). Myxoid liposarcomas may also be sparsely cellular with abundant background myxoid material, but can be distinguished by their delicate arborizing vasculature (Figure 10.41). Other sarcomas that may present with myxoid features include myxoid leiomyosarcomas and myxoid variant of SFT, dermatofibrosarcoma protuberans (DFSP), and MPNST.

Myoepithelial tumors of soft tissue (myoepithelioma or mixed tumor) are composed of epithelial and/or myoepithelial cellular elements. They have chondromyxoid to hyalinized stroma. Foci may show ductal differentiation. Their cytomorphology resembles mixed tumors seen in the parotid gland. There may be varying proportions of epithelioid, spindled, plasmacytoid, or clear cells (Figure 10.70). These cells may form clusters, cords, or ductules. There may also be divergent differentiation (e.g., squamous, fatty, cartilaginous, osseous regions). Most of these tumors have a benign behavior. Tumors with dedifferentiation to myoepithelial carcinoma display more significant atypia. Immunohistochemistry shows that these tumor cells are positive for both cytokeratin and S100, but may also stain with EMA, GFAP, calponin, p63, smooth muscle actin, and desmin. Cases with t(1;22)(q23;q12) translocation with *EWSR1-PBX1* fusion have been reported.

LGFMS, or Evans tumor, usually occurs in the deep soft tissues of the extremities and trunk. They have alternating collagenized and myxoid zones, which is difficult to appreciate in cytology samples. They contain deceptively bland fibroblast-like spindled cells, proliferating small vessels, and background myxoid material (59). Tumor cells may stain with EMA (up to 80% of cases), p63 and MUC4. They may also show aberrant DOG1 expression. FISH and/or PCR for the *FUS-CREB3L2* fusion transcript are useful tools for confirming the diagnosis of LGFMS.

Myxofibrosarcoma is a common sarcoma of older patients. They typically arise in the deep dermis and subcutaneous fat of the limbs and limb girdles. Of note, other myxoid soft tissue lesions tend to occur in deeper locations. Also, these tumors can metastasize to lymph nodes. Specimens procured from these tumors show variable cellularity and pleomorphism. Low-grade sarcomas are hypocellular and contain mostly spindled cells with mild to moderate atypia (Figure 10.71). High-grade myxofibrosarcomas are hypercellular and show spindled and pleomorphic tumor cells, atypical vacuolated cells (pseudolipoblasts) that often cling to curvilinear vessels, along with necrosis in a myxoid background (Figure 10.72) (60). They may also have bizarre, multinucleated giant cells. Ancillary studies are not helpful, except to exclude other myxoid neoplasms.

EMC is another myxoid sarcoma that may present in the deep soft tissues of the lower extremities in adults. They are aggressive sarcomas with a high risk of local recurrence that respond poorly to chemotherapy. These sarcomas are composed of spindle and epithelioid tumor cells associated with abundant myxoid and sometimes cartilaginous matrix. Touch preparations usually show spindled-shaped cells, sometimes forming short anastomosing cords, and a myxoid background (Figure 10.73). There may also be single cells or small cell clusters.

The cells are monotonous in appearance, have a moderate amount of vacuolated cytoplasm, and contain bland nuclei with evenly dispersed chromatin and variably sized nucleoli (61). Cellularity and matrix composition depends on the grade of neoplasm; high-grade (poorly differentiated) tumors demonstrate increased cellularity and less matrix (Figure 10.74). Necrosis may be identified. Immunostains show that the tumor cells are positive for S100, neuroendocrine markers in some cases (chromogranin, NSE), and rarely cytokeratin or EMA. Molecular or genetic studies can confirm the diagnosis by detecting the t(9;22) (EWS:NR4A3) translocation (Figure 10.75).

Epithelioid Tumors

Several neoplasms with epithelioid morphology may be encountered in soft tissue including benign mesenchymal neoplasms (rhabdomyoma, granular cell tumor) and malignant mesenchymal neoplasms (epithelioid sarcoma, clear cell sarcoma, alveolar soft part sarcoma, PEComa, myoepithelial carcinoma). The differential includes epithelioid variants of other sarcomas such as leiomyosarcoma (Figure 10.76), RMS, MPNST (Figure 10.77), hemangioendothelioma (Figure 10.78), and angiosarcoma. Nonmesenchymal tumors such as metastases (melanoma (Figure 10.79), carcinoma, mesothelioma), and hematolymphoid tumors (lymphoma, plasmacytoma, myeloid sarcoma) may also present as a soft tissue mass.

Granular cell tumor is a neoplasm of Schwann cell origin. They may occur in a wide variety of locations. The majority of granular cell tumors are benign. Cytology specimens are characterized by having large, polygonal cells with abundant, granular cytoplasm and indistinct cell borders (Figure 10.80). Their nuclei are typically uniform, small, and round with only occasional nucleoli evident. The background is usually granular. Cytoplasmic granules are PAS+. Granular cell tumors are typically S-100 and CD68 positive.

Epithelioid sarcoma is an uncommon soft tissue tumor that usually presents in the distal extremities of young adults. Proximal/axial epithelioid sarcomas have a poorer prognosis. These tumors have a high propensity for metastasis, usually to other skin sites, lymph nodes, or lungs. They are difficult to diagnose in cytology specimens alone. Histopathology is often required to demonstrate the presence of epithelioid tumor cells proliferating in a granuloma-like fashion around areas of necrosis and central hyalinization is characteristic. Variable cytopathologic features that may be identified include polygonal (Figure 10.81) as well as spindled cells, rhabdoid-like intracytoplasmic inclusions, and giant cells (62). Positive immunostains include cytokeratin, EMA, vimentin, and in some cases CD34, ERG, and FLI1 with loss of INI1.

Clear-cell sarcoma (malignant melanoma of soft parts) is a rare sarcoma that affects mainly young adults around 30 to 40 years. Most of these tumors are located in the extremities near the ankle or foot. Metastases occur mainly to regional lymph nodes and lungs. Cytology specimens show a predominance of single epithelioid cells, but sometimes these may form loosely cohesive cell groups with a microacinar arrangement (Figure 10.82). The tumor cells are round to oval and may have bi- and/or multinucleation. Their cytoplasm is moderately abundant, occasionally vacuolated, and individual cells may contain melanin pigment. Their nuclei are round or oval, eccentric, and contain one or more nucleoli. Occasional intranuclear inclusions may be seen. The background can be tigroid. These tumors demonstrate immunopositivity for S100, HMB45, MITF, and MelanA. Clear cell sarcoma can be differentiated from metastatic melanoma with FISH to demonstrate their characteristic t(12;22)(q13;q12) translocation. The EWS-ATF1 fusion product can also be detected by PCR in 90% of cases.

Alveolar soft part sarcoma is a rare soft tissue sarcoma seen mainly in older children and young adults. They are commonly located on the extremities in adults and head and neck area in children. They grow slowly and have a low recurrence rate, but are well known for having early and frequent metastases to the lungs, bones, and brain. Cytomorphology shows a mix of single cells, small clusters, and bare nuclei. Clusters may show syncytial or acinar-like morphology. The tumor cells are large and polygonal and have abundant fragile, granular, or vacuolated cytoplasm. Their nuclei are large and centrally located with prominent nucleoli (Figure 10.83). These tumor cells mimic clear cell renal cell carcinoma. Some cells may show bi- and multinucleation. Characteristic rod-shaped or rhomboid crystals seen in histology are rarely seen in cytology specimens. Tumor cells are positive for PAS, desmin, MyoD1, and TFE3.

Giant Cell Lesions

Giant cell containing lesions can be reactive or neoplastic. They can be benign (e.g., multinucleated giant cell of Langhans type seen with granulomas or tophaceous gout [Figure 10.84]) or neoplastic (e.g., giant-cell tumor). Neoplastic giant cells are more pleomorphic and have atypical, hyperchromatic nuclei. However, the presence of bland appearing giant cells does not exclude malignancy, as certain high-grade malignancies such as giant cell–rich osteosarcoma may contain reactive osteoclast-like giant cells that appear cytologically bland. Soft tissue tumors that show a predominance of giant cells include benign lesions (e.g., tenosynovial GCT, nodular fasciitis) and malignant tumors (e.g., GCT, myxofibrosarcoma, undifferentiated pleomorphic sarcoma) (63). The differential also includes nonmesenchymal lesions such as metastatic giant cell carcinoma, anaplastic large cell lymphoma, and Reed–Sternberg cells in Hodgkin lymphoma (Figure 10.85).

Tenosynovial GCT may be of localized type (so-called GCT of tendon sheath) or diffuse type (so-called pigmented villonodular synovitis). These are locally aggressive tumors that arise from the synovium of joints, tendon sheath, or bursae. They may be intra- or extra-articular. Extra-articular soft tissue masses may present with or without involvement of the adjacent joint; typically the major joints (e.g., hip, knee, ankle, shoulder). Cytology preparations may show a single cell arrangement, clusters, or papillary configurations (Figure 10.86). These tumors consist of mononuclear synovial-like cells accompanied by a variable number of multinucleated osteoclast-like giant cells, foamy macrophages, hemosiderin-laden histiocytes, and scant inflammatory cells (Figure 10.87). The multinucleated giant cells have uniform nuclei similar to the mononuclear cells. Nuclear grooves and intranuclear pseudo-inclusions may be present in stromal cells (64,65). Prussian blue staining of iron in hemosiderin can help differentiate pigment from melanin. Tumor cells demonstrate immunoreactivity for vimentin, CD68, and often desmin.

Pleomorphic Tumors

Several sarcomas can present with an abundance of pleomorphic tumor cells such as pleomorphic variants of liposarcoma, RMS, and leiomyosarcoma (Figure 10.88). These tumors are usually cellular and have a loosely cohesive pleomorphic and/or spindle tumor cell population. There may be a mixture of mononucleated, binucleated, and multinucleated cells that show marked pleomorphism with nuclear atypia that includes coarse chromatin, prominent nucleoli and macronucleoli. Mitoses are often frequent. They commonly have a granular, myxoid, or necrotic background. The differential diagnosis includes giant-cell carcinoma, malignant melanoma, and anaplastic lymphoma. Immunostains may be helpful, such as smooth muscle markers to diagnose leiomyosarcoma or skeletal muscle markers to confirm RMS. Sometimes these soft tissue sarcomas reveal no identifiable line of differentiation. In such cases, a diagnosis of undifferentiated pleomorphic sarcoma (akin to pleomorphic malignant fibrous histiocytoma or MFH) can be rendered (Figure 10.89).

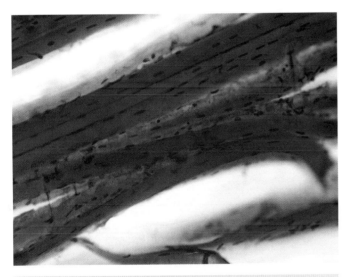

FIGURE 10.32 Normal skeletal muscle. TP showing longitudinal skeletal muscle fibers with multiple peripheral, small, bland nuclei, and cross striations (DQ-stained TP, low power). DQ, Diff-Quik; TP, touch preparation.

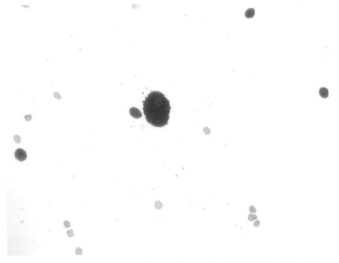

FIGURE 10.33 Mast cell. TP from a neurofibroma showing a mast cell with dense cytoplasmic granules (DQ-stained TP, high power). DQ, Diff-Quik; TP, touch preparation.

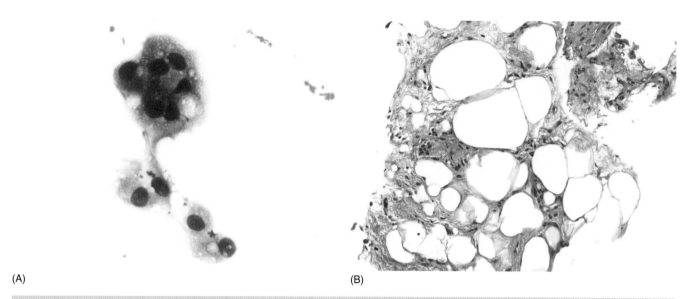

(A)   (B)

FIGURE 10.34 Fat necrosis. (A) TP showing reactive foamy macrophages. (B) Corresponding core biopsy showing mature adipocytes with intervening foamy histiocytes. ((A) DQ-stained TP, high power; (B) H&E-stained core biopsy, low power.) DQ, Diff-Quik; H&E, hematoxylin and eosin; TP, touch preparation.

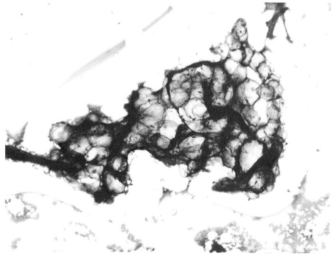

FIGURE 10.35 Spindle cell/pleomorphic lipoma. TP showing several bland spindle cells, stripped nuclei, and a floret-like multinucleated stromal cell (DQ-stained TP, low power). DQ, Diff-Quik; TP, touch preparation.

FIGURE 10.36 Angiolipoma. TP showing a group of mature adipocytes with many intermingled blood vessels (DQ-stained TP, low power). DQ, Diff-Quik; TP, touch preparation.

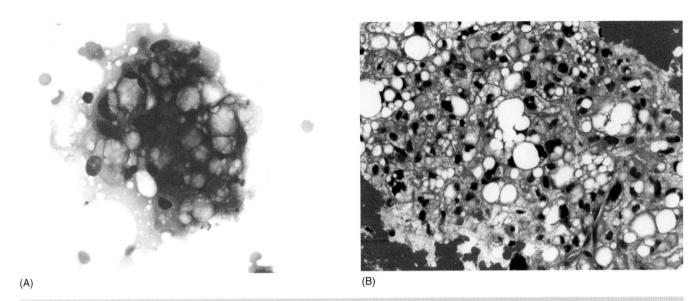

(A)

(B)

FIGURE 10.37 Liposarcoma. (A) TP showing mono- and multivacuolated lipoblasts with pleomorphic hyperchromatic nuclei. (B) Corresponding core biopsy showing similar lipoblasts. ((A) DQ-stained TP, high power; (B) H&E-stained core biopsy, medium power.) DQ, Diff-Quik; H&E, hematoxylin and eosin; TP, touch preparation.

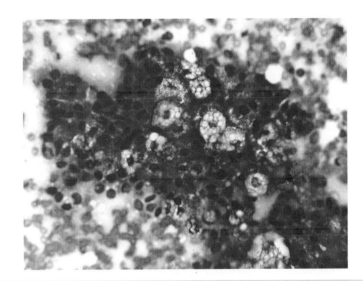

FIGURE 10.38 Sebaceous carcinoma. TP showing multivacuolated malignant sebocytes that mimic lipoblastoma (DQ-stained TP, medium power). DQ, Diff-Quik; TP, touch preparation.

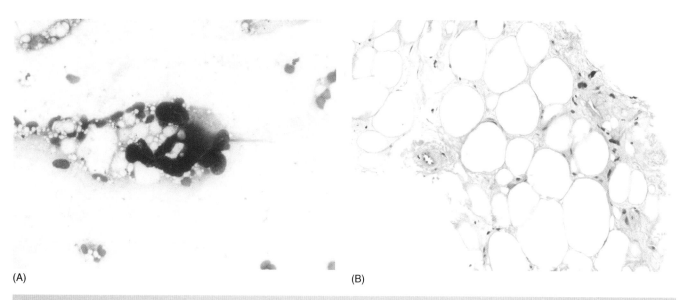

(A)   (B)

FIGURE 10.39 ALT. (A) TP showing atypical stromal cells with hyperchromatic nuclei. (B) Corresponding core biopsy showing a lipoma-like well-differentiated liposarcoma characterized by adipocytes of varying size and scattered atypical stromal cells. ((A) DQ-stained TP, high power; (B) H&E-stained core biopsy, medium power.) ALT, atypical lipomatous tumor; DQ, Diff-Quik; H&E, hematoxylin and eosin; TP, touch preparation.

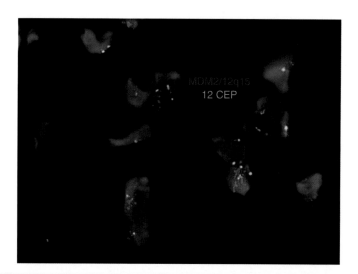

FIGURE 10.40 ALT. FISH showing gene amplification of both the *MDM2* (red) gene locus (12q15) and chromosome 12 centromere (green) signals, indicative of ALT. ALT, atypical lipomatous tumor; FISH, fluorescence in-situ hybridization.

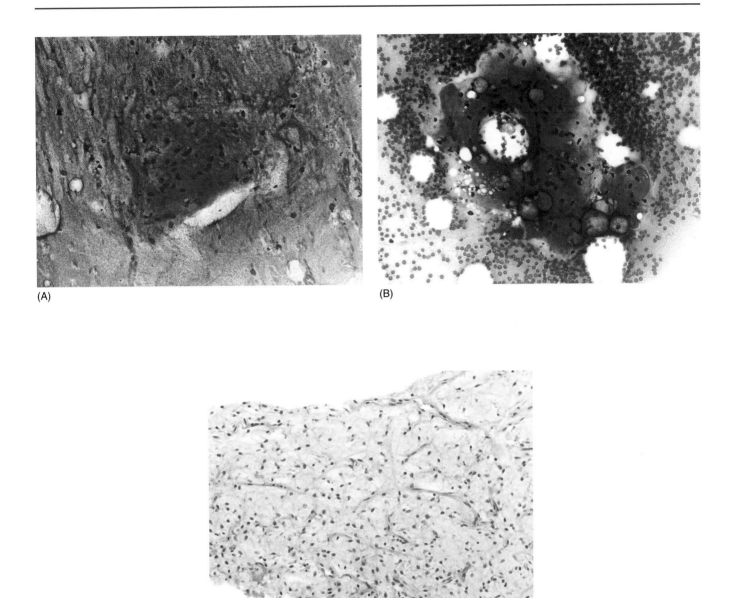

FIGURE 10.41 Myxoid liposarcoma. (A) TP showing predominantly myxoid material with several embedded nonlipogenic round to oval tumor cells. (B) TP showing delicate branching vessels with a few lipoblasts and associated myxoid stroma. (C). Corresponding core biopsy showing branching networks of capillary vessels with abundant myxoid stroma. ((A) and (B) DQ-stained TP, high power; (C) H&E-stained core biopsy, medium power.) DQ, Diff-Quik; H&E, hematoxylin and eosin; TP, touch preparation.

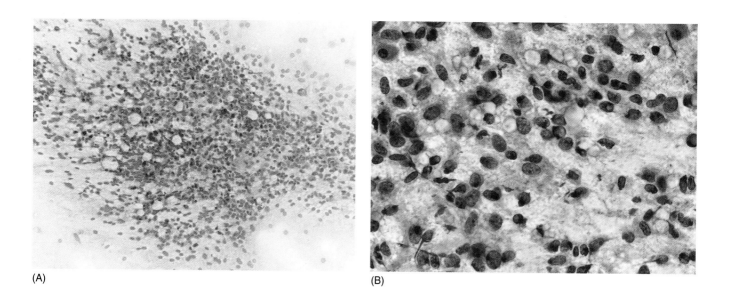

(A)   (B)

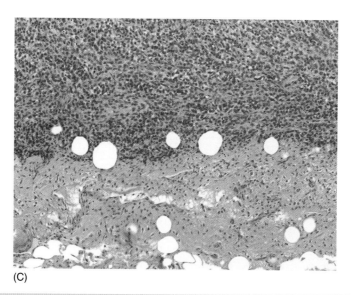

(C)

FIGURE 10.42 High-grade (round cell) myxoid liposarcoma. (A) Intraoperative TP showing predominantly small round cells admixed with erythrocytes. A myxoid background is not evident. (B) The round tumor cells have variable amounts of cytoplasm, high N:C ratios, and rounded atypical nuclei with occasional nucleoli. (C) The corresponding tumor resection shows an abrupt transition from low-grade myxoid liposarcoma with pools of myxoid stroma to high-grade myxoid liposarcoma characterized by a solid sheet of primitive round cells. ((A) and (B) H&E-stained TP, high power; (C) H&E-stained resection, low power.) DQ, Diff-Quik; H&E, hematoxylin and eosin; N:C, nuclear:cytoplasmic; TP, touch preparation.

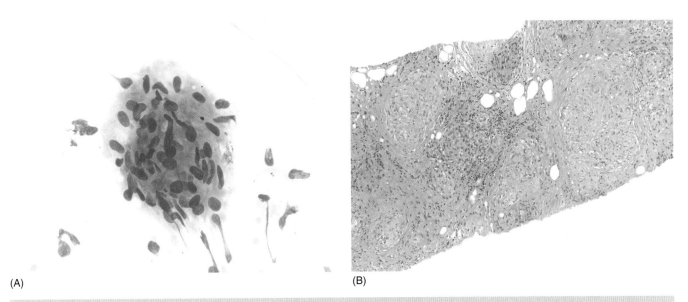

(A)

(B)

FIGURE 10.43 Sarcoidosis. (A) TP showing an aggregate of spindled histiocytes. (B) Corresponding core biopsy showing deep-seated nonnecrotizing granulomas. ((A) DQ-stained TP, medium power; (B) H&E-stained core biopsy, low power.) DQ, Diff-Quik; H&E, hematoxylin and eosin; TP, touch preparation.

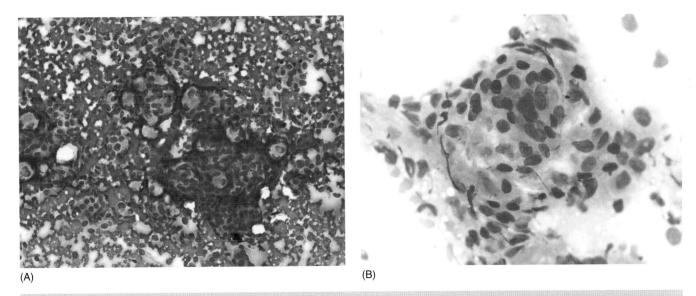

(A)

(B)

FIGURE 10.44 Ectopic meningioma. (A) TP showing meningeal cells forming characteristic whorls. (B) Spindled-shaped meningeal cells are shown with uniform bland nuclei. ((A) DQ-stained TP, medium power; (B) DQ-stained TP, high power.) DQ, Diff-Quik; TP, touch preparation. Refer to Figure 11.21 for comparison to dural-based meningioma.

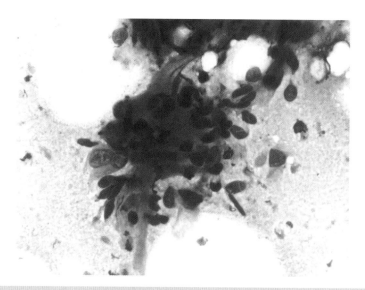

FIGURE 10.45 Nodular fasciitis. TP showing mixed spindled-shaped and more plump fibroblasts associated with collagen stroma (DQ-stained TP, high power). DQ, Diff-Quik; TP, touch preparation.

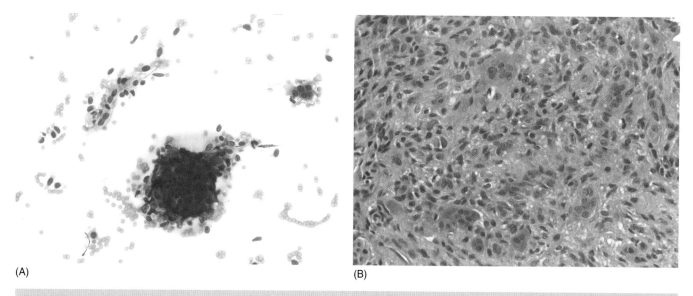

(A)   (B)

FIGURE 10.46 Myositis ossificans. (A) TP showing bland spindle-shaped fibroblasts present as single cells and in clusters. Note the mitotic figure on the left and osteoclast-like multinucleated giant cell on the right. (B) Corresponding core biopsy showing admixed spindle-shaped fibroblasts and multinucleated giant cell. This biopsy also contained trabeculae of woven bone. ((A) DQ-stained TP, medium power; (B) H&E-stained core biopsy, low power.) DQ, Diff-Quik; H&E, hematoxylin and eosin; TP, touch preparation.

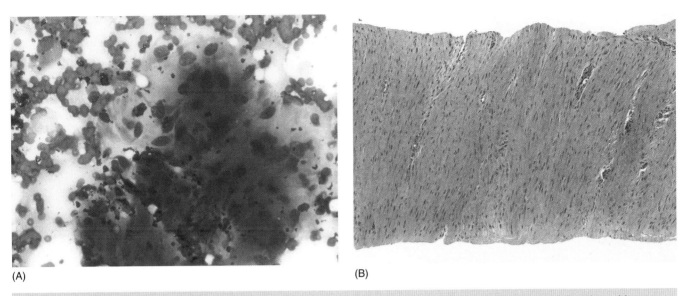

FIGURE 10.47 Desmoid-type fibromatosis. (A) TP from a 37-year-old woman with Lynch syndrome presenting with an abdominal mass showing a sheet of uniform, bland spindle cells associated with collagen stroma. (B) Corresponding core biopsy showing proliferating elongated spindled-cells set in collagenous stoma. ((A) DQ-stained TP, low power; (B) H&E-stained core biopsy, low power.) DQ, Diff-Quik; H&E, hematoxylin and eosin; TP, touch preparation.

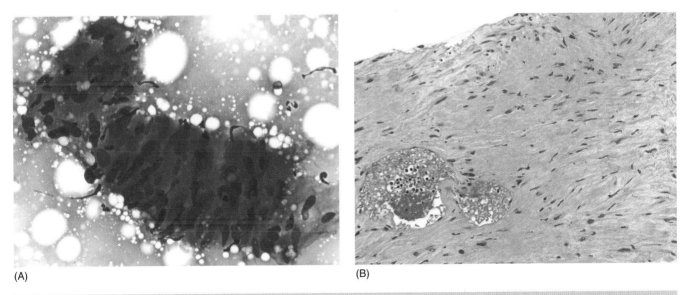

FIGURE 10.48 Schwannoma. (A) TP showing a tumor fragment comprised of bland spindle cells with indistinct cytoplasm and comma- as well as bullet-shaped nuclei with pointed ends. (B) Corresponding core biopsy showing spindled Schwann cells. ((A) DQ-stained TP, medium power; (B) H&E-stained core biopsy, medium power.) DQ, Diff-Quik; H&E, hematoxylin and eosin; TP, touch preparation.

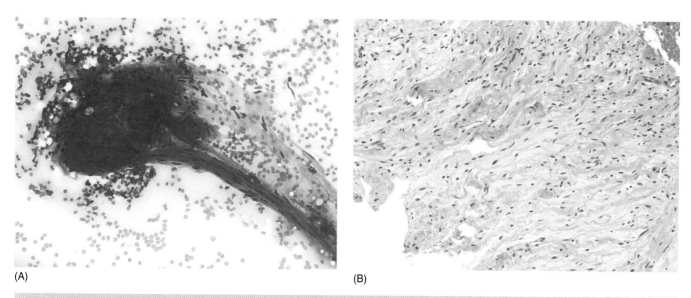

(A)

(B)

FIGURE 10.49   Neurofibroma. (A) TP showing spindle cells with comma-shaped nuclei that have pointed ends.
(B) Corresponding core biopsy showing bland spindled cells within fibrillary stroma and "shredded" collagen fibers.
((A) DQ-stained TP, medium power; (B) H&E-stained core biopsy, medium power.) DQ, Diff-Quik; H&E, hematoxylin and
eosin; TP, touch preparation.

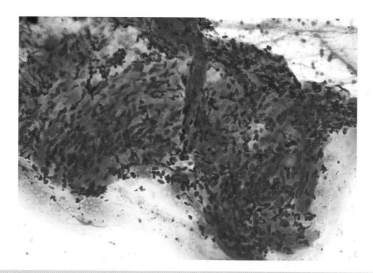

FIGURE 10.50   Cellular schwannoma. Hypercellular tissue fragment showing predominantly comma-shaped and
occasional oval cells (DQ-stained TP, medium power). DQ, Diff-Quik; TP, touch preparation.

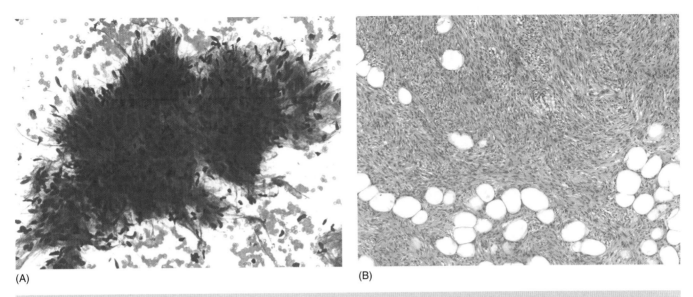

(A)

(B)

FIGURE 10.51   DFSP. (A) Hypercellular TP showing spindled cells with mild nuclear atypia. (B) Corresponding histopathology showing spindled cells infiltrating deeply into and entrapping subcutaneous fat. ((A) DQ-stained TP, medium power; (B) H&E-stained tissue section, low power.) DFSP, dermatofibrosarcoma protuberans; DQ, Diff-Quik; H&E, hematoxylin and eosin; TP, touch preparation.

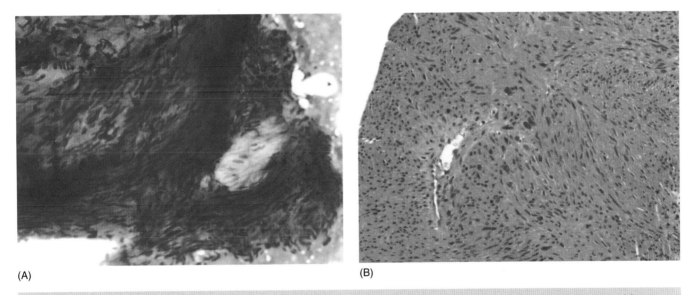

(A)

(B)

FIGURE 10.52   Leiomyosarcoma. (A) TP showing spindle cells with cigar-shaped nuclei. (B) Corresponding core biopsy showing fascicles of smooth muscle cells with notable nuclear atypia. ((A) DQ-stained TP, medium power; (B) H&E-stained core biopsy, low power.) DQ, Diff-Quik; H&E, hematoxylin and eosin; TP, touch preparation.

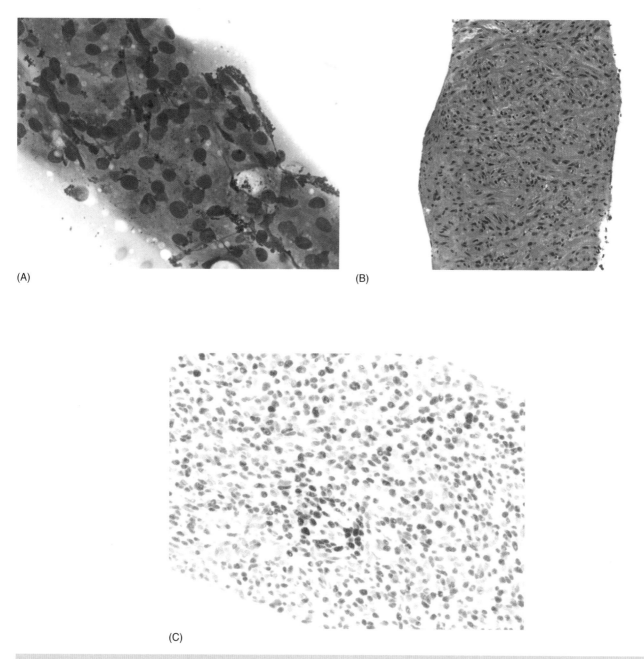

FIGURE 10.53 EBV-associated smooth muscle tumor. (A) TP from a transplant patient showing spindle cells with bland oval nuclei. (B) Corresponding core biopsy showing proliferating smooth muscle cells with minimal nuclear atypia. (C) Smooth muscle tumor cells are positive for EBER in situ hybridization. ((A) DQ-stained TP, medium power; (B) H&E-stained core biopsy, low power; (C) EBER in situ hybridization, medium power.) EBER, EBV-encoded small RNA; EBV, Epstein–Barr virus; DQ, Diff-Quik; H&E, hematoxylin and eosin; TP, touch preparation.

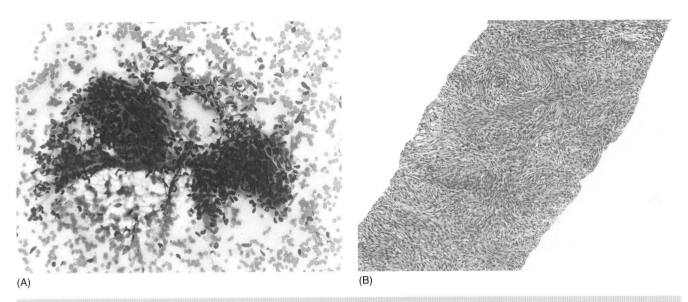

(A)

(B)

FIGURE 10.54 Monophasic synovial sarcoma. (A) Hypercellular TP showing many closely packed short spindle cells. (B) Corresponding core biopsy showing a dense sheet of spindle cells with sparse cytoplasm, hyperchromatic nuclei and inconspicuous nucleoli. ((A) DQ-stained TP, low power; (B) H&E-stained core biopsy, low power.) DQ, Diff-Quik; H&E, hematoxylin and eosin; TP, touch preparation.

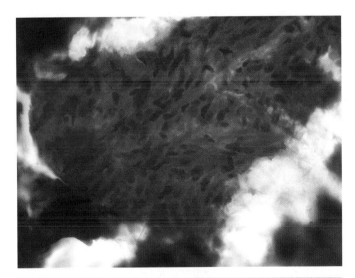

FIGURE 10.55 MPNST. (A) Hypercellular TP showing numerous spindle cells with hyperchromatic nuclei and mild nuclear atypia (DQ-stained TP, medium power). DQ, Diff-Quik; MPNST, malignant peripheral nerve sheath tumor; TP, touch preparation.

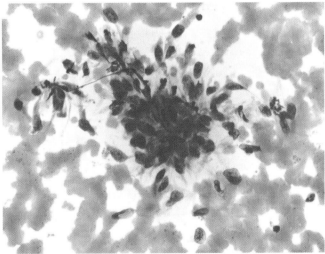

FIGURE 10.56 Kaposi sarcoma. TP from an HIV-positive patient showing atypical spindle cells with a bloody background (DQ-stained TP, medium power). DQ, Diff-Quik; TP, touch preparation.

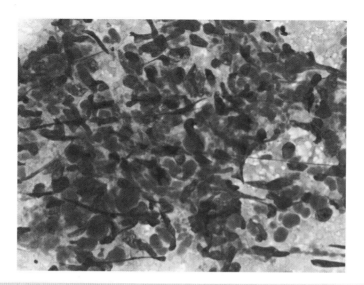

FIGURE 10.57 Angiosarcoma. Atypical spindled cells are shown associated with striking eosinophilic globules (DQ-stained TP, medium power). DQ, Diff-Quik; TP, touch preparation.

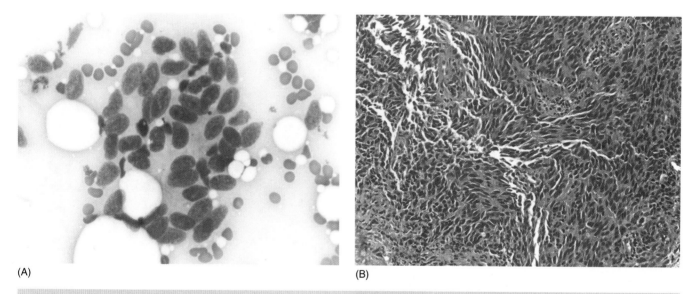

(A)   (B)

FIGURE 10.58 Spindle cell melanoma. (A) TP showing atypical spindle cells. (B) Corresponding core biopsy showing sheets of infiltrating spindle melanoma cells. ((A) DQ-stained TP, high power; (B) H&E-stained core biopsy, medium power.) DQ, Diff-Quik; H&E, hematoxylin and eosin; TP, touch preparation.

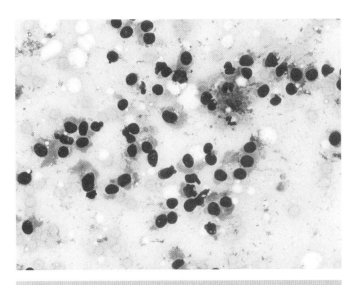

FIGURE 10.59 Malignant SFT. TP showing predominantly small rounded cells, instead of the spindled-shaped cells typically seen in SFT (DQ-stained TP, medium power). DQ, Diff-Quik; SFT, solitary fibrous tumor; TP, touch preparation.

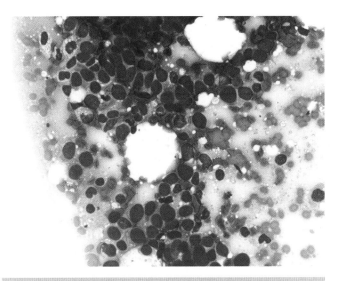

FIGURE 10.60 Small cell osteosarcoma. TP showing predominantly small pleomorphic rounded cells. Malignant osteoid, not shown in this field, is helpful to make this diagnosis (DQ-stained TP, medium power). DQ, Diff-Quik; TP, touch preparation.

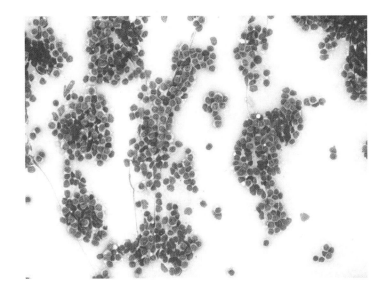

FIGURE 10.61 Extranodal marginal zone lymphoma of soft tissue. TP of a soft tissue mass from a 64-year-old male shows abundant monomorphous small lymphocytes. Immunophenotyping confirmed the diagnosis of a B-cell non-Hodgkin lymphoma (DQ-stained TP, low power). DQ, Diff-Quik; TP, touch preparation.

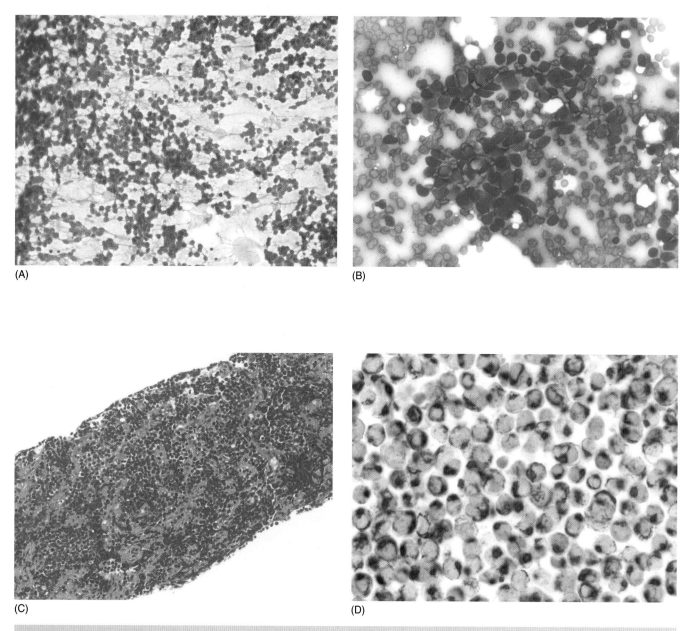

FIGURE 10.62 Merkel cell carcinoma. (A) Intraoperative TP showing predominantly small rounded cells. (B) Merkel tumor cells are shown with minimal cytoplasm and nuclei with finely granular "salt and pepper" chromatin. (C) Corresponding core biopsy showing infiltrating neuroendocrine carcinoma. (D) Tumor cells show CK20 perinuclear dot-like immunoreactivity. ((A) H&E-stained TP, low power; (B) DQ-stained TP, high power; (C) H&E-stained core biopsy, medium power; (D) CK20 stain, high power.) DQ, Diff-Quik; H&E, hematoxylin and eosin; TP, touch preparation.

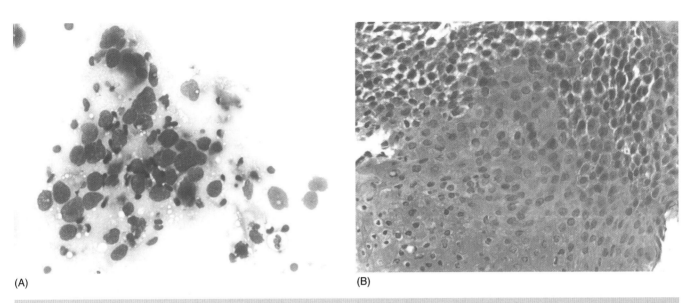

(A)

(B)

FIGURE 10.63 Pilomatricoma. (A) TP showing predominantly basaloid cells. (B) Corresponding core biopsy shows proliferating germinative matrical cells. ((A) DQ-stained TP, high power; (B) H&E-stained core biopsy, medium power.) DQ, Diff-Quik; H&E, hematoxylin and eosin; TP, touch preparation.

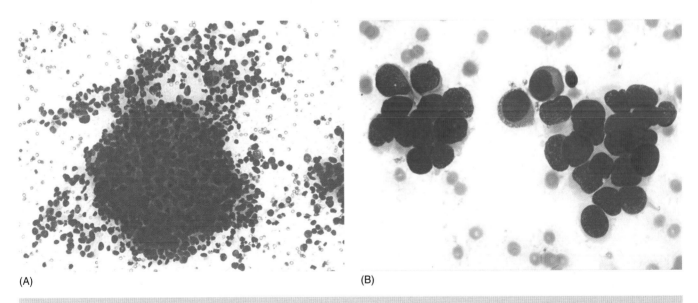

(A)

(B)

FIGURE 10.64 Alveolar RMS. (A) Hypercellular TP showing many single cells and large clusters of small round tumor cells. Note the rare multinucleated giant cell, which is a characteristic feature of this tumor. (B) TP showing small cohesive clusters of small- to medium-sized rounded cells with scant vacuolated cytoplasm, coarse chromatin, and indistinct nucleoli. ((A) DQ-stained TP, medium power; (B) DQ-stained TP, high power.) DQ, Diff-Quik; RMS, rhabdomyosarcoma; TP, touch preparation.

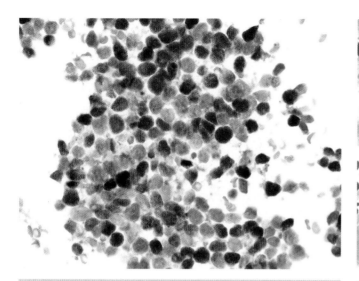

FIGURE 10.65 Alveolar RMS. Tumor cells show myogenin nuclear immunoreactivity. Although MyoD1 shows similar nuclear positivity there is often also nonspecific cytoplasmic staining with RMS (Myogenin stain, medium power). RMS, rhabdomyosarcoma.

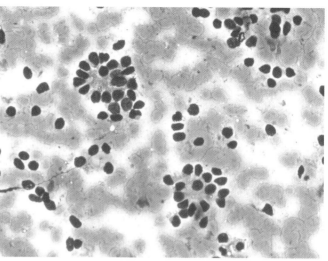

FIGURE 10.67 Ewing sarcoma/PNET. TP showing Homer–Wright rosette formations. Nuclei are arranged around central areas of neuropil (DQ-stained TP, medium power). DQ, Diff-Quik; PNET, primitive neuroectodermal tumor; TP, touch preparation.

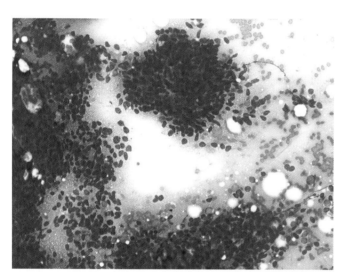

FIGURE 10.66 Ewing sarcoma/PNET. Hypercellular TP showing clusters of small round tumor cells. Note the focal tigroid background near these cell groups (DQ-stained TP, low power). DQ, Diff-Quik; PNET, primitive neuroectodermal tumor; TP, touch preparation.

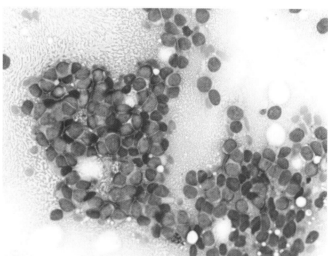

FIGURE 10.68 Ewing sarcoma/PNET. TP showing a dual population of large light cells with moderate cytoplasm and smaller dark cells with scant cytoplasm. Note the presence of nuclear molding, slight anisonucleosis, even chromatin with inconspicuous nucleoli, and lacy (tigroid) background (DQ-stained TP, medium power). DQ, Diff-Quik; PNET, primitive neuroectodermal tumor; TP, touch preparation.

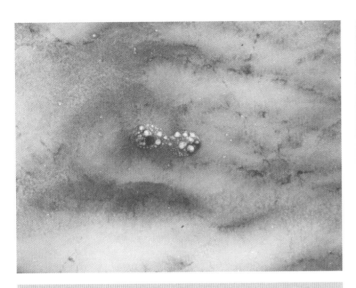

FIGURE 10.69 Intramuscular myxoma. TP showing only scant foamy macrophages with abundant background granular myxoid material (DQ-stained TP, high power). DQ, Diff-Quik; TP, touch preparation.

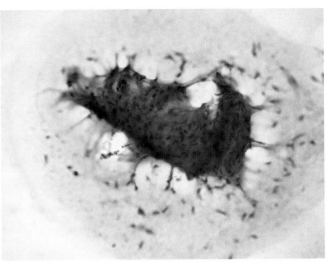

FIGURE 10.70 Myoepithelial tumor of soft tissue. A fragment of bland spindled cells with fusiform nuclei is shown associated with myxoid stroma (H&E-stained TP, medium power). H&E, hematoxylin and eosin; TP, touch preparation.

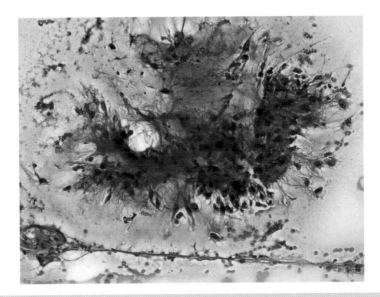

FIGURE 10.71 Myxofibrosarcoma, low-grade. A tissue fragment of atypical fibroblast-like spindle and histiocyte-like epithelioid cells is shown associated with abundant myxoid stroma (H&E-stained TP, medium power). H&E, hematoxylin and eosin; TP, touch preparation.

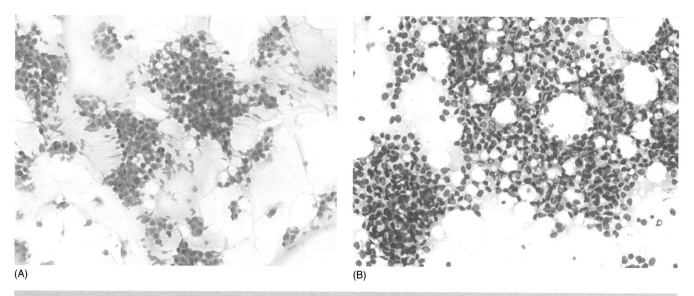

(A)   (B)

FIGURE 10.72 Myxofibrosarcoma, high-grade. (A) Intraoperative imprint showing abundant pleomorphic epithelioid cells with a myxoid background. (B) This hypercellular TP shows predominantly small rounded tumor cells without a myxoid background. ((A) H&E-stained imprint, medium power; (B) DQ-stained TP, medium power.) DQ, Diff-Quik; H&E, hematoxylin and eosin; TP, touch preparation.

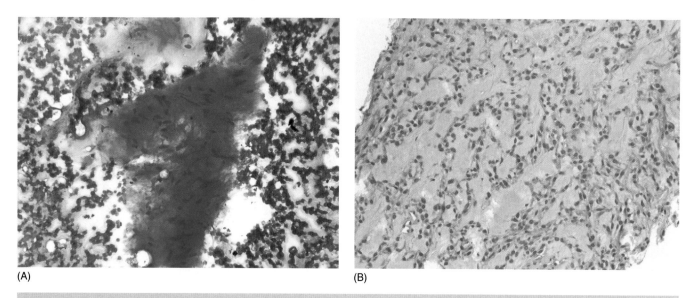

(A)   (B)

FIGURE 10.73 Extraskeletal myxoid chondrosarcoma, conventional type. (A) TP showing a tumor fragment with uniform spindled-shaped cells and myxoid stroma. (B) Corresponding core biopsy showing interconnecting cells forming cords within abundant pale blue myxoid matrix. ((A) DQ-stained TP, medium power; (B) H&E-stained core biopsy, medium power.) DQ, Diff-Quik; H&E, hematoxylin and eosin; TP, touch preparation.

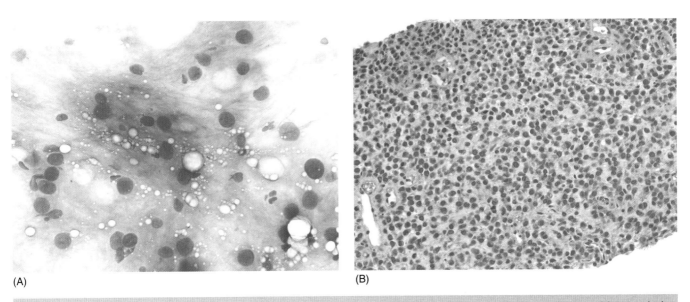

(A)

(B)

FIGURE 10.74 Extraskeletal myxoid chondrosarcoma, high-grade. (A) This hypercellular TP shows pleomorphic rounded tumor cells with a myxoid background. (B) The corresponding core biopsy shows a sheet of round tumor cells in a myxoid matrix. ((A) DQ-stained TP, high power; (B) H&E-stained core biopsy, medium power.) DQ, Diff-Quik; H&E, hematoxylin and eosin; TP, touch preparation.

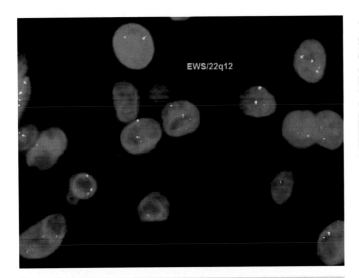

FIGURE 10.75 Extraskeletal myxoid chondrosarcoma. This FISH study is positive for *EWSR1* translocation. Hybridization with the *EWSR1* (22q12) break apart probe in this tumor identifies a chromosomal rearrangement in the *EWSR1* gene region, but not the specific gene-fusion partner. FISH, fluorescence in-situ hybridization.

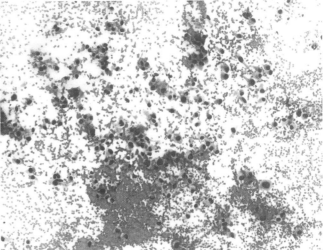

FIGURE 10.76 Epithelioid leiomyosarcoma. TP showing epithelioid smooth muscle tumor cells with abundant cytoplasm and pleomorphic round to oval nuclei. Positive immunohistochemistry for smooth muscle markers was required to confirm the diagnosis (DQ-stained TP, medium power). DQ, Diff-Quik; TP, touch preparation.

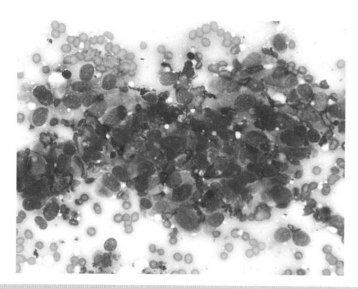

FIGURE 10.77   Epithelioid MPNST. TP showing large epithelioid cells with abundant cytoplasm and large vesicular nuclei with macronucleoli (DQ-stained TP, medium power). DQ, Diff-Quik; MPNST, malignant peripheral nerve sheath tumor; TP, touch preparation.

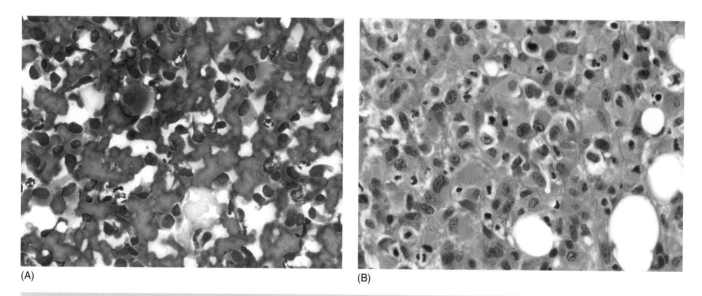

(A)   (B)

FIGURE 10.78   Epithelioid hemangioendothelioma. (A) TP showing discohesive pleomorphic epithelioid cells and a bloody background. Binucleated cells as shown in this specimen are a frequent finding. (B) Corresponding core biopsy showing a sheet of epithelioid cells. Note the scattered cells containing cytoplasmic vacuoles and intracytoplasmic endothelial lumina containing erythrocytes. ((A) DQ-stained TP, medium power; (B) H&E-stained core biopsy, medium power.) DQ, Diff-Quik; H&E, hematoxylin and eosin; TP, touch preparation.

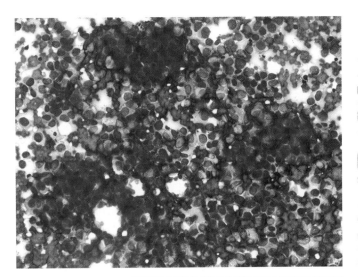

FIGURE 10.79 Metastatic melanoma. TP of this gluteus maximus mass shows numerous epithelioid melanoma cells. Clustering of tumor cells as in this case may mimic carcinoma (DQ-stained TP, medium power). DQ, Diff-Quik; TP, touch preparation.

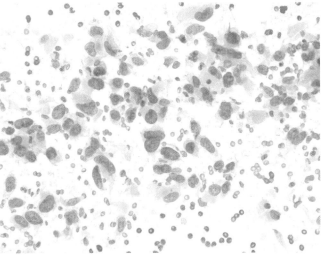

FIGURE 10.81 Epithelioid sarcoma. Multiple single, large epithelioid cells are shown with moderate cytoplasm and enlarged eccentric nuclei with irregular nuclear contours and vesicular chromatin (Pap-stained TP, medium power). TP, touch preparation.

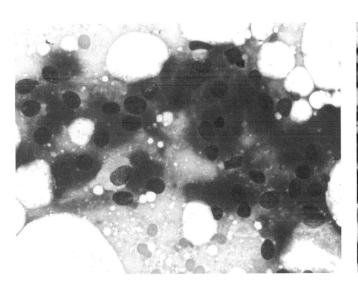

FIGURE 10.80 Granular cell tumor. TP showing several cells with indistinct cytoplasmic borders, abundant granular cytoplasm, and round to oval bland nuclei with an even dark chromatin pattern. There are also several naked nuclei present with a dirty granular background (DQ-stained TP, high power). DQ, Diff-Quik; TP, touch preparation.

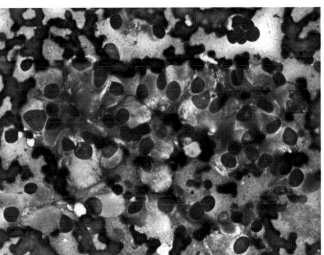

FIGURE 10.82 Clear cell sarcoma. TP showing noncohesive polygonal cells with abundant clear vacuolated cytoplasm and round, pleomorphic nuclei containing large nucleoli. Occasional naked nuclei are also seen in the background (DQ-stained TP, medium power). DQ, Diff-Quik; TP, touch preparation.

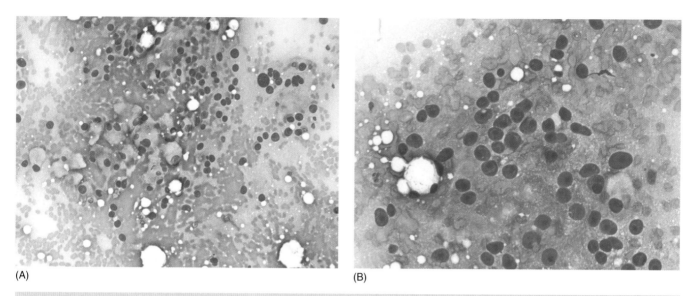

(A)

(B)

FIGURE 10.83 Alveolar soft part sarcoma. (A) TP showing dispersed cells with abundant cytoplasm and many naked nuclei. Binucleated cells can be identified. (B) Tumor cells have rounded nuclei with prominent central nucleoli. The bloody background also contains cytoplasmic debris. ((A) DQ-stained TP, low power; (B) DQ-stained TP, medium power.) DQ, Diff-Quik; TP, touch preparation.

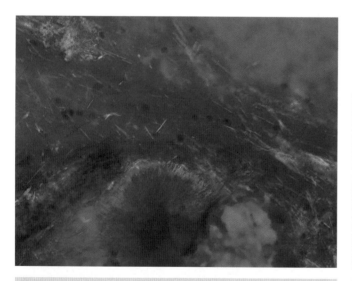

FIGURE 10.84 Tophaceous gout. Polarized touch preparation showing birefringent needle-shaped monosodium urate crystals.

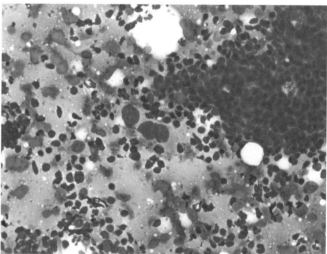

FIGURE 10.85 Classical Hodgkin lymphoma. TP of a chest wall soft tissue mass showing enlarged Reed–Sternberg cells associated with abundant lymphocytes and a few eosinophils (DQ-stained TP, medium power). DQ, Diff-Quik; TP, touch preparation.

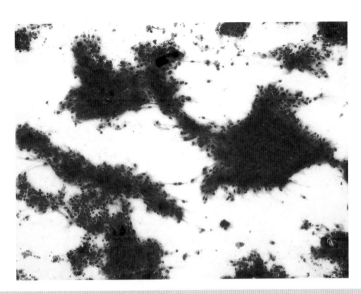

FIGURE 10.86 Tenosynovial giant cell tumor, diffuse type. Papillary structures containing mononuclear stromal features are a characteristic finding in PVNS (DQ-stained TP, medium power). DQ, Diff-Quik; PVNS, pigmented villonodular synovitis; TP, touch preparation.

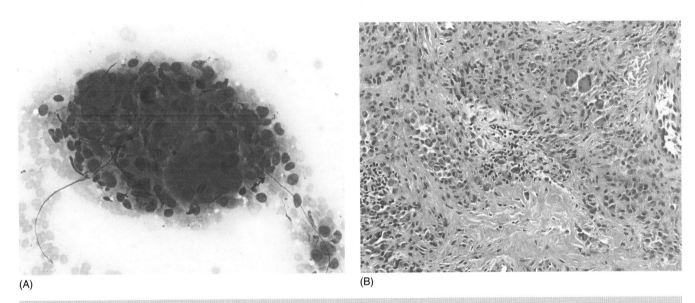

(A)

(B)

FIGURE 10.87 Tenosynovial giant cell tumor, diffuse type. (A) Cluster of cells showing mixed mononuclear stromal cells with an osteoclastic giant cell. Note the presence of brown hemosiderin pigment. (B) Corresponding histopathology showing mixed histiocytic stromal cells, osteoclast-like giant cells, fibrosis, and hemosiderin pigment. ((A) DQ-stained TP, high power; (B) H&E-stained core biopsy, medium power.) DQ, Diff-Quik; H&E, hematoxylin and eosin; TP, touch preparation.

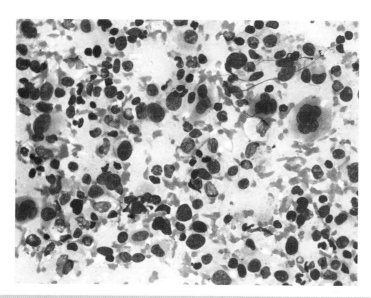

FIGURE 10.88 Pleomorphic leiomyosarcoma. TP showing many pleomorphic tumor cells of varying size (DQ-stained TP, medium power). DQ, Diff-Quik; TP, touch preparation.

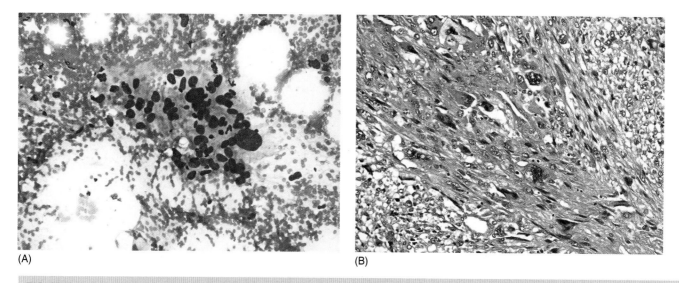

(A)   (B)

FIGURE 10.89 Undifferentiated pleomorphic sarcoma. (A) TP showing markedly pleomorphic tumor cells with stripped hyperchromatic nuclei. (B) Resected tumor showing a high-grade sarcoma with fascicles of pleomorphic tumor cells and scattered bizarre giant tumor cells. ((A) DQ-stained TP, medium power; (B) H&E-stained section, medium power.) DQ, Diff-Quik; H&E, hematoxylin and eosin; TP, touch preparation.

REFERENCES

1. Arora HL, Solanki RL, Poònia IJ. The role of imprint cytology in diagnosis of various bone and joint diseases. *Indian J Cancer.* 1990;27:38-45.
2. Kubik MJ, Bovbel A, Goli H, et al. Diagnostic value and accuracy of imprint cytology evaluation during image-guided core needle biopsies: review of our experience at a large academic center. *Diagn Cytopathol.* 2015;43:773-779.
3. Adams SC, Potter BK, Pitcher DJ, Temple HT. Office-based core needle biopsy of bone and soft tissue malignancies: an accurate alternative to open biopsy with infrequent complications. *Clin Orthop Relat Res.* 2010;468:2774-2780.
4. Huang AJ, Kattapuram SV. Musculoskeletal neoplasms: biopsy and intervention. *Radiol Clin North Am.* 2011;49:1287-1305.
5. Koscick RL, Petersilge CA, Makley JT, Abdul-Karim FW. CT-guided fine needle aspiration and needle core biopsy of skeletal lesions. Complementary diagnostic techniques. *Acta Cytol.* 1998;42:697-702.
6. Domanski HA, Akerman M, Carlén B, et al. Core-needle biopsy performed by the cytopathologist: a technique to complement fine-needle aspiration of soft tissue and bone lesions. *Cancer.* 2005;105:229-239.
7. Kubik MJ, Mohammadi A, Rosa M. Diagnostic benefits and cost-effectiveness of onsite imprint cytology adequacy evaluation of

core needle biopsies of bone lesions. *Diagn Cytopathol.* 2014;42:506-513.

8. Kim BK, Mooney NC, Mulcahy H, et al. Rapid onsite evaluation (ROSE) of touch preprarations from CT-guided bone biopsies: retrospective evaluation reveals that cases accompanied by ROSE have a higher diagnostic yield. *Mod Pathol* 2014;27:108A.

9. Bokun R. Correlation of imprint cytology and histopathologic findings in bone tumors. *J BUON.* 2002;7:257-260.

10. Bui MM, Smith P, Agresta SV, et al. Practical issues of intraoperative frozen section diagnosis of bone and soft tissue lesions. *Cancer Control.* 2008;15:7-12.

11. Wisanuyotin T, Mitchai J, Sirichativapee W, et al. Tissue imprint for intra-operative evaluation of musculoskeletal tumors. *J Med Assoc Thai.* 2009;92:654-659.

12. Bhaker P, Mohan H, Handa U, Kumar S. Role of intraoperative pathology consultation in skeletal tumors and tumor-like lesions. *Sarcoma.* 2014;2014:902104.

13. Paker IO, Sezak M, Doganavsargil B, et al. The value of touch imprint cytology of core needle biopsy in the diagnosis of spinal lesions. *Turk Neurosurg.* 2013;23:183-117.

14. Fletcher CDM, Bridge JA, Hogendoorn PCW, Mertens F. *WHO Classification of Tumours of Soft Tissue and Bone.* Lyon, France: IARC; 2013.

15. Cabay RJ, Reddy V, David O, et al. Cytologic features of primary chondroid tumors of bone in crush preparations. *Diagn Cytopathol.* 2008;36:758-761.

16. Fukuda T, Saito M, Nakajima T. Imprint cytology of chondroblastoma of bone. A case report. *Acta Cytol.* 1998;42:403-406.

17. VandenBussche CJ, Sathiyamoorthy S, Wakely PE Jr, Ali SZ. Chondroblastic osteosarcoma: cytomorphologic characteristics and differential diagnosis on FNA. *Cancer Cytopathol.* 2016;124:493-500.

18. Chhabra S, Chopra R, Handa U, et al. Cytomorphologic features of chondroid neoplasms: a comparative study. *Acta Cytol.* 2010;54:1101-1110.

19. Rinas AC, Ward WG, Kilpatrick SE. Potential sampling error in fine needle aspiration biopsy of dedifferentiated chondrosarcoma: a report of 4 cases. *Acta Cytol.* 2005;49:554-559.

20. Jiang XS, Pantanowitz L, Bui MM, et al. Clear cell chondrosarcoma: cytologic findings in six cases. *Diagn Cytopathol.* 2014;42:784-791.

21. Bhatia A, Ashokraj G. Cytological diversity of osteosarcoma. *Indian J Cancer.* 1992;29:56-60.

22. Sathiyamoorthy S, Ali SZ. Osteoblastic osteosarcoma: cytomorphologic characteristics and differential diagnosis on fine-needle aspiration. *Acta Cytol.* 2012;56:481-486.

23. Mehdi G, Siddiqui F, Maheshwari V, Khan AQ. Imprint smear cytology of chondroblastic osteosarcoma: a case report. *Diagn Cytopathol.* 2009;37:446-449.

24. Cabral LA, Werkman C, Brandão AA, Almeida JD. Imprint cytology of osteosarcoma of the jaw: a case report. *J Med Case Rep.* 2009;3:9327.

25. Nagira K, Yamamoto T, Akisue T, et al. Scrape and fine-needle aspiration cytology of extraskeletal osteosarcoma. *Diagn Cytopathol.* 2002;27:177-180.

26. Mokhtari M, Kumar PV, Rezazadeh S. Confusing cytological findings in myositis ossificans. *Acta Cytol.* 2012;56:565-570.

27. Huening MA, Reddy S, Dodd LG. Fine-needle aspiration of fibrous dysplasia of bone: a worthwhile endeavor or not? *Diagn Cytopathol.* 2008;36:325-330.

28. Bishop JA, Shum CH, Sheth S, et al.. Small cell osteosarcoma: cytopathologic characteristics and differential diagnosis. *Am J Clin Pathol.* 2010;133:756-761.

29. Akerman M, Domanski HA, Jonsson K. Cytological features of bone tumours in FNA smears V: giant-cell lesions. *Monogr Clin Cytol.* 2010;19:55-61.

30. Vetrani A, Fulciniti F, Boschi R, et al. Fine needle aspiration biopsy diagnosis of giant-cell tumor of bone. An experience with nine cases. *Acta Cytol.* 1990;34:863-867.

31. Crapanzano JP, Ali SZ, Ginsberg MS, Zakowski MF. Chordoma: a cytologic study with histologic and radiologic correlation. *Cancer.* 2001;93:40-51.

32. Layfield LJ. Cytologic differential diagnosis of myxoid and mucinous neoplasms of the sacrum and parasacral soft tissues. *Diagn Cytopathol.* 2003;28:264-271.

33. Jo VY, Hornick JL, Qian X. Utility of brachyury in distinction of chordoma from cytomorphologic mimics in fine-needle aspiration and core needle biopsy. *Diagn Cytopathol.* 2014;42:647-652.

34. Bishop JA, Ali SZ. Primary tibial adamantinoma diagnosed by fine needle aspiration. *Diagn Cytopathol.* 2010;38:198-201.

35. Woodard A, Jaffe R, Monaco S, et al. Cytopathology of osseous and non-osseous Langerhans cell histiocytosis. *J Am Soc Cytopathol.* 2012;1(1S):S117.

36. Deshpande V, Rosenberg AE, Nielsen GP. Metastatic tumors. In: Nielsen GP, Rosenberg AE, et al., eds. *Diagnostic Pathology: Bone.* Altona, Canada: Amirsys; 2013:14-2–14-7.

37. Khalbuss WE, Parwani AV. *Cytopathology of Soft Tissue and Bone Lesions.* New York, NY: Springer; 2011.

38. Klijanienko J, Caillaud JM, Lagacé R. Fine-needle aspiration in liposarcoma: cytohistologic correlative study including well-differentiated, myxoid, and pleomorphic variants. *Diagn Cytopathol.* 2004;30:307-312.

39. Ocque R, Khalbuss WE, Monaco SE, et al. Cytopathology of extracranial ectopic and metastatic meningiomas. *Acta Cytol.* 2014;58:1-8.

40. Allison DB, Wakely PE Jr, Siddiqui MT, Ali SZ. Nodular fasciitis: a frequent diagnostic pitfall on fine-needle aspiration. *Cancer.* 2017;125:20-29.

41. Shin C, Low I, Ng D, et al. USP6 gene rearrangement in nodular fasciitis and histological mimics. *Histopathology.* 2016;69:784-791.

42. Klijanienko J, Caillaud JM, Lagacé R. Cytohistologic correlations in schwannomas (neurilemmomas), including "ancient," cellular, and epithelioid variants. *Diagn Cytopathol.* 2006;34:517-522.

43. Gupta N, Barwad A, Katamuthu K, et al. Solitary fibrous tumour: a diagnostic challenge for the cytopathologist. *Cytopathology.* 2012;23:250-255.

44. Khairwa A, Dey P, Nada R. Fine needle aspiration cytology of malignant solitary fibrous tumour. *Cytopathology.* 2015;26:391-393.

45. Domanski HA, Akerman M, Rissler P, Gustafson P. Fine-needle aspiration of soft tissue leiomyosarcoma: an analysis of the most common cytologic findings and the value of ancillary techniques. *Diagn Cytopathol.* 2006;34:597-604.

46. Akerman M, Domanski HA. The complex cytological features of synovial sarcoma in fine needle aspirates, an analysis of four illustrative cases. *Cytopathology.* 2007;18:234-240.

47. Gamborino E, Carrilho C, Ferro J, et al. Fine-needle aspiration diagnosis of Kaposi's sarcoma in a developing country. *Diagn Cytopathol.* 2000;23:322-325.

48. Klijanienko J, Caillaud JM, Lagacé R, Vielh P. Cytohistologic correlations in angiosarcoma including classic and epithelioid variants: Institut Curie's experience. *Diagn Cytopathol.* 2003;29:140-145.

49. Thapliyal N, Joshi U, Vaibhav G, et al. Pilomatricoma mimicking small round cell tumor on fine needle aspiration cytology: a case report. *Acta Cytol.* 2008;52:627-630.

50. Das DK. Fine-needle aspiration (FNA) cytology diagnosis of small round cell tumors: value and limitations. *Indian J Pathol Microbiol.* 2004;47:309-318.

51. Rajwanshi A, Srinivas R, Upasana G. Malignant small round cell tumors. *J Cytol.* 2009;26:1-10.

52. Klijanienko J, Caillaud JM, Orbach D, et al. Cyto-histological correlations in primary, recurrent and metastatic rhabdomyosarcoma: the institut Curie's experience. *Diagn Cytopathol.* 2007;35:482-487.

53. Atahan S, Aksu O, Ekinci C. Cytologic diagnosis and subtyping of rhabdomyosarcoma. *Cytopathology.* 1998;9:389-397.

54. Renshaw AA, Perez-Atayde AR, Fletcher JA, Granter SR. Cytology of typical and atypical Ewing's sarcoma/PNET. *Am J Clin Pathol.* 1996;106:620-624.

55. Guiter GE, Gamboni MM, Zakowski MF. The cytology of extraskeletal Ewing sarcoma. *Cancer.* 1999;87:141-148.

56. Klijanienko J, Colin P, Couturier J, et al. Fine-needle aspiration in desmoplastic small round cell tumor: a report of 10 new tumors in 8 patients with clinicopathological and molecular correlations with review of the literature. *Cancer Cytopathol.* 2014;122:386-393.

57. González-Cámpora R, Otal-Salaverri C, Hevia-Vázquez A, et al. Fine needle aspiration in myxoid tumors of the soft tissues. *Acta Cytol.* 1990;34:179-191.

58. Wakely PE Jr. Myxomatous soft tissue tumors: correlation of cytopathology and histopathology. *Ann Diagn Pathol.* 1999;3:227-242.

59. Evans HL. Low-grade fibromyxoid sarcoma: a clinicopathologic study of 33 cases with long-term follow-up. *Am J Surg Pathol.* 2011;35:1450-1462.

60. Olson MT, Ali SZ. Myxofibrosarcoma: cytomorphologic findings and differential diagnosis on fine needle aspiration. *Acta Cytol.* 2012;56:15-24.

61. Jakowski JD, Wakely PE Jr. Cytopathology of extraskeletal myxoid chondrosarcoma: report of 8 cases. *Cancer.* 2007;111:298-305.

62. Rekhi B, Singh N. Spectrum of cytopathologic features of epithelioid sarcoma in a series of 7 uncommon cases with immunohistochemical results, including loss of INI1/SMARCB1 in two test cases. *Diagn Cytopathol.* 2016;44:636-642.

63. Gupta K, Dey P, Goldsmith R, Vasishta RK. Comparison of cytologic features of giant-cell tumor and giant-cell tumor of tendon sheath. *Diagn Cytopathol.* 2004;30:14-18.

64. Batra VV, Jain S, Singh DK, Kumar N. Cytomorphologic spectrum of giant cell tumor of tendon sheath. *Acta Cytol.* 2008;52:152-158.

65. Ho CY, Maleki Z. Giant cell tumor of tendon sheath: cytomorphologic and radiologic findings in 41 patients. *Diagn Cytopathol.* 2012;40(suppl 2):E94-E98.

CHAPTER 11

Central Nervous System

Julia Kofler

INTRODUCTION

In surgical neuropathology, cytological preparations are primarily used in the context of intraoperative evaluations. They have several distinct advantages over frozen sections including elimination of freezing artifact, better nuclear and cytoplasmic detail, sampling of different specimen areas, faster turnaround time, and minimal tissue use permitting tissue preservation for permanent sections and ancillary studies (1,2). Frozen sections are superior for evaluation of architectural features, for cohesive tumors and assessment of tumor margins.

Different types of cytological preparations are used for intraoperative diagnostic evaluation of neuropathology cases, depending on tumor location and anticipated differential diagnosis. The most commonly used technique for intra-axial lesions is the smear preparation, which provides important information about cell processes and tumor matrix. Touch preparations are valuable for evaluation of discohesive lesions and are most commonly employed for evaluation of pituitary lesions, but may also be useful in the assessment of abscesses, lymphomas, plasma cell neoplasms, some metastatic tumors, or meningiomas. Lastly, touch or smear preparations may be helpful in the evaluation of bone-infiltrating lesions such as epidural tumors when frozen sections are not feasible.

If specimen size permits, touch preparations should be performed on the freshly cut surface after bisecting the tissue sample. With smaller specimens, the entire tissue sample is touched to the glass slide, attempting to preferentially examine noncauterized and nonhemorrhagic specimen areas.

SELLAR REGION

The most commonly encountered sellar region specimen in the frozen section room is the pituitary adenoma with the surgeon requesting a determination between adenoma and normal pituitary tissue. Touch preparations are ideally suited for this distinction. Rarely, other nonneoplastic and neoplastic lesions are encountered.

Normal Pituitary

Distinction between normal pituitary and adenoma relies primarily on architectural characteristics and much less on cytological features. The acinar architecture of normal pituitary with its reticulin-rich fibrovascular septa will restrict release of cells onto the slide during a touch preparation resulting in a paucicellular preparation (Figure 11.1). Occasionally, when mapping the extent of an adenoma, a fragment of normal neurohypophysis is submitted by the neurosurgeon. Given the glial nature of the posterior pituitary, the tissue is more cohesive and little is usually released onto the slide during a touch prep (Figure 11.2).

Pituitary Adenoma

Pituitary adenomas are characterized by effacement of the normal pituitary acinar architecture and decreased reticulin network resulting in increased shedding of cells during a touch preparation, usually permitting easy distinction from normal pituitary gland (Figures 11.3–11.5). Occasionally, when an adenoma has infiltrated fibroconnective tissue (e.g., capsule), this architectural feature may be lost resulting in a paucicellular touch prep. The adenoma cells are usually uniform in appearance with round nuclei, scant cytoplasm, and fine salt-and-pepper chromatin (3). In pituitary apoplexy, an adenoma undergoes infarction, which can be recognized on a touch prep by the presence of necrotic cells (Figure 11.6) and occasionally admixed neutrophils.

Other Neoplastic and Nonneoplastic Lesions of the Sellar Region

A variety of other neoplastic and nonneoplastic lesions may be occasionally encountered in the sellar region. Granular cell tumor, spindle cell oncocytoma, and pituicytoma arise from the neurohypophysis including infundibulum and are thought to represent a spectrum of a single nosological entity characterized by nuclear TTF-1 (thyroid transcription factor 1) expression (4,5). The cytological features of these lesions are better appreciated on a smear than a touch preparation, which is usually hypocellular due to the cohesive nature of the tissue. Pituicytomas are composed of bland spindle cells, whereas granular cell tumors consist of spindle or plump cells with a granular cytoplasm, and spindle cell oncocytomas exhibit an oncocytic cytoplasm (Figures 11.7 and 11.8). A definitive distinction between these three entities may be difficult during intraoperative evaluation.

Two variants of craniopharyngioma can be distinguished based on histomorphological and molecular features. Adamantinomatous craniopharyngiomas are characterized by cohesive sheets of basaloid epithelial cells with peripheral palisading and wet keratin (Figures 11.9 and 11.10) and may be accompanied by degenerative changes with foamy macrophages, multinucleated giant cells, inflammation, and cholesterol clefts (Figures 11.11 and 11.16). The intervening stellate reticulum is better appreciated on permanent sections than intraoperative touch or smear preparations. Papillary craniopharyngiomas are composed of mature nonkeratinizing squamous epithelium and lack wet keratin (Figure 11.12). On a molecular level, adamantinomatous craniopharyngiomas are characterized by WNT (Wingless-related integration site) signaling activation due to beta–catenin mutations leading to nuclear beta–catenin accumulation detectable by immunohistochemical staining. On the other hand, the majority of papillary craniopharyngiomas harbor a *BRAF* V600E mutation (4,6).

Although rare, metastatic tumors may be occasionally encountered in the sellar region. Metastatic squamous cell carcinomas exhibit a higher degree of nuclear pleomorphism (Figure 11.13) than the mature squamous epithelium in craniopharyngiomas or squamous metaplasia in Rathke's cleft cysts. Epidermoid cysts and teratomas may also enter the differential diagnosis of squamous lesions in this region.

Rathke's cleft cysts are lined by ciliated respiratory epithelium, contain goblet cells or squamous metaplasia in some cases, and are filled with amorphous cyst contents (Figures 11.14 and 11.15). It is important to keep in mind that many sellar region surgeries are performed using an endonasal approach, resulting in occasional nasal respiratory epithelium contaminants on the slide.

Several lesions in the sellar region may undergo degenerative changes with a xanthogranulomatous reaction, including craniopharyngiomas, pituitary adenomas, and ruptured Rathke's cleft cysts. In these instances, foamy macrophages, degenerating cells, and multinucleated giant cells may be encountered (Figure 11.16).

Central nervous system (CNS) germ cell tumors occur most frequently in pineal and pituitary regions. Similar to their counterparts outside the CNS, germinomas arising in the CNS are characterized by dual cell populations (Figure 11.17). The tumor cells are large with prominent nucleoli and are admixed with small reactive lymphocytes and sometimes granulomatous inflammation with multinucleated giant cells.

After involvement of craniofacial bones and skull base, the sellar region is the most common location for intracranial Langerhans cell histiocytosis (LCH). Similar to LCH elsewhere in the body, the cytologic features include the presence of Langerhans cells and a mixed inflammatory infiltrate (Figure 11.18).

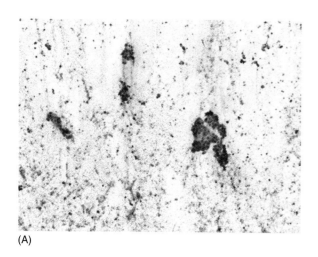

(A)

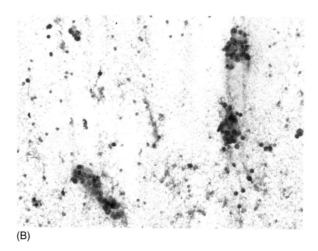

(B)

FIGURE 11.1 Normal adenohypophysis. Normal anterior pituitary gland is characterized by an acinar architecture with reticulin-rich fibrovascular septa that restrict release of cells on to a glass slide. A TP of normal pituitary will only show a few small clusters of cells with neuroendocrine features. The mixed cell types of normal adenohypophysis are often not apparent. ((A) and (B) H&E-stained, low power.) H&E, hematoxylin and eosin; TP, touch preparation.

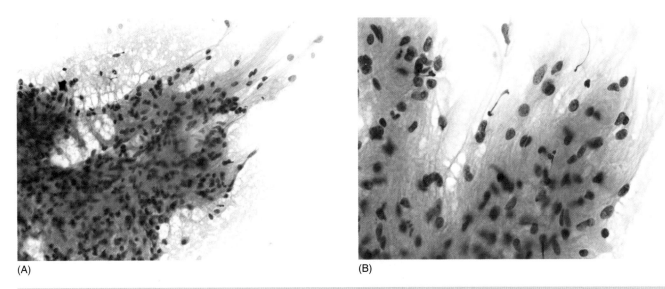

(A)
(B)

FIGURE 11.2 Normal infundibulum/neurohypophysis. The glial tissue of normal posterior pituitary is composed of elongated cells in a fibrillary background, which is usually better appreciated in a smear preparation. A pituicytoma is characterized by higher cellularity and somewhat lower fibrillarity, but distinction from normal posterior pituitary may be difficult in the frozen section room. (H&E-stained, (A) low power; (B) high power.) H&E, hematoxylin and eosin.

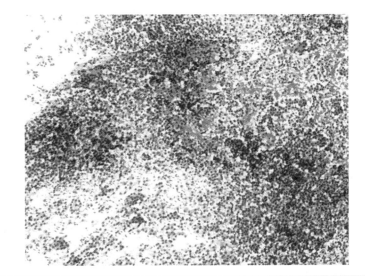

FIGURE 11.3 Pituitary adenoma. Unlike nonneoplastic anterior pituitary, touch preparations of an adenoma demonstrate abundant cells filling the entire microscopic field (H&E-stained, low power). H&E, hematoxylin and eosin.

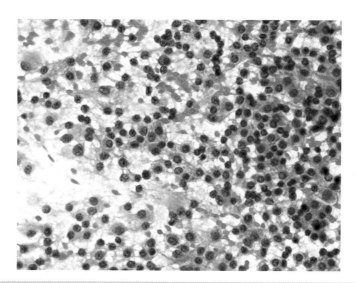

FIGURE 11.4 Pituitary adenoma. Higher magnification demonstrates a rather monotonous population of cells with round nuclei and salt-and-pepper chromatin. Nucleoli are usually small and inconspicuous. Some nuclear pleomorphism and occasional binucleation may be seen, but these features may also be encountered in nonneoplastic pituitary and do not allow a definitive distinction (H&E-stained, high power). H&E, hematoxylin and eosin.

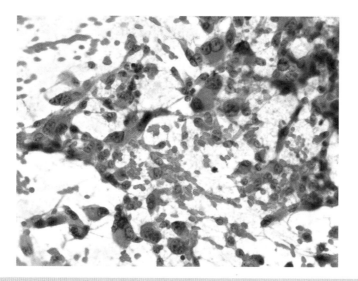

FIGURE 11.5 Pituitary adenoma. In rare instances, a higher degree of nuclear pleomorphism may be present (H&E-stained, high power). H&E, hematoxylin and eosin.

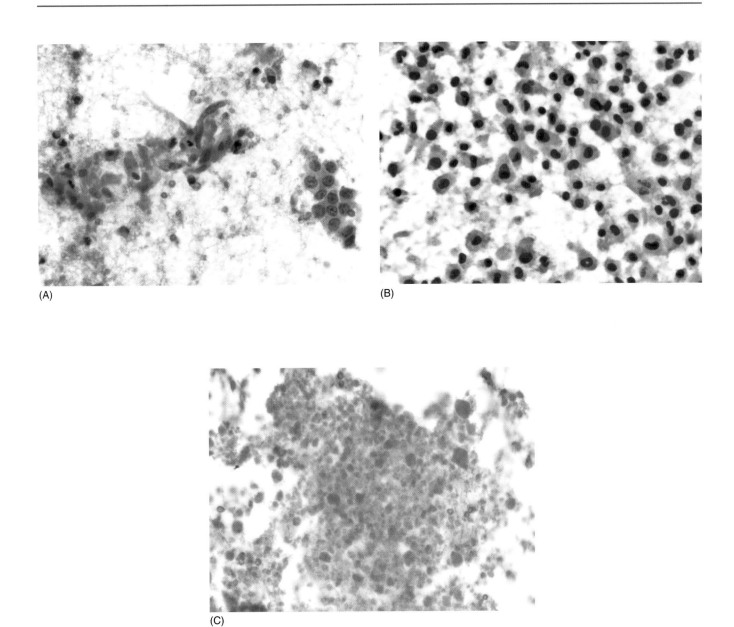

FIGURE 11.6 Pituitary apoplexy. Pituitary adenomas may undergo infarction resulting in nuclear pyknosis and cytoplasmic eosinophilia (A and B) and, eventually, anuclear necrotic cells (C). Admixed neutrophils may be seen in some cases. ((A)–(C) H&E-stained, high power.) H&E, hematoxylin and eosin.

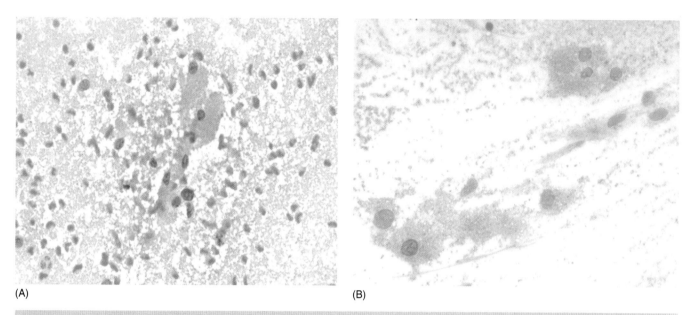

(A)   (B)

FIGURE 11.7 Granular cell tumor. Both pituicytomas and granular cell tumors derive from pituicytes and may present as intra- or suprasellar lesions. Unlike pituicytomas, granular cell tumors do not appear astrocytic but are composed of polygonal cells with granular cytoplasm and bland nuclei. ((A) and (B) H&E-stained, high power.) Note that these fragile cells disrupt easily when manipulated, resulting in a granular background when their cytoplasmic contents get spilled on to the slide. H&E, hematoxylin and eosin.

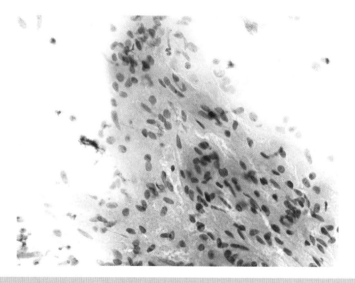

FIGURE 11.8 Spindle cell oncocytoma. These pituitary neoplasms are composed of eosinophilic spindle cells rich in mitochondria (H&E-stained, low power). H&E, hematoxylin and eosin.

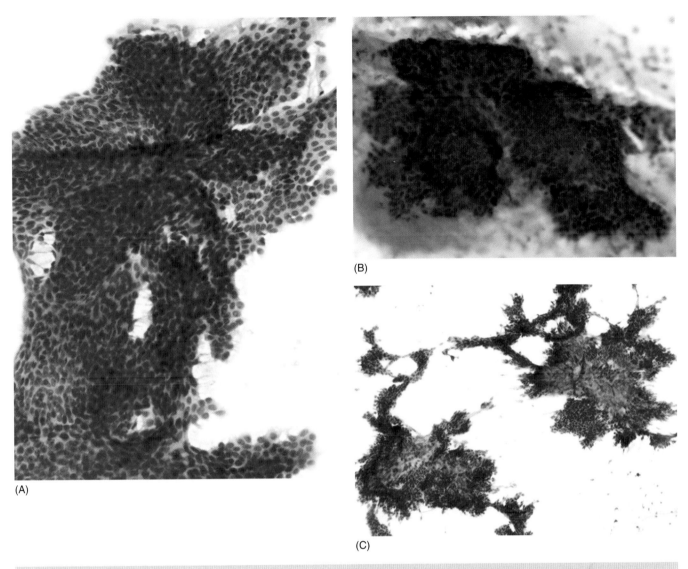

FIGURE 11.9 Adamantinomatous craniopharyngioma. This more common craniopharyngioma subtype is composed of cohesive sheets of basaloid epithelial cells with peripheral palisading. The epithelial sheets often form complex folds on intraoperative touch and smear preparations. ((A)–(C) H&E-stained, low power.) H&E, hematoxylin and eosin.

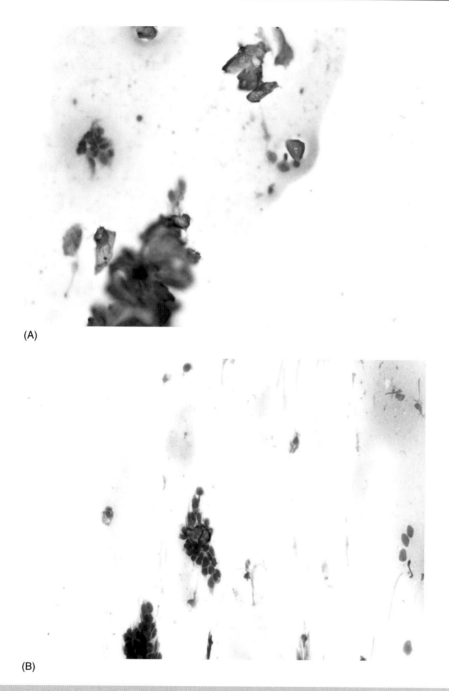

(A)

(B)

FIGURE 11.10 Adamantinomatous craniopharyngioma. The presence of "wet keratin" is a characteristic feature of adamantinomatous craniopharyngioma and consists of anuclear squamous cells, which may become calcified. ((A) and (B) H&E-stained, low power.) H&E, hematoxylin and eosin.

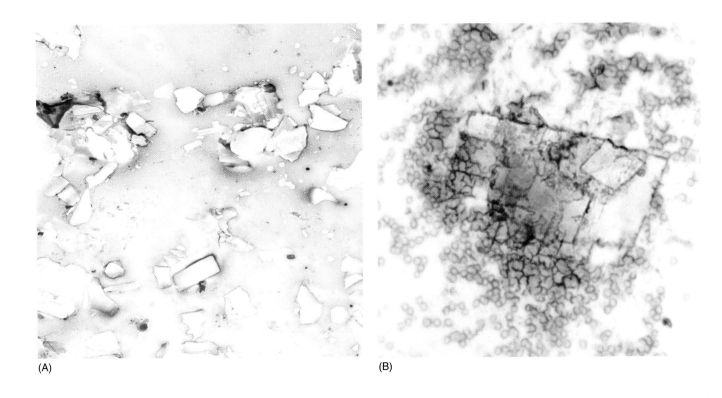

(A)

(B)

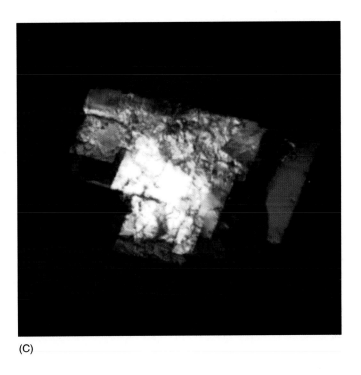

(C)

FIGURE 11.11 Adamantinomatous craniopharyngioma. Cystic areas are filled with "machine oil-like" fluid containing numerous polygonal cholesterol crystals. ((A) H&E-stained, low power; (B) unstained, high power; (C) same area as in image (B), viewed under polarizing filter, high power.) H&E, hematoxylin and eosin.

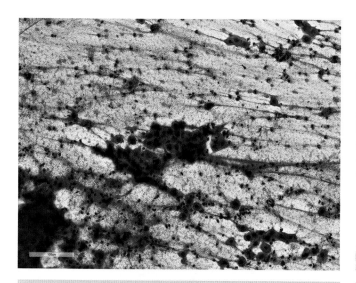

FIGURE 11.12 Papillary craniopharyngioma. This variant is composed of squamous epithelium with more distinct cell borders. It lacks the basaloid features, wet keratin, and stellate reticulum of adamantinomatous variants (H&E-stained, low power). H&E, hematoxylin and eosin.

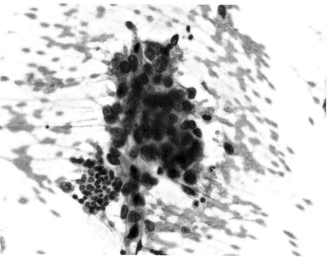

FIGURE 11.13 Metastatic squamous cell carcinoma. Metastatic squamous cell carcinomas usually demonstrate a higher degree of cellular pleomorphism (H&E-stained, high power). H&E, hematoxylin and eosin.

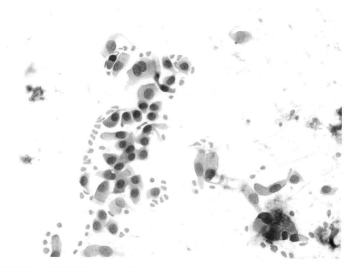

FIGURE 11.14 Rathke's cleft cyst. The cyst lining consists of ciliated respiratory epithelium, admixed with goblet cells and squamous metaplasia in some cases (H&E-stained, high power). H&E, hematoxylin and eosin.

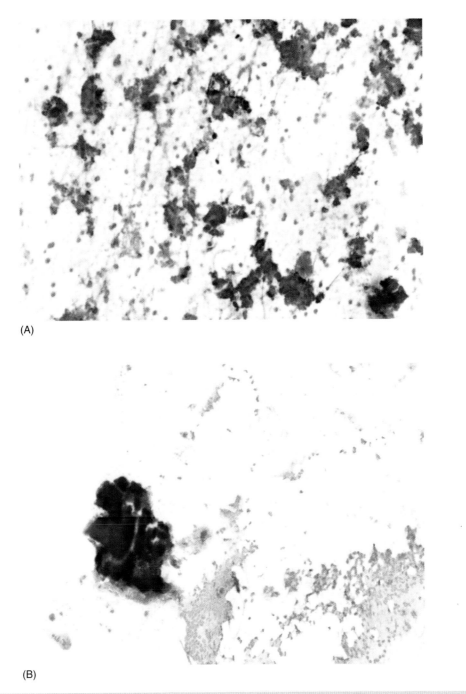

(A)

(B)

FIGURE 11.15 Rathke's cleft cyst. In some cases, only amorphous cyst contents may be seen. ((A) and (B) H&E-stained, low power.) H&E, hematoxylin and eosin.

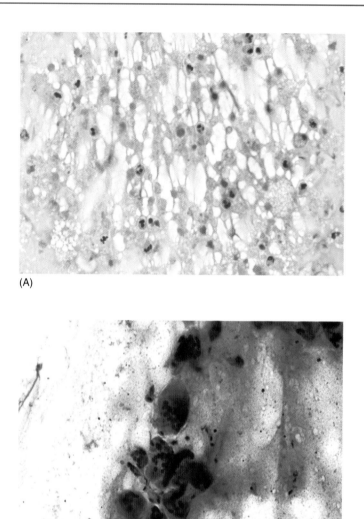

(A)

(B)

FIGURE 11.16 Xanthogranulomatous change. Degenerative changes with a xanthogranulomatous reaction may be present focally or extensively in several sellar lesions, including craniopharyngiomas, pituitary adenomas, and ruptured Rathke's cleft cysts. On a TP, only a few foamy macrophages and degenerating cells may be seen (A). Sometimes, foreign-type, multinucleated giant cells may be visualized (B). (H&E-stained, (A) high power; (B) low power.) H&E, hematoxylin and eosin; TP, touch preparation.

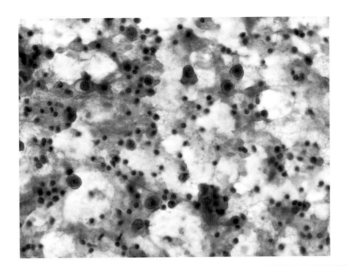

FIGURE 11.17 Germinoma. These tumors are typically composed of large round tumor cells with prominent nucleoli, admixed with a population of small reactive lymphocytes (H&E-stained, high power). H&E, hematoxylin and eosin.

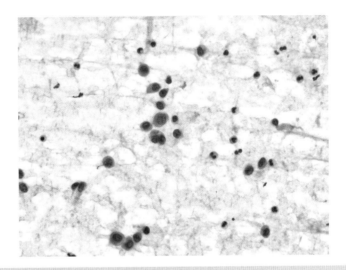

FIGURE 11.18 LCH. LCH is composed of Langerhans cells with irregular grooved and clefted "coffee bean" nuclei, variably admixed with eosinophils, lymphocytes, histiocytes, and multinucleated cells. Eosinophils may not appear very eosinophilic on touch and smear preparations (H&E-stained, high power). H&E, hematoxylin and eosin; LCH, Langerhans cell histiocytosis.

EXTRA-AXIAL LESIONS

Touch preparations are of variable value in the evaluation of extra-axial lesions. Many meningiomas and metastatic tumors release sufficient cellular material on to the slide for diagnostic evaluation. On the other hand, touch preparations of many other neoplastic spindle-cell lesions only yield some blood, but no diagnostic cells or tissue fragments, therefore requiring smear preparations or frozen sections instead for evaluation.

Meningioma

Meningiomas are the most common dural-based neoplasms. They can exhibit a variety of different morphologic growth patterns (4), but the vast majority of tumors show distinctive cytologic features on intraoperative touch preparations (1,2,7). Typically, slides show cohesive clusters of cells with indistinct cell borders, wispy cytoplasm, and broad-based processes. Nuclei are ovoid with delicate chromatin and small nucleoli, and often exhibit nuclear pseudoinclusions. Whorls are diagnostic of meningothelial lesions, but are not seen in all meningiomas (Figures 11.19–11.23).

Although most meningiomas are World Health Organization (WHO) grade 1 lesions, increased mitotic activity, brain invasion, specific growth patterns, or atypical features indicate higher grade lesions (Figures 11.24 and 11.25). These atypical features include necrosis, high nuclear:cytoplasmic (N:C) ratio, small cell change, prominent nucleoli, and sheeting for grade 2 atypical meningiomas. Frankly malignant cytology is present in grade 3 anaplastic meningiomas. The latter may be indistinguishable from metastatic neoplasms on intraoperative evaluation. While definitive grading is usually performed on permanent sections, sometimes higher grade features may be recognized on intraoperative touch preparations.

Other Extra-axial Neoplasms

A wide spectrum of mesenchymal tumors can rarely present as dural-based or extra-axial masses (3). Their detailed discussion is beyond the scope of this chapter. Touch preparations are usually of very limited value in the evaluation of these tumors as most of them are very cohesive and do not shed diagnostic material on to the slide (Figures 11.26 and 11.27). Depending on tumor location, the differential diagnosis of a spindle cell neoplasm may include fibrous meningioma, solitary fibrous tumor/hemangiopericytoma,

schwannoma, and other uncommon neoplasms. Frozen section evaluation, and in many cases permanent sections, and immunohistochemical staining are required for definitive diagnosis.

Chordomas are one of the few mesenchymal neoplasms that exhibit characteristic features on intraoperative cytological preparations (Figure 11.28). They typically present as clival or sacral midline masses and are composed of epithelioid cells arranged in cords and lobules admixed with a myxoid matrix. Chordomas are composed of large cells with clear to eosinophilic cytoplasm and contain characteristic physaliphorous cells, which are typified by abundant vacuolated cytoplasm (1,8). Immunohistochemical reactivity for cytokeratins, epithelial membrane antigen (EMA), S100, and specifically brachyury allows definitive distinction from chondrosarcomas and chordoid meningiomas.

Metastatic tumors are one of the main considerations in the differential diagnosis of meningiomas. Metastatic carcinomas often present as tissue fragments composed of cells with higher N:C ratios compared to meningiomas, larger nuclei, sharp cell borders and no distinct cell processes, and often display mitotic activity (Figure 11.29). The presence of intra- or extracellular mucin or intracellular pigment provides further support for a diagnosis of metastatic adenocarcinoma or melanoma, respectively.

Dermoid cysts are distinguished from the more prevalent epidermoid cysts by the presence of adnexal structures in the cyst wall. They also show a different preferential distribution within the CNS. Epidermoid cysts are frequently seen in the cerebellopontine angle or suprasellar region, whereas dermoid cysts commonly occur along the posterior fossa midline. Both cyst types are lined by keratinizing squamous epithelium and contain flaky "dry" keratin (Figure 11.30), which is often the predominant material on intraoperative touch preparations and distinctively different from the wet keratin seen with adamantinomatous craniopharyngiomas (Figure 11.10).

Spinal Epidural Tumors

Frequently encountered extra-axial spinal lesions include meningiomas, nerve sheath tumors, hematopoietic neoplasms (Figures 11.31 and 11.32), and metastatic tumors (Figure 11.33). Touch preparations may be particularly useful in situations where a predominantly bony specimen is submitted by the surgeon.

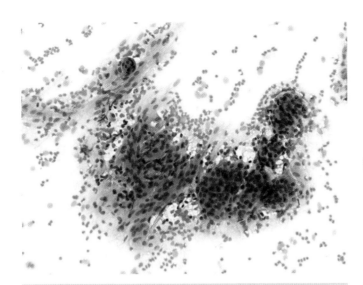

FIGURE 11.19 Meningioma. TP of a meningioma showing typical small cell clusters and tissue fragments in a lobular arrangement (H&E-stained, medium power). H&E, hematoxylin and eosin; TP, touch preparation.

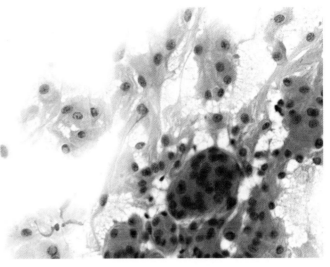

FIGURE 11.20 Meningioma. The cytologic features of meningothelial tumor cells are best appreciated in individual cells or at the edge of tissue fragments. Meningioma cells have ovoid nuclei with delicate chromatin, small nucleoli, and occasional nuclear pseudoinclusions. The cytoplasm is wispy with indistinct cell borders and broad-based processes, unlike the fibrillary processes of gliomas (H&E-stained, high power). H&E, hematoxylin and eosin.

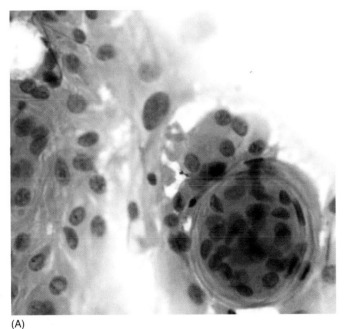

(A)

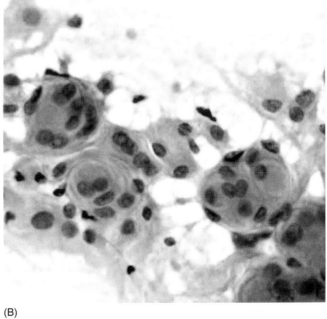

(B)

FIGURE 11.21 Meningioma. TP of a meningioma demonstrating diagnostic whorls ((A) and (B) H&E-stained, high power.) H&E, hematoxylin and eosin; TP, touch preparation.

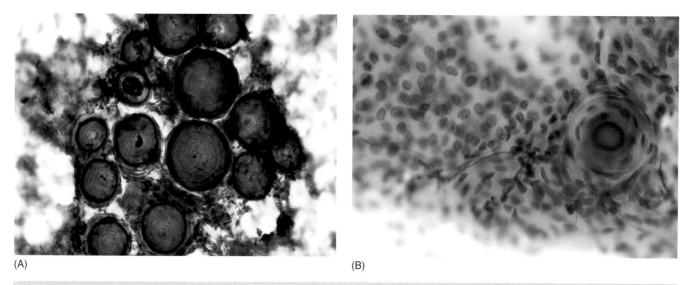

(A)   (B)

FIGURE 11.22 Meningioma. Psammoma bodies can be seen in many meningiomas with variable frequency. At the extreme end with the psammomatous meningioma variant, psammoma bodies are the predominant feature. Their characteristic concentric nature is best viewed under the microscope without a condenser. (H&E-stained, (A) medium power, viewed without condenser; (B) high power, viewed with condenser.) H&E, hematoxylin and eosin.

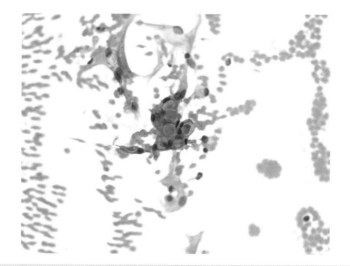

FIGURE 11.23 Secretory meningioma. Some meningioma variants can be readily identified on touch or smear preparations. Secretory meningiomas contain characteristic cytoplasmic eosinophilic inclusions (pseudopsammoma bodies). While secretory meningiomas are typically WHO grade 1 lesions, they may be associated with a significant amount of edema in adjacent brain tissue (H&E-stained, high power). H&E, hematoxylin and eosin; WHO, World Health Organization.

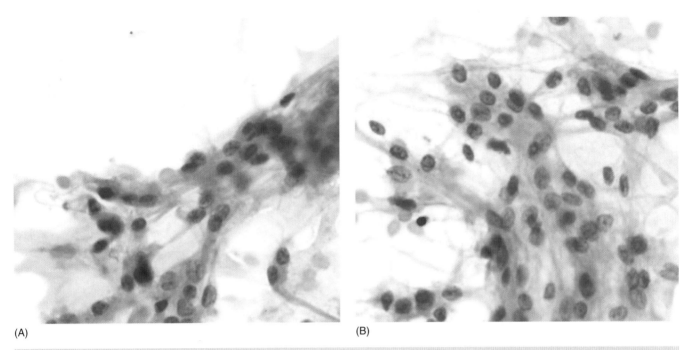

(A)

(B)

FIGURE 11.24 Chordoid meningioma. This meningioma subtype is characterized by cords of tumor cells embedded in a myxoid background. Chordoid features can be seen focally in some meningiomas. If chordoid features predominate, the meningioma is by definition classified as a WHO grade 2 lesion. Evaluation of permanent sections is required for assessment of extent of chordoid morphology and definitive grading. Chordoma is the main differential diagnosis of a chordoid meningioma near the midline of the skull base. The absence of physaliphorous cells (see Figure 11.28) and the recognition of meningothelial cytologic features aid in the distinction between these two entities. ((A) and (B) H&E-stained, high power.) H&E, hematoxylin and eosin; WHO, World Health Organization.

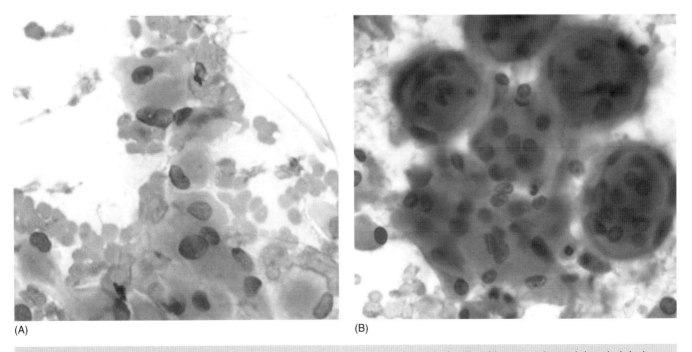

(A)

(B)

FIGURE 11.25 Rhabdoid meningioma. This meningioma variant is composed of cells with eccentric nuclei and globular eosinophilic cytoplasmic inclusions (A). If rhabdoid morphology is the predominant feature, the meningioma is by definition a WHO grade 3 tumor. Rhabdoid cells can be admixed with more conventional meningioma cells (B), aiding in establishing the diagnosis of meningioma. ((A) and (B) H&E-stained, high power.) H&E, hematoxylin and eosin; WHO, World Health Organization.

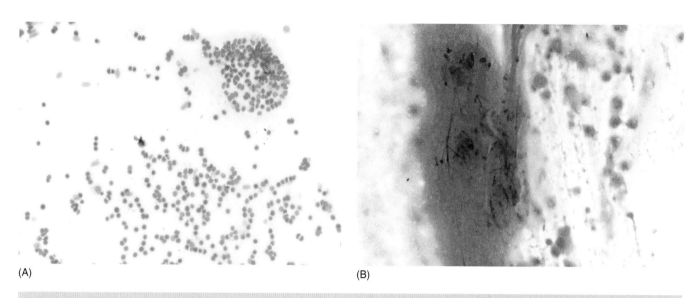

(A)   (B)

FIGURE 11.26 Nondiagnostic TP. In many instances, TPs of cohesive mesenchymal neoplasms only show blood (A) or scant, nondiagnostic tissue fragments as in this example of a schwannoma (B). (H&E-stained, (A) medium power; (B) low power.) H&E, hematoxylin and eosin; TP, touch preparation.

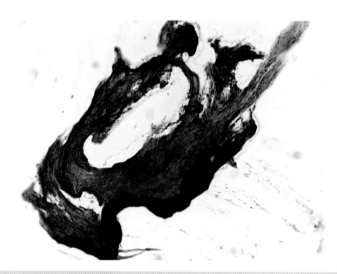

FIGURE 11.27 Spindle cell neoplasm. In this example of an SFT, a spindle cell tissue fragment was released during TP (H&E-stained, low power). H&E, hematoxylin and eosin; SFT, solitary fibrous tumor; TP, touch preparation.

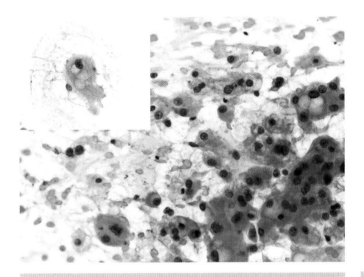

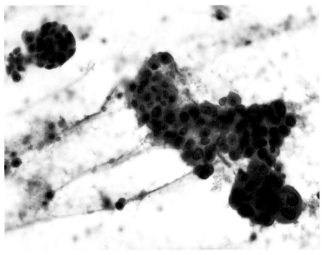

FIGURE 11.28 Chordoma. The cells have eosinophilic, variably vacuolated cytoplasm with distinct cell borders and usually bland nuclei, but variable nuclear pleomorphism may be encountered in some cases. Physaliphorous cells (inset) are the hallmark feature of chordomas but may be difficult to find (H&E-stained, high power). H&E, hematoxylin and eosin.

FIGURE 11.29 Metastatic carcinoma. These are typically composed of cohesive clusters of cells with distinct cell borders, high N:C ratio, and prominent nucleoli as in this example (H&E-stained, high power; see also sections "Spinal Epidural Tumors" and "Metastatic Neoplasms"). H&E, hematoxylin and eosin; N:C, nuclear:cytoplasmic.

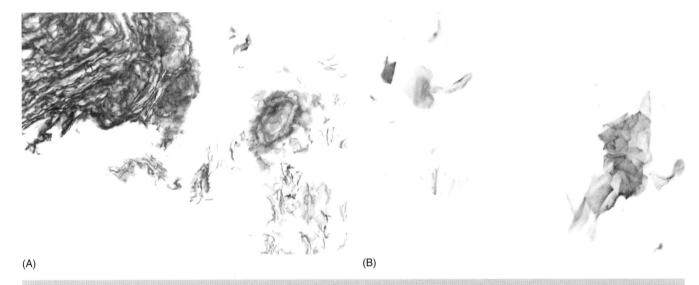

(A)   (B)

FIGURE 11.30 Epidermoid cyst. The predominant finding on TP is cyst contents composed of anucleate squamous cells and flaky "dry" keratin. The cyst lining of keratinizing squamous epithelium with keratohyaline granules may be absent or only focally present. The differential diagnosis includes a dermoid cyst (with adnexal structures in the cyst wall) and teratomas. (H&E-stained, (A) low power; (B) medium power.) H&E, hematoxylin and eosin; TP, touch preparation.

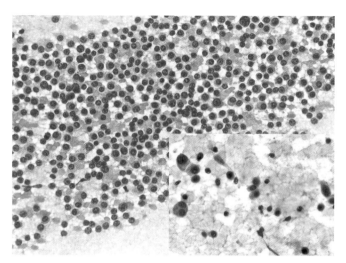

FIGURE 11.31 Plasmacytoma. Plasma cell neoplasms can show varying morphologies. The main image demonstrates a lesion composed of rather mature appearing discohesive plasma cells, which can be recognized by their eccentric nuclei and perinuclear clearing (hof). In some cases, bi- or multinucleation and increased atypia may be present (inset) (H&E-stained, high power). H&E, hematoxylin and eosin.

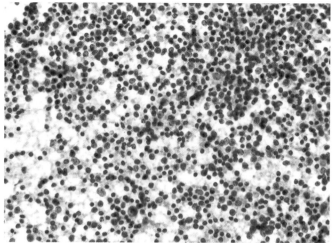

FIGURE 11.32 Lymphoma. Unlike primary CNS lymphoma, which most commonly presents as a diffuse large B-cell lymphoma, the epidural space can be involved by a wide range of small and large cell lymphomas. TPs demonstrate discohesive sheets of rather monomorphous round cells with scant cytoplasm as seen in this example of a follicular lymphoma. If lymphoma is suspected based on the intraoperative findings and there is an adequate amount of material, some of the tissue should be submitted for flow cytometry studies (H&E-stained, high power). CNS, central nervous system; H&E, hematoxylin and eosin; TP, touch preparation.

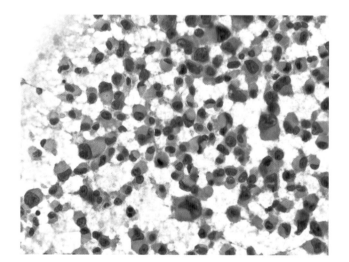

FIGURE 11.33 Metastatic carcinoma. Like this example of a metastatic breast carcinoma, some carcinomas may exhibit plasmacytoid features and may be difficult to distinguish from plasma cell lesions on intraoperative preparations (H&E-stained, high power; see also sections "Other Extra-axial Neoplasms" and "Metastatic Neoplasms"). H&E, hematoxylin and eosin.

INTRA-AXIAL LESIONS

Smear preparations are the primary cytological technique employed in the evaluation of intra-axial lesions as they provide unrivaled information about cell processes. Touch preparations are frequently paucicellular due to the cohesiveness of the tissue but may provide diagnostic information in nonneoplastic/inflammatory lesions, nonglial neoplasms, and some glial tumors. Cytologic preparations are particularly useful in the evaluation of small surgical specimens such as stereotactic biopsies. In these instances, the primary goal is to confirm that adequate material has been obtained for diagnostic evaluation and only secondarily to provide information about the nature of the lesion. Following the recent transition of CNS tumor classification to an integrated histological-molecular system, the issue of adequacy is more important than ever to assure that sufficient material is present for ancillary studies (3).

Normal

Normal CNS tissue only releases very limited material during a touch preparation and is much better evaluated on smears. It is characterized by an admixture of the various cell types of the CNS including neurons, astrocytes, oligodendrocytes, and microglia (Figure 11.34). Reactive gliosis is characterized by astrocytes with abundant eosinophilic cytoplasm (Figure 11.35). Reactive changes need to be interpreted in the context of radiologic and clinical findings and may be indicative of a "near-miss" biopsy. One of the most commonly encountered normal brain regions is the cerebellum, a common site of metastatic neoplasms and primary CNS tumors. The densely cellular granular layer of the cerebellar cortex should not be mistaken for hypercellular tumor tissue (Figure 11.36).

Nonneoplastic Lesions

Several infectious, inflammatory, demyelinating or ischemic processes may either prompt a biopsy for diagnostic confirmation or enter the differential diagnosis of a neoplastic process. The appearance of an abscess will depend on the evolutionary stage and location of the biopsy. Numerous neutrophils and macrophages are the most prominent feature of an acute abscess (Figure 11.37). The causative organisms are rarely identified. However, neutrophils are not specific to an abscess and can be seen in organizing blood clots, acute infarcts, and necrotic neoplasms. Further evaluation of the tissue sample by smear may help better evaluate underlying tissue morphology.

Over time, an abscess becomes organized and separated from the surrounding brain tissue by a wall of reactive gliosis and fibroblast-rich granulation tissue. Smear preparations in these cases will demonstrate cohesive fragments of spindle cells, reactive astrocytes, and often only scant inflammatory cells, whereas touch preps from this region will likely be paucicellular and nondiagnostic (Figure 11.38)

Biopsies of some brain lesions yield a preparation predominantly composed of macrophages, which are identified by their abundant foamy cytoplasm and bland eccentric nuclei. The main differential diagnoses of these macrophage-rich lesions are demyelinating lesions and evolving infarcts (Figures 11.39–11.42). The presence of admixed lymphocytes would favor an inflammatory demyelinating lesion, whereas the presence of ischemic neurons would suggest an infarct. However, these features may be subtle or absent and a definitive distinction is usually deferred to permanent sections. The presence of bizarre astrocytes may suggest a diagnosis of progressive multifocal leukoencephalopathy.

Primary CNS Neoplasms

The classification of primary CNS tumors has recently undergone significant changes (3,9). For many entities, ancillary studies are now required for an integrated histologic–molecular diagnostic designation. Although this development has limited immediate impact on the diagnostic impression rendered at the time of intraoperative evaluation, it is important to assure that adequate tissue has been obtained for complete permanent section evaluation.

As indicated earlier, touch preparations are of limited value in the evaluation of primary CNS neoplasms. Smear preparations are superior in demonstrating the cell processes and other characteristic features of a glial tumor. A few examples of touch preparations of low- and high-grade primary CNS tumors are presented. For more detailed description of characteristic features on smear preparations and frozen sections, the reader is referred to other excellent resources (1,2,10). Cellularity, nuclear morphology, cell processes, pleomorphism, mitotic activity, necrosis, and perivascular structuring are some of the main features evaluated in the assessment of a glial neoplasm (Figures 11.43–11.52). The presence of tumor cells with round nuclei and scant cytoplasm favors an oligodendroglioma over an astrocytic neoplasm, which typically shows more ovoid to elongated nuclei and more prominent fibrillary processes. Higher-grade neoplasms are characterized by increased cellularity, pleomorphism, mitotic activity, and presence of necrosis. Not all of these features may be present on intraoperative evaluation, and definitive grading is often deferred to permanent sections.

Embryonal tumors of the CNS have also undergone significant changes in classification and nomenclature. The designation CNS primitive neuroectodermal tumor (PNET) has been abandoned in favor of more genetically defined entities (3,9,11,12). On cytologic preparations, embryonal CNS tumors show similar features to "small round blue cell tumors" elsewhere in the body with predominantly round nuclei, scant cytoplasm, variable atypia, and variable apoptotic/mitotic activity (Figures 11.53–11.55).

Primary CNS lymphomas are predominantly of the diffuse large B-cell type. Cytologic features include discohesive cells with scant cytoplasm, mostly round nuclei, and prominent nucleoli (Figure 11.56). A second population of reactive lymphocytes may be present. Pretreatment of CNS lymphomas with steroids may result in prominent apoptotic tumor cell death with numerous foamy macrophages. This may lead to the cytologic appearance of a macrophage-rich lesion without a diagnostic lymphoma cell population. Lymphomas may be difficult to distinguish from glioblastomas with a prominent small cell component with sparse cell processes and from some metastatic lesions (e.g., metastatic small cell carcinoma).

Metastatic Neoplasms

Metastatic tumors are one of the main differential diagnoses in the evaluation of a ring-enhancing brain lesion. The tumor cells are typically more cohesive than in glial neoplasms, often forming small clusters or lobules with distinct cell borders. The presence of intracellular mucin, glandular structures, or the presence of melanin pigment may aid in the differential diagnosis (Figures 11.57–11.59).

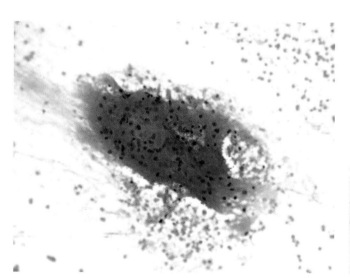

FIGURE 11.34 Normal brain tissue. Small tissue fragment of white matter, composed of admixed cell types with a predominance of bland appearing oligodendrocytes (H&E-stained, medium power). H&E, hematoxylin and eosin.

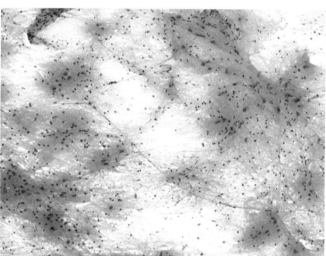

FIGURE 11.35 Brain tissue with reactive changes. This smear preparation, compared to a touch prep, much better demonstrates the fibrillary nature of brain tissue. Also evident in this image are scattered reactive astrocytes with abundant eosinophilic cytoplasm (H&E-stained, low power). H&E, hematoxylin and eosin.

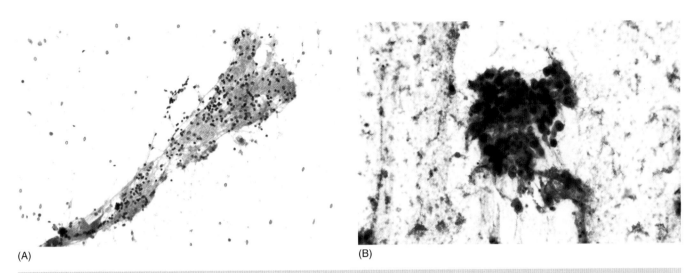

(A)

(B)

FIGURE 11.36 Cerebellar cortex with metastatic carcinoma. The cerebellum is a common site of metastatic and primary CNS tumors, and it is important not to mistake the densely cellular granular layer of the cerebellar cortex with hypercellular tumor tissue. In this figure, image A demonstrates a fragment of cerebellar cortex with its small round granular cells. Image B shows a different field of the same touch prep slide demonstrating a fragment of metastatic carcinoma with larger and more pleomorphic overlapping nuclei. In this side-by-side comparison, the different cytologic features are readily apparent, but in other cases the distinction may be more challenging and require a frozen section to reveal the typical architectural features of cerebellar cortex (H&E-stained, medium power). CNS, central nervous system; H&E, hematoxylin and eosin.

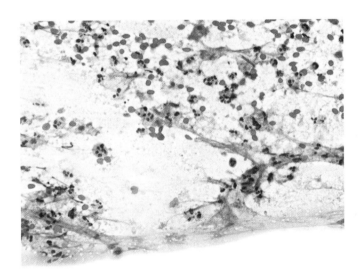

FIGURE 11.37 Acute abscess. A biopsy taken from the center of an acute abscess may yield numerous neutrophils and admixed macrophages on a TP and should prompt a recommendation of tissue cultures to the surgeon (H&E-stained, high power). H&E, hematoxylin and eosin; TP, touch preparation.

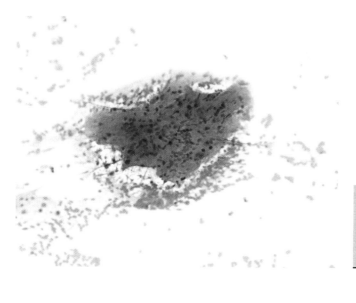

FIGURE 11.38 Abscess wall. When this area is biopsied by the surgeon, cohesive tissue fragments may be seen, and inflammatory cells may be scarce. The proliferating fibroblasts may mimic a glial neoplasm (H&E-stained, medium power). H&E, hematoxylin and eosin.

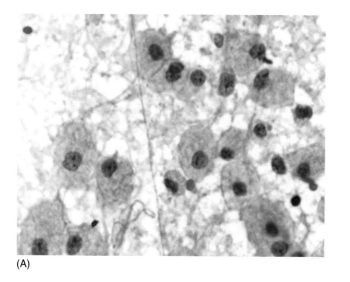

(A)

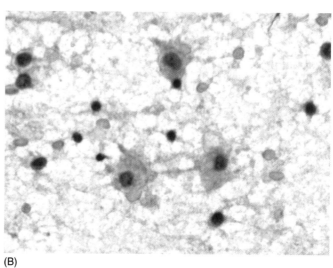

(B)

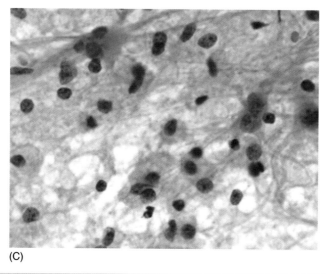

(C)

FIGURE 11.39 Demyelinating lesion. Macrophages are well recognized on a TP by their abundant foamy cytoplasm and eccentric bland nuclei. While macrophages may easily touch off (A and B), the accompanying reactive glial changes are usually better appreciated on a smear preparation (C). Inflammatory demyelinating lesions show a variable presence of admixed lymphocytic infiltrates (B). ((A)–(C) H&E-stained, high power.) H&E, hematoxylin and eosin; TP, touch preparation.

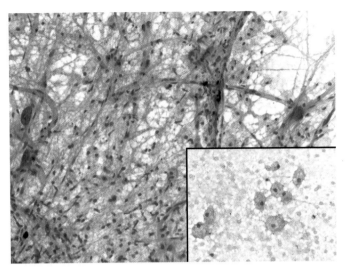

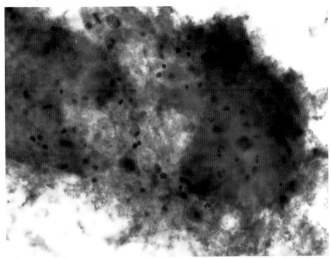

FIGURE 11.40 Progressive multifocal leukoencephalopathy. While a TP may only show foamy macrophages with minimal accompanying lymphocytic infiltrate (inset), the characteristic bizarre astrocytes of PML are often seen on a smear preparation and are suggestive of the diagnosis (H&E-stained, medium power (inset), high power). H&E, hematoxylin and eosin; PML, progressive multifocal leukoencephalopathy; TP, touch preparation.

FIGURE 11.41 Infarct. Occasionally, an atypical clinical and radiographic presentation of an infarct will prompt a brain biopsy for diagnostic purposes. TPs of infarcts often yield predominantly blood, but scattered admixed macrophages and inflammatory cells may suggest an underlying macrophage-rich lesion and should be followed up by a smear for further diagnostic evaluation to rule out an underlying neoplasm and to assure that diagnostic tissue material has been obtained (H&E-stained, high power). H&E, hematoxylin and eosin; TP, touch preparation.

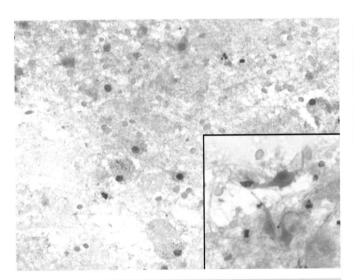

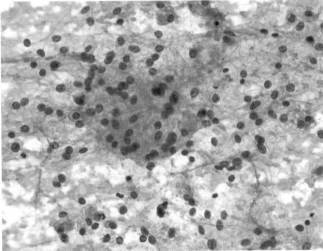

FIGURE 11.42 Infarct. In some instances, the necrotic tissue releases degenerating cells during a TP. The combination of ischemic "dead red" neurons, foamy and hemosiderin-laden macrophages, and admixed inflammatory cells is highly suggestive of an ischemic lesion. The inset highlights the features of an ischemic neuron with increased cytoplasmic eosinophilia and shrunken nucleus (H&E-stained, high power). H&E, hematoxylin and eosin; TP, touch preparation.

FIGURE 11.43 Oligodendroglioma. Oligodendrogliomas are composed of cells with round nuclei and scant cytoplasm and typically lack the fibrillary processes seen in astrocytomas (H&E-stained, high power). H&E, hematoxylin and eosin.

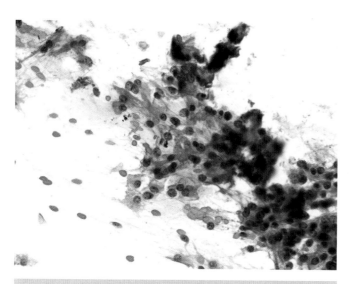

FIGURE 11.44 Oligodendroglioma. Oligodendrogliomas often have a myxoid background, which can sometimes be recognized on intraoperative preparations. However, this is a nonspecific finding and can also be seen in other glial and nonglial neoplasms (H&E-stained, high power). H&E, hematoxylin and eosin.

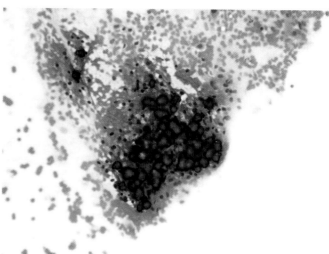

FIGURE 11.45 Oligodendroglioma. Microcalcifications are commonly seen in oligodendrogliomas and occasionally encountered on intraoperative preparations. In severe cases as this one, the tissue may have a notable gritty texture (H&E-stained, medium power). H&E, hematoxylin and eosin.

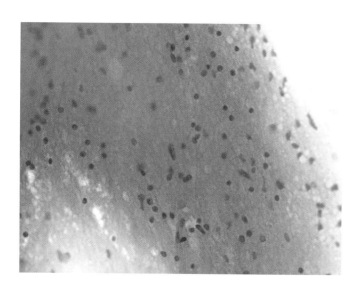

FIGURE 11.46 Astrocytoma. Since astrocytomas are infiltrative tumors, biopsies usually contain admixed neoplastic and nonneoplastic glial cells. Samples of less involved areas may only show subtle increases in overall cellularity with scattered atypical nuclei (H&E-stained, high power). H&E, hematoxylin and eosin.

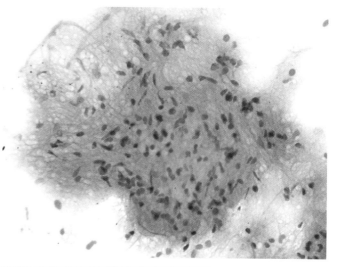

FIGURE 11.47 Astrocytoma. Biopsies of more solid tumor areas will show increased cellularity and a more uniform population of atypical cells with elongated and irregular nuclei. Definitive grading of infiltrating gliomas is usually deferred to permanent sections (H&E-stained, high power). H&E, hematoxylin and eosin.

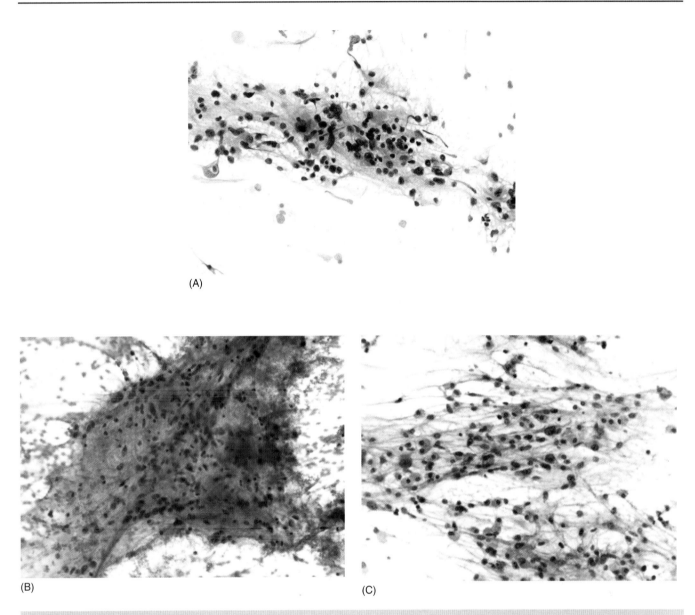

(A)

(B)

(C)

FIGURE 11.48 High-grade glioma. Infiltrating high-grade gliomas are typically hypercellular lesions composed of small elongated to variably pleomorphic cells with indistinct cell borders. The finely fibrillary background is best appreciated in smear preparations but can sometimes be discerned in small tissue fragments on a touch prep. ((A)–(C) H&E-stained, medium power.) H&E, hematoxylin and eosin.

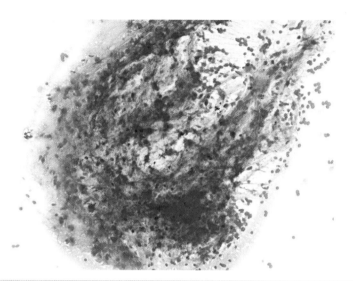

FIGURE 11.49 High-grade glioma. Necrosis and vascular proliferation are the hallmark features distinguishing glioblastoma from an anaplastic astrocytoma. As shown in the image, necrosis is usually easy to recognize and frequently encountered. On the other hand, true vascular proliferation may be difficult to distinguish from thickened vessels and should be evaluated with caution. When definitive glioblastoma features are lacking in the touch and smear preparations, an intraoperative diagnosis of high-grade glioma can be rendered based on cytologic features with definitive grading deferred to permanent sections (H&E-stained, medium power). H&E, hematoxylin and eosin.

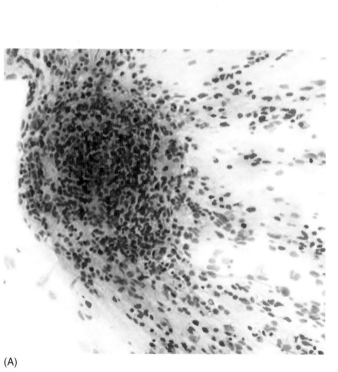

(A)

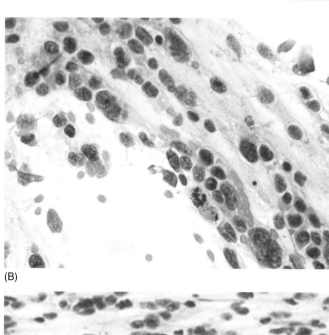

(B)

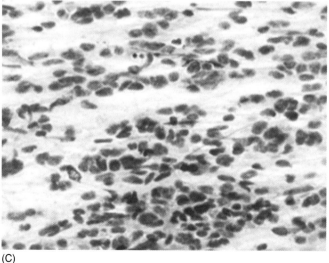

(C)

FIGURE 11.50 High-grade glioma with PNET-like features. Some glioblastomas demonstrate a PNET-like morphology with naked pleomorphic nuclei or scant cytoplasm. Cellular processes may be scarce or absent, even on smear preparations. In the absence of more typical glioma areas with distinct cytologic features, tumor typing is best deferred to permanent sections (H&E-stained, (A) low power; (B) high power; (C) smear preparation, medium power.) H&E, hematoxylin and eosin; PNET, primitive neuroectodermal tumor.

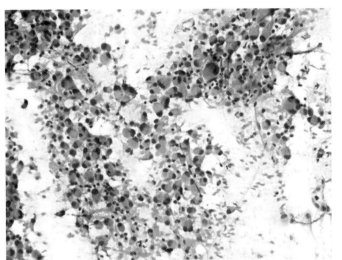

FIGURE 11.51 High-grade glioma with rhabdoid features. In rare cases, glioblastomas can exhibit a rhabdoid or epithelioid morphology with scant or absent glial processes, making a distinction from metastatic carcinoma or other rhabdoid tumors (e.g., meningioma) challenging (H&E-stained, medium power). H&E, hematoxylin and eosin.

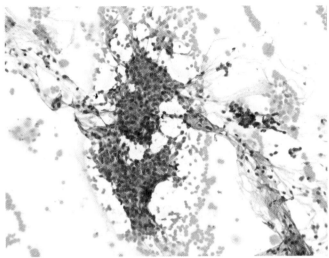

FIGURE 11.52 Ependymoma. These very fibrillary tumors usually do not release much material during a touch preparation and are better evaluated with smears and frozen sections. Ependymomas are composed of uniform cells with oval nuclei. In the absence of characteristic perivascular pseudorosettes, they may be difficult to distinguish from other glial and nonglial neoplasms on TP (H&E-stained, medium power). H&E, hematoxylin and eosin; TP, touch preparation.

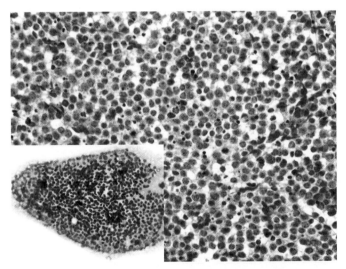

FIGURE 11.53 Medulloblastoma. Classic medulloblastomas have the typical appearance of a small round blue cell tumor on TPs, consisting of discohesive sheets of round cells with scant cytoplasm. Apoptotic bodies and mitotic figures are variable in density. Nuclear pleomorphism may be pronounced in large cell/anaplastic medulloblastoma variants (H&E-stained, high power). H&E, hematoxylin and eosin; TP, touch preparation.

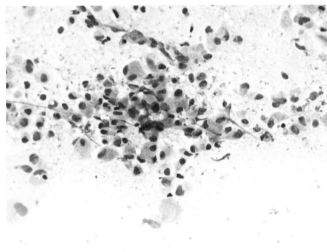

FIGURE 11.54 ATRT. ATRT is characterized by rhabdoid cells with an epithelioid appearance, but in some cases small undifferentiated cells predominate precluding a definitive intraoperative diagnosis (H&E-stained, high power). ATRT, atypical teratoid rhabdoid tumor; H&E, hematoxylin and eosin.

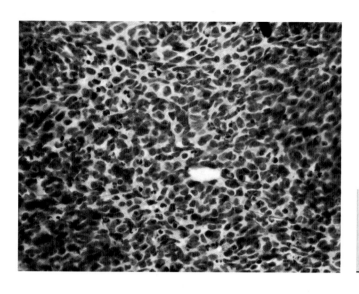

FIGURE 11.55 Pineoblastoma. These malignant pineal neoplasms are characterized by variably pleomorphic cells with scant cytoplasm, nuclear molding, mitotic figures, and apoptotic bodies (H&E-stained, high power). H&E, hematoxylin and eosin.

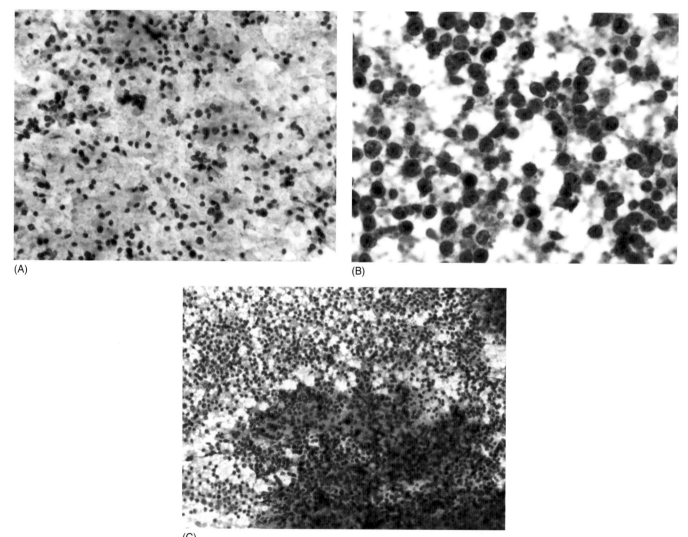

(A)

(B)

(C)

FIGURE 11.56 Primary CNS lymphoma. TPs of primary CNS lymphomas may show variable cellularity ranging from bloody imprints with a few admixed lymphoid cells (A) to discohesive sheets of rounded cells with scant cytoplasm, variable nuclear pleomorphism, and prominent nucleoli (B). Note the presence of pale lymphoglandular bodies in the background. The characteristic angiocentric growth pattern may be better appreciated on smear preparations (C) or frozen sections. (H&E-stained, (A) medium power; (B) high power; (C) smear preparation, medium power.) CNS, central nervous system; H&E, hematoxylin and eosin; TP, touch preparation.

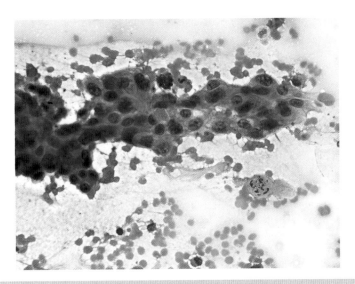

FIGURE 11.57 Metastatic carcinoma. On TP, metastases typically present as cohesive tissue fragments with distinct cell borders and lack the distinct fibrillary processes of glial neoplasms. Mitotic figures may be variably identified (H&E-stained, high power; see also sections "Other Extra-axial Neoplasms" and "Spinal Epidural Tumors"). H&E, hematoxylin and eosin; TP, touch preparation.

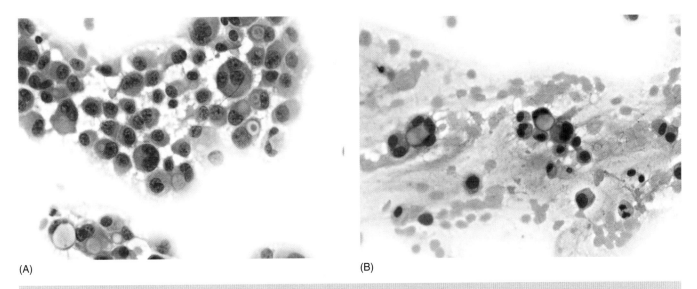

(A)   (B)

FIGURE 11.58 Metastatic carcinoma. Intra- and extracellular mucin and signet ring morphology can be seen in some adenocarcinomas. ((A) and (B) H&E-stained, high power.) H&E, hematoxylin and eosin.

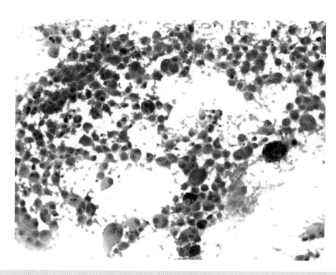

FIGURE 11.59 Metastatic melanoma. The diagnosis of melanoma is straightforward in the presence of pigmented tumor cells as seen in this example, but may be more challenging in the absence of melanin pigment. Given the wide variety of morphologic appearances of melanoma, a definitive distinction from metastatic carcinoma or, in the case of a melanoma with spindle cells from a glial tumor, may be difficult or impossible on intraoperative evaluation (H&E-stained, medium power). H&E, hematoxylin and eosin.

REFERENCES

1. Burger PC. *Smears and Frozen Sections in Surgical Neuropathology. A Manual.* Baltimore, MD: PB Medical Publishing; 2009.
2. Joseph JT. *Diagnostic Neuropathology Smears.* Philadelphia, PA: Lippincott Williams and Wilkins; 2007.
3. Afroz N, Khan N, Hassan J, Huda MF. Role of imprint cytology in the intraoperative diagnosis of pituitary adenomas. *Diagn Cytopathol.* 2011;39:138-140.
4. Louis DN, Perry A, Reifenberger G, et al., eds. *WHO Classification of Tumours of the Central Nervous System.* Revised 4th ed. Lyon, France: International Agency for Research on Cancer; 2016.
5. Lee EB, Tihan T, Scheithauer BW, et al. Thyroid transcription factor 1 expression in sellar tumors: a histogenetic marker? *J Neuropathol Exp Neurol.* 2009;68:482-488.
6. Larkin SJ, Preda V, Karavitaki N, et al. BRAF V600E mutations are characteristic for papillary craniopharyngioma and may coexist with CTNNB1-mutated adamantinomatous craniopharyngioma. *Acta Neuropathol.* 2014;127:927-929.
7. Siddiqui MT, Mahon BM, Cochran E, Gattuso P. Cytologic features of meningiomas on crush preparations: a review. *Diagn Cytopathol.* 2008;36:202-206.
8. Fletcher CDM, Bridge JA, Hogendoorn P, Mertens F., eds. *WHO Classification of Tumours of Soft Tissue and Bone.* 4th ed. Lyon, France: International Agency for Research on Cancer; 2013.
9. Louis DN, Perry A, Reifenberger, G, et al. The 2016 World Health Organization classification of tumors of the central nervous system: a summary. *Acta Neuropathol.* 2016;131:803-820.
10. Sharma S, Deb P. Intraoperative neurocytology of primary central nervous system neoplasia: a simplified and practical diagnostic approach. *J Cytol.* 2011;28:147-158.
11. Sturm D, Orr BA, Toprak UH, et al. New brain tumor entities emerge from molecular classification of CNS-PNETs. *Cell.* 2016; 164:1060-1072.
12. Taylor MD, Northcott PA, Korshunov A, et al. Molecular subgroups of medulloblastoma: the current consensus. *Acta Neuropathol.* 2012;123:465-472.

CHAPTER 12

Mediastinum, Retroperitoneum, and Adrenal Glands

Juan Xing

INTRODUCTION

A wide variety of mass lesions can arise from the mediastinum. Three factors that are useful to narrow the differential diagnosis are tumor location, age of the patient, and the presence or absence of symptoms. Anterior mediastinal tumors and lesions seen in young patients or symptomatic patients are more likely to be malignant (1). The most common cause of an anterior mediastinal mass includes lymphoma, in addition to lesions arising from the thymus, thyroid, or germ cells (e.g., teratoma). Congenital cystic lesions usually arise from the central mediastinum, whereas neurogenic tumors arise more often from the posterior compartment. Metastatic malignancies are more frequent than primary mediastinal malignancies and the lung is the most common site of origin. One study has shown the diagnostic accuracy of cytology imprints to be 93.6% for rapid intraoperative evaluation of mediastinal lymphadenopathy and tumors of the lung and mediastinum (2).

Although a wide diversity of pathology can arise from the retroperitoneum, primary retroperitoneal tumors are rare entities. Malignant neoplasms are more common than benign ones, and metastatic malignancies to the retroperitoneum are far more common than primary retroperitoneal malignancies. The adrenal glands are paired retroperitoneal endocrine organs. The main etiology of adrenal gland masses includes benign and malignant adrenal cortical tumors, adrenal medullary tumors, hyperplasia, and metastasis. The diagnostic approach for adrenal masses is multidisciplinary. Cytology evaluation of adrenal mass lesions is rarely requested, and usually reserved for cases with suspected metastases (3). However, intraoperative cytology imprints demonstrate unique value in certain disease entities such as pheochromocytoma and myelolipoma, in addition to metastatic malignancies.

NORMAL

Touch imprints of the normal mediastinum and retroperitoneum are typically hypocellular. Normal mesothelial cells (Figure 12.1) and occasional benign fibroadipose tissue fragments can be seen on imprints. Reactive mesothelial cells can show atypical features and may accordingly be misinterpreted as malignant cells.

Normal adrenal gland imprints show single cells, in addition to cords and clusters of adrenal cortical cells in a "frothy" lipid background. Naked nuclei are common and can mimic lymphoma or small cell carcinoma (Figure 12.2).

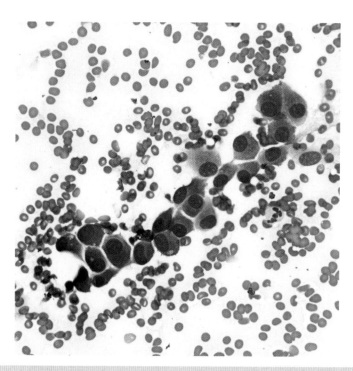

FIGURE 12.1 Normal mesothelial cells. The TP shows a flat monolayered sheet of cells with round nuclei and single nucleoli. The dense cytoplasm shows a characteristic lighter outer rim. "Windows" can be appreciated between adjacent cells (DQ-stained TP, high power). DQ, Diff-Quik; TP, touch preparation.

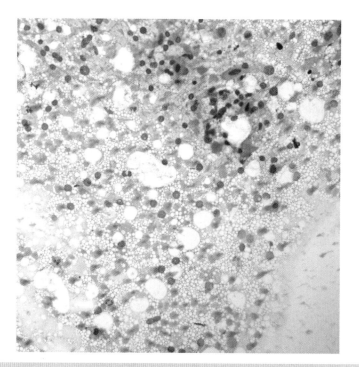

FIGURE 12.2 Normal adrenal gland. Many naked round nuclei are shown in a "frothy" lipid background. Mild nuclear size variation ("neuroendocrine atypia") can be seen. Rare cells have intact vacuolated cytoplasm, and only a few cells have dense cytoplasm (H&E-stained, high power). H&E, hematoxylin and eosin.

BENIGN ENTITIES

Mediastinum and Retroperitoneum

Cytology imprints are seldom used to evaluate reactive changes in the mediastinal and retroperitoneal regions. One entity that may be encountered is fat necrosis, which can present as a mass lesion and mimic malignancy (Figure 12.3). Cytology imprints of mediastinal and retroperitoneal lymphadenopathy due to infection are occasionally seen. Lymphadenopathy from mycobacterial infection can be seen in immunocompromised patients such as those with solid organ transplantation or HIV infection. The differential diagnosis includes reactive lymphadenopathy and lymphoproliferative disorders. Diff Quik–stained air-dried imprints are a valuable tool for rapid detection of microorganisms and appropriate specimen triage (Figure 12.4).

Thymoma is the most common primary neoplasm of the anterior mediastinum and occurs mainly in adults older than 40 years. Parathymic syndromes including myasthenia gravis, hypogammaglobulinemia, and pure red cell aplasia can be seen in up to one half of the patients (4). Thymomas are epithelial neoplasms with mixed epithelial cells and mature lymphocytes that lack overtly malignant cytological features. The proportion of epithelial cells and lymphocytes varies according to the different thymoma subtypes (Table 12.1). Type A thymoma shows purely spindle epithelial cells with few or no lymphocytes (Figure 12.5). The differential diagnosis includes spindle cell mesothelioma and a variety of other benign soft tissue spindle cell neoplasms. Type AB thymoma shows mixed spindle epithelial cells and polymorphous lymphocytes (Figure 12.6). The diagnosis of type B1, B2, and B3 thymoma by cytology imprints is challenging. The most challenging part is to identify the epithelial cells. The epithelial cells form small tight clusters in type B1 thymoma (Figure 12.7) and larger loose aggregates or just occur singly in type B2 and B3 thymoma. Useful clues for identifying epithelial cells include the presence of cells with a spindle shape or those with small distinct nucleoli, as well as clusters of cells with indistinct cell borders, and nuclear overlapping (5). Benign teratoma is the most common mediastinal germ cell tumor. It occurs predominantly in children and young adults. Males and females are equally affected. Most arise within or adjacent to the thymus. Mature teratoma is encapsulated and consists of cystic and solid areas. These tumors are composed of tissues that arise from more than one of three primitive germ cell layers. Rarely, touch imprints are used intraoperatively to facilitate their diagnosis (Figure 12.8).

Adrenal Gland

Adrenal cortical adenoma is 60 times more common than adrenal cortical carcinoma (3). As with fine needle aspiration, imprints of hyperplastic nodules, adrenal adenomas, and even well-differentiated adrenal cortical carcinomas show similar cytomorphology. Myelolipoma is an uncommon benign neoplasm that occurs almost exclusively in the adrenal gland. It is composed of adipose tissue and trilineage hematopoietic elements. Because of the presence of adipose tissue, intraoperative frozen sections may impose technical difficulty and hence touch imprints are particularly valuable in this situation (Figure 12.9).

TABLE 12.1 WHO Classification of Thymoma

Thymoma Type	Synonym	Cytomorphology
A	Spindle cell or medullary	Bland spindle/oval epithelial cells No/few lymphocytes
AB	Mixed	Mixed features Some lymphocytes
B1	Lymphocyte-rich, lymphocytic, predominantly cortical, or organoid	Abundant lymphocytes Scant, small bland epithelial cells
B2	Cortical	Numerous lymphocytes Large, polygonal epithelial cells
B3	Epithelial, atypical, squamoid, or well-differentiated thymic carcinoma	Few lymphocytes Predominantly round/polygonal epithelial cells with atypia

WHO, World Health Organization.

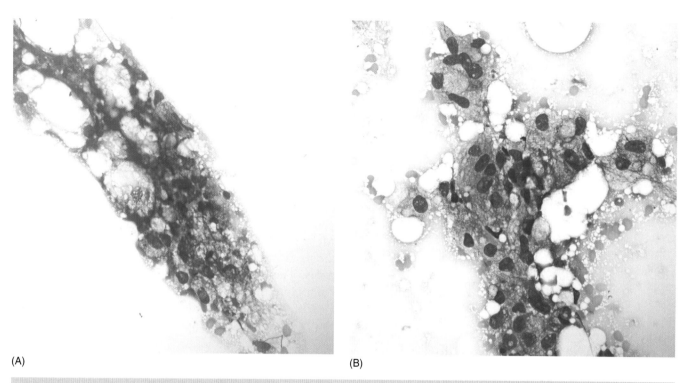

(A)

(B)

FIGURE 12.3 Fat necrosis. (A) Touch imprint shows enlarged and distorted adipocytes with foamy macrophages (DQ-stained TP, high power). (B) Foamy macrophages may show atypical features such as nuclear pleomorphism, irregular nuclear contours, and one or more prominent nucleoli, mimicking malignant cells (DQ-stained TP, high power). DQ, Diff-Quik; TP, touch preparation.

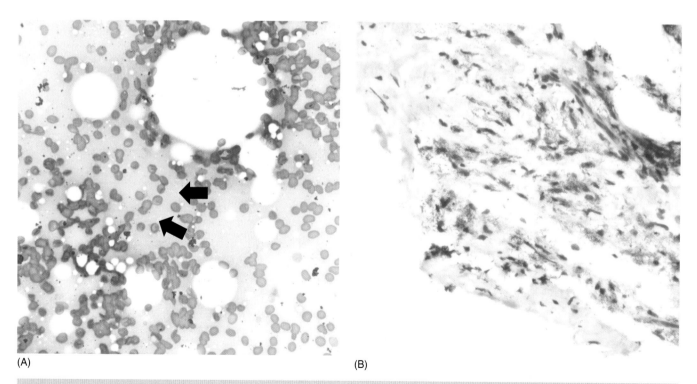

(A)

(B)

FIGURE 12.4 Mycobacterium avium-intracellulare infection. (A) The imprint shows many "negative images" (arrows) and a few macrophages (DQ-stained TP, high power). (B) Acid Fast (AFB) special stain highlights numerous mycobacteria (AFB stain, high power). DQ, Diff-Quik; TP, touch preparation.

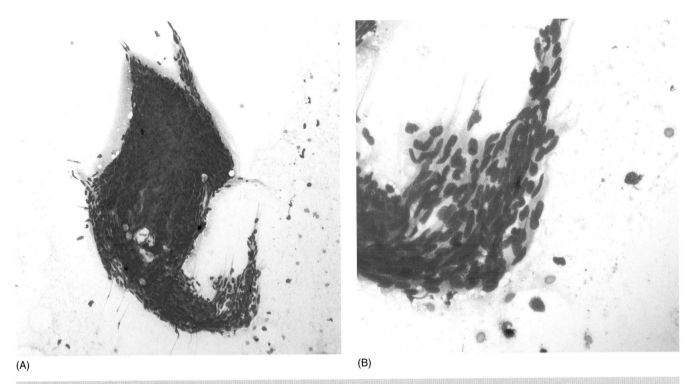

(A)

(B)

FIGURE 12.5 Type A thymoma (spindle cell thymoma). (A and B) The TP shows a syncytial fragment of bland spindle cells with rare background lymphocytes (DQ-stained TP, medium and high power). DQ, Diff-Quik; TP, touch preparation.

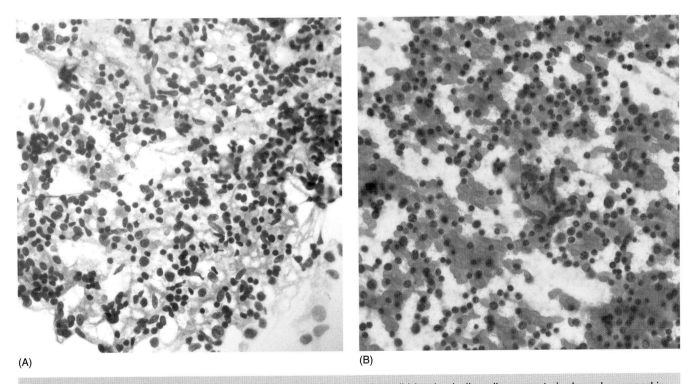

(A)

(B)

FIGURE 12.6 Type AB thymoma. (A and B) The TP shows mixed small bland spindle cells present singly and arranged in small clusters admixed with background small polymorphous lymphocytes (H&E-stained, high power). H&E, hematoxylin and eosin; TP, touch preparation.

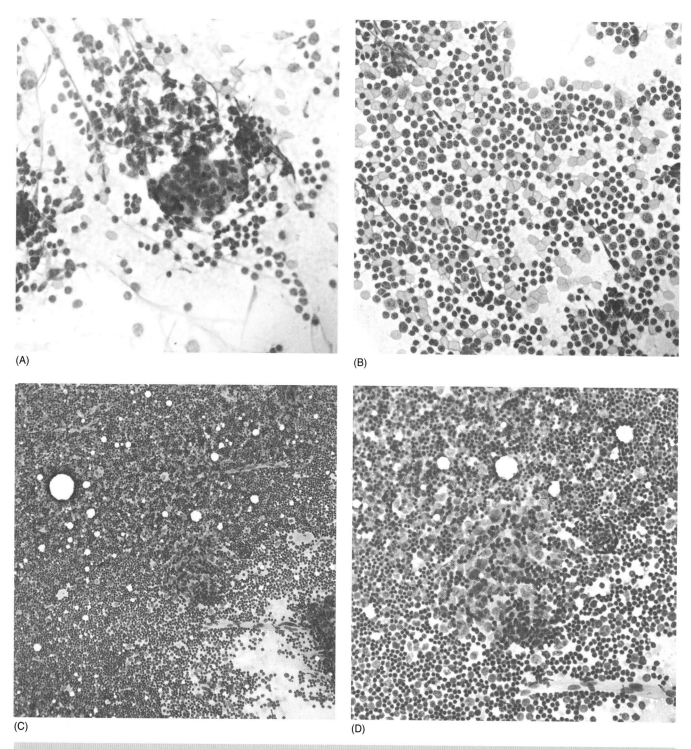

FIGURE 12.7 Type B1 thymoma. (A) A small tight cluster of epithelial cells is shown in a background of polymorphous lymphocytes (H&E-stained, high power). (B) Numerous background lymphocytes resemble a reactive lymph node (H&E-stained, high power). (C) On low power, the impression is of a reactive lymph node, (D) but an aggregate of epithelial cells can be seen in the center of the image on high power magnification (DQ-stained TP, low and medium power). DQ, Diff-Quik; H&E, hematoxylin and eosin; TP, touch preparation.

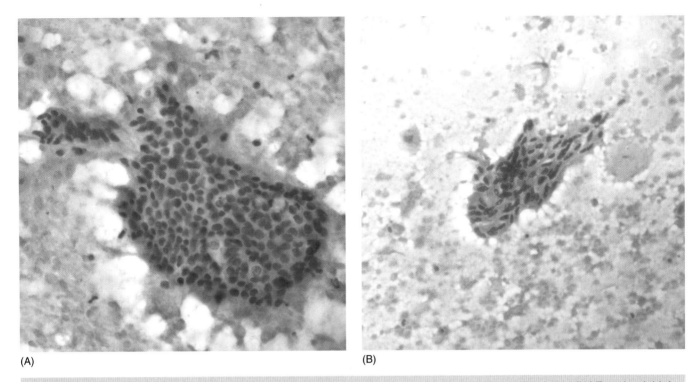

(A)

(B)

FIGURE 12.8 Mature mediastinal teratoma. (A) A cluster of benign respiratory epithelial cells is shown (H&E-stained, high power). (B) A cluster of benign squamous cells is shown with abundant dense eosinophilic cytoplasm (H&E-stained, high power). H&E, hematoxylin and eosin.

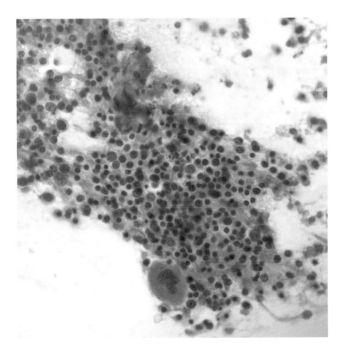

FIGURE 12.9 Myelolipoma. (A) This TP shows benign trilineage hematopoietic cells with a rare megakaryocyte, numerous nucleated erythrocytes, and myeloid cells (H&E-stained, high power). H&E, hematoxylin and eosin; TP, touch preparation.

MALIGNANT ENTITIES

Mediastinum and Retroperitoneum

Thymic carcinoma is rare and occurs mainly in middle-aged men. It is a heterogeneous group of aggressive epithelial malignancies arising from the thymus. Squamous cell carcinoma and lymphoepithelioma-like carcinoma are the most common cell types. It can be differentiated from thymoma by the presence of overt malignant cytological features, necrosis, and mitoses. Metastasis from an occult lung primary malignancy must be excluded, and hence ancillary studies are necessary to render an accurate diagnosis. Primary mediastinal seminoma is uncommon, but comprises 25% to 50% of malignant mediastinal germ cell tumors (1). It commonly occurs in men between the ages 20 to 40 years. Touch imprints from seminomas show large dispersed monotonous neoplastic cells with scant finely vacuolated cytoplasm and reactive lymphocytes in a tigroid background (Figure 12.10). Primary mediastinal (thymic) large B-cell lymphoma accounts for 2% to 4% of non-Hodgkin lymphomas and occurs predominantly in young adult females. It shows a wide cytological spectrum from case to case. Therefore, clinical history and ancillary studies are required to make the correct diagnosis. The tumor cells express B-cell antigens, and typically have thin lace-like fibrous bands within the lymphoid proliferation. CD30 is positive in more than 80% of cases, but is usually weak and heterogeneous (Figure 12.11). This is an important entity to consider in young patients, given the significant overlap with classical Hodgkin lymphoma, which also occurs in a similar age group, can have fibrotic bands, and shows CD30 positivity.

Malignant mesothelioma is a rare, but very aggressive malignancy arising from the serosa. The most important risk factor is exposure to asbestos. It occurs four times more commonly in the pleural cavity than the peritoneal cavity. The cytology diagnosis of malignant mesothelioma shows high specificity but low sensitivity. The features that help to differentiate malignant mesothelial cells from benign or reactive mesothelial cells include hypercellularity, morula-papillary structures, cytological atypia with enlarged nuclei, macronucleoli, and frequent cytoplasmic vacuoles (Figure 12.12) (6). Metastases to the mediastinum and retroperitoneum are far more common than primary malignancies. The most common metastases are from carcinomas involving adjacent organs. Cytology imprints in these cases typically show cells with overt malignant features, and allocation of material for cell block is critical in order to have material for immunohistochemical studies for subclassification or theranostic studies (Figure 12.13).

Adrenal Glands

Adrenal cortical carcinoma is a rare primary adrenal gland malignancy. These tumors are large (>5 cm in size) and 80% of them are functional. Histologically, they range from well-differentiated to poorly differentiated tumors. It is difficult to reliably differentiate adrenal cortical adenoma from adrenal cortical carcinoma by cytology alone, especially the well differentiated tumors. Useful cytologic criteria for making a diagnosis of carcinoma include the presence of numerous isolated cells with intact granular or vacuolated cytoplasm, enlarged and pleomorphic nuclei, and the presence of mitoses or necrosis (Figure 12.14). This is in contrast to adenoma, which contains numerous naked nuclei in a "frothy" lipid background, and lacks necrosis. Pheochromocytoma is a catecholamine-producing neuroendocrine tumor, of which the majority arise from the adrenal medulla. Pheochromocytoma can be sporadic or hereditary with about 10% to 20% of cases associated with familial neoplastic syndromes such as multiple endocrine neoplasia syndromes 2a and 2b, neurofibromatosis, and the von Hippel–Lindau (VHL) syndrome. Aspirate cytology is generally avoided due to episodic hypertension, hemorrhage, and even death. Intraoperative touch imprints are invaluable, because of their quick turnaround time (Figure 12.15). As with most organ systems, metastatic malignancies are more common than primary ones in adrenal glands. The most common malignancies that metastasize to the adrenal glands are lung cancers (Figure 12.16), melanoma, and renal cell carcinoma (Figure 12.17). Clinical history and ancillary studies are essential to make the correct diagnosis.

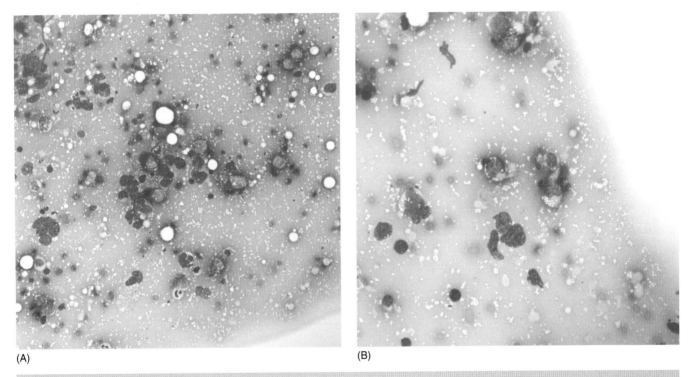

FIGURE 12.10 Mediastinal seminoma. The TP shows dispersed, large monotonous, neoplastic cells with scant vacuolated cytoplasm and prominent nucleoli together with scattered small lymphocytes in a tigroid background (DQ-stained TP, high power). DQ, Diff-Quik; TP, touch preparation.

(A)

(B)

FIGURE 12.11 Primary mediastinal (thymic) large B-cell lymphoma. (A and B) The TP demonstrates large atypical lymphoid cells with irregular nuclear contours, immature chromatin, and cytoplasmic vacuoles. The presence of cytoplasmic vacuoles mimics Burkitt lymphoma, but Burkitt lymphoma by comparison has round smooth nuclei (DQ-stained TP, high power). DQ, Diff-Quik; TP, touch preparation. (*continued*)

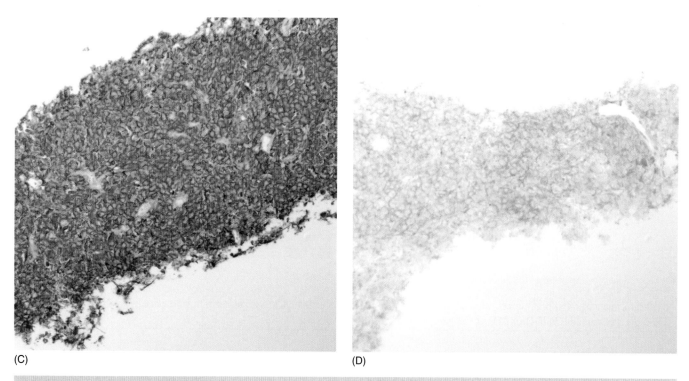

(C)   (D)

FIGURE 12.11 (continued) (C) The cells are positive for CD20, confirming their B-cell origin (CD20 stain, medium power). (D) The cells are also weakly positive for CD30, which may be seen in 80% of such cases (CD30 stain, medium power).

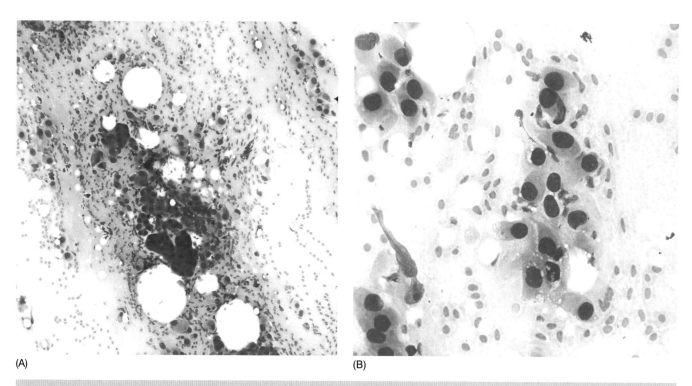

(A)   (B)

FIGURE 12.12 Malignant mesothelioma. (A) A hypercellular cluster of mesothelial cells with a vague papillary architecture is seen. (B) in addition to loosely cohesive cells with enlarged, hyperchromatic nuclei and many intracytoplasmic vacuoles. (*continued*)

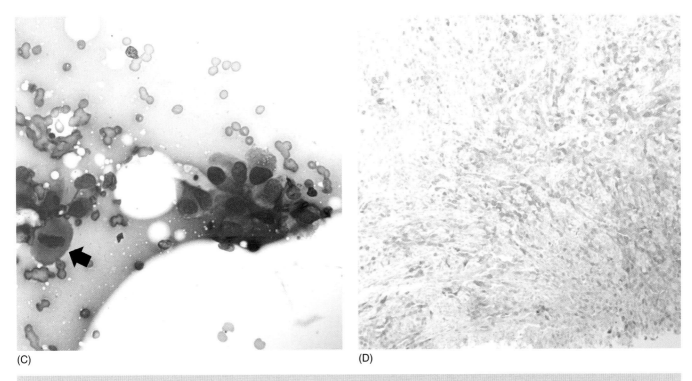

(C)

(D)

FIGURE 12.12 (*continued*) (C) Touch imprint in this case shows a mitotic figure (arrow) and cells with macronucleoli (DQ-stained TP, high power). (D) Mesothelial cells are weakly positive for calretinin on the corresponding core biopsy (Immunohistochemical stain, medium power). DQ, Diff-Quik; TP, touch preparation.

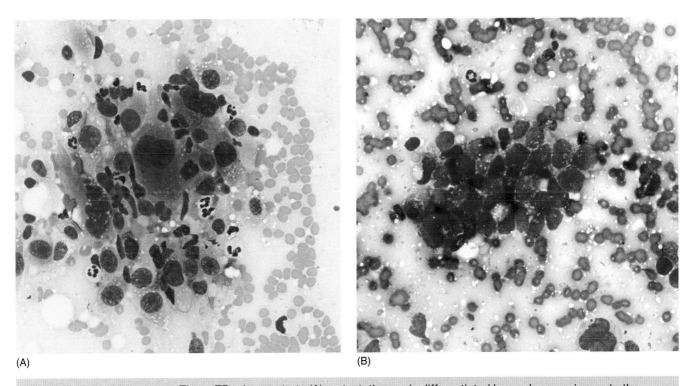

(A)

(B)

FIGURE 12.13 Metastases. These TPs demonstrate (A) metastatic poorly differentiated lung adenocarcinoma to the mediastinum (DQ-stained TP, high power) and (B) metastatic ovarian carcinoma to the retroperitoneum (DQ-stained TP, high power). DQ, Diff-Quik; TP, touch preparation.

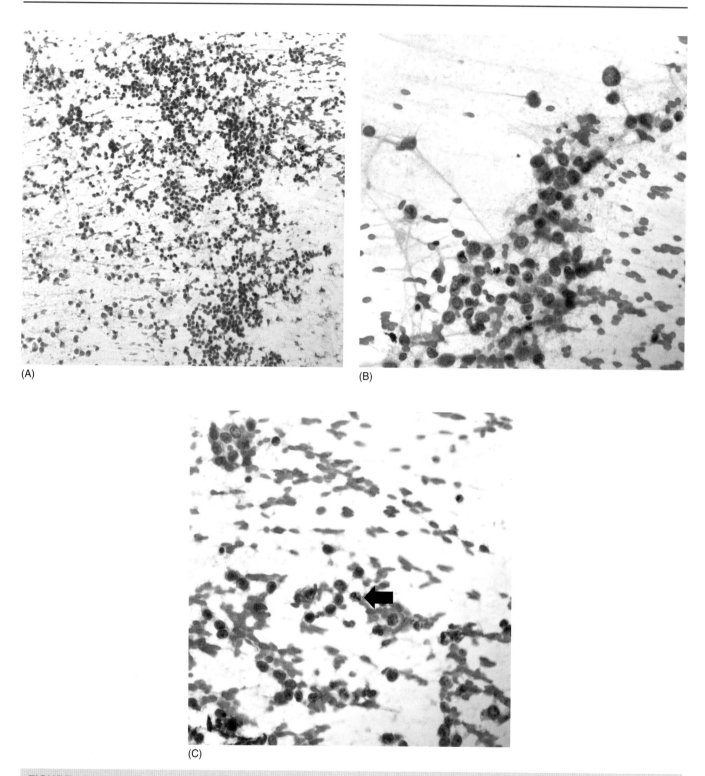

FIGURE 12.14 Adrenal cortical carcinoma. (A) The imprint is cellular and (B and C) contains cells demonstrating nuclear pleomorphism, thin rims of cytoplasm, and mitoses (arrow). (H&E-stained, low (A) and high (B and C) power.) H&E, hematoxylin and eosin.

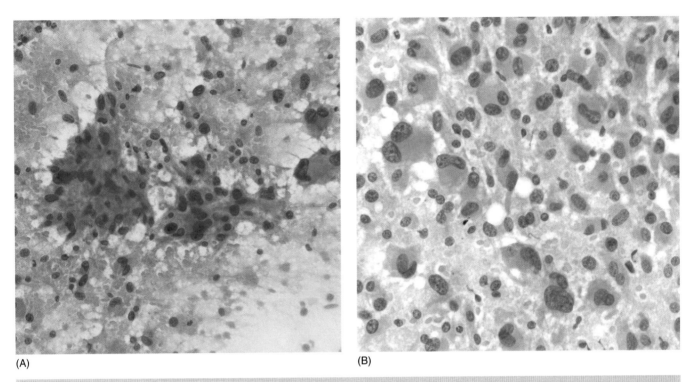

FIGURE 12.15 Pheochromocytoma (A and B). The imprints show loose clusters and single epithelioid and some spindled cells with marked nuclear pleomorphism and characteristic basophilic granular cytoplasm (H&E-stained, high power). The atypia does not necessarily correlate with malignancy. H&E, hematoxylin and eosin.

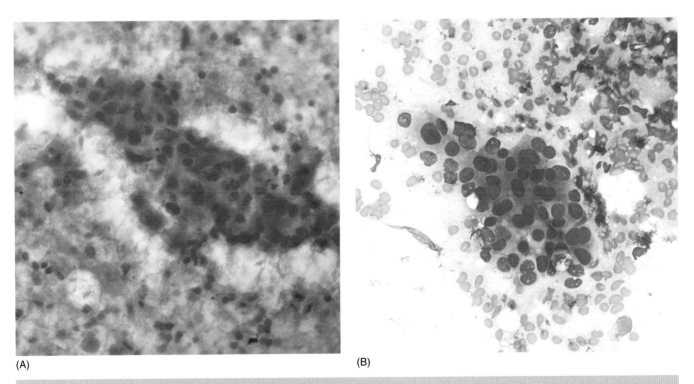

FIGURE 12.16 Metastatic lung adenocarcinoma to the adrenal gland. (A and B) These TPs show cohesive clusters of malignant epithelial cells and background benign naked cortical cell nuclei. ((A) H&E-stained, high power; (B) DQ-stained TP, high power.) (C) The morphology is similar on the corresponding histology section (H&E-stained, high power). (*continued*)

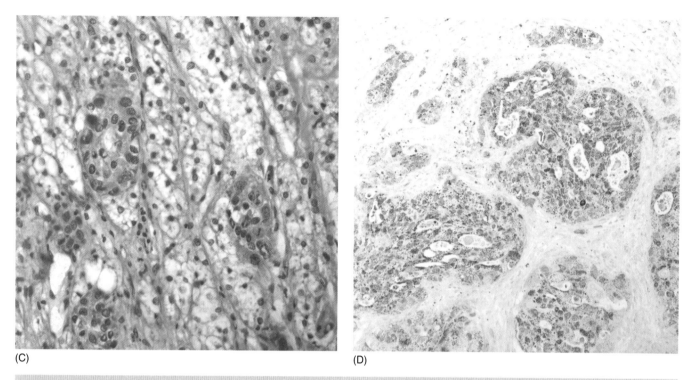

(C)   (D)

FIGURE 12.16 (*continued*) (D) These tumor cells are positive for thyroid transcription factor 1 (TTF-1) and Napsin A (Dual immunohistochemical stain with red chromogen (Napsin A) and brown chromogen (TTF-1), medium power). DQ, Diff-Quik; H&E, hematoxylin and eosin; TP, touch preparation.

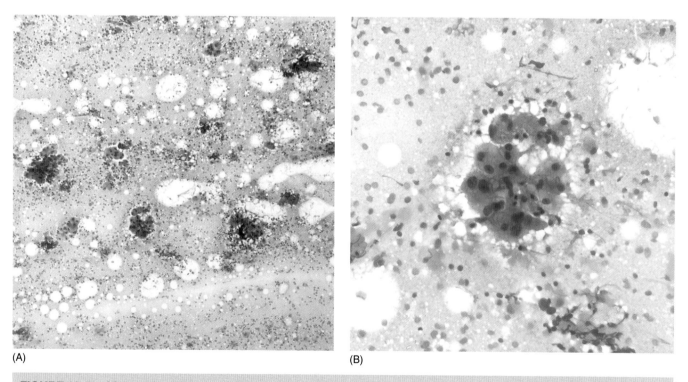

(A)   (B)

FIGURE 12.17 Metastatic renal cell carcinoma to the adrenal gland. (A and B) The TP shows clusters of cells with abundant cytoplasm in a background of benign adrenal cortical cells (H&E-stained, low and high power). (*continued*)

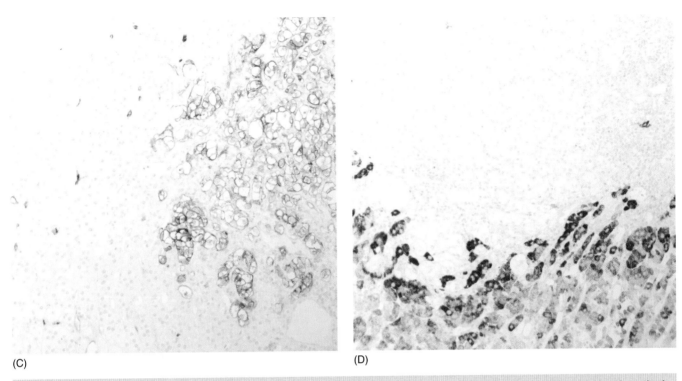

(C)

(D)

FIGURE 12.17 *(continued)* (C) The tumor cells are positive for CD10 and (D) negative for inhibin, while the adrenal cortical tissue is positive for inhibin and negative for CD10. ((C), CD10 immunostain, medium power; (D) Inhibin immunostain, medium power.) H&E, hematoxylin and eosin; TP, touch preparation.

REFERENCES

1. Duwe BV, Sterman DH, Musani AI. Tumors of the mediastinum. *Chest.* 2005;128(4):2893-2909.

2. Tatomirović Z, Bokun R, Stoiljković B, Stepić V. Value of cytologic diagnosis in rapid intraoperative diagnosis of mediastinal lymphadenopathy and tumors of the lung and mediastinum. *Mil Med Pharmaceut Rev.* 2002;59(5):493-497.

3. Moreira SG Jr, Pow-Sang JM. Evaluation and management of adrenal masses. *Cancer Control.* 2002;9(4):326-334.

4. Strollo DC, Rosado de Christenson ML, Jett JR. Primary mediastinal tumors. Part 1: tumors of the anterior mediastinum. *Chest.* 1997;112(2):511-522.

5. Kornstein MJ, Max LD, Wakely PE Jr. Touch imprints in the intraoperative diagnosis of anterior mediastinal neoplasms. *Arch Pathol Lab Med.* 1996;120(12):1116-1122.

6. Henderson DW, Reid G, Kao SC, et al. Challenges and controversies in the diagnosis of mesothelioma: part 1. Cytology-only diagnosis, biopsies, immunohistochemistry, discrimination between mesothelioma and reactive mesothelial hyperplasia, and biomarkers. *J Clin Pathol.* 2013;66(10):847-853.

CHAPTER 13

Ancillary Testing

Sara E. Monaco

INTRODUCTION

Core needle biopsies (CNBs) are often used to supplement fine-needle aspiration (FNA) specimens in order to obtain architectural information and to provide additional material for ancillary studies. In today's modern era of personalized medicine, performance of ancillary studies is the main goal of many biopsies, particularly in patients with a known history of malignancy, and this is a major change from the past when having a diagnosis alone was sufficient (1,2). Touch preparations can help in providing a preliminary diagnosis, triaging the specimen, and confirming that lesional material is present for the necessary tests. This chapter addresses some of the key issues to consider when submitting a core biopsy specimen for ancillary studies, and highlights some of the diagnostic challenges.

MATERIAL FOR ANCILLARY TESTING

Core biopsies can provide material for ancillary studies directly, or can be used to prepare alternative material such as touch preparations for special studies (Table 13.1). In some situations, concurrent FNA specimens may provide material for special studies when the core is less than optimal or nonrepresentative.

Unstained Touch Preparations

Dedicated unstained slides prepared at the time of specimen collection can be a valuable source of material for ancillary studies. These slides are particularly advantageous for fluorescence in-situ hybridization (FISH) studies as touch imprints, scrapes, and aspirate smears contain the entire nucleus on the slide, opposed to the truncation artifact seen with tissue sections, and avoids artifacts associated with formalin fixation (3). This allows for more accurate signal counting in FISH evaluation. FISH studies have been applied to cytological specimens for the assessment of characteristic translocations in soft tissue/bone tumors, and for the assessment of *IgH* gene and other rearrangements in hematolymphoid malignancies (3,4). Furthermore, touch

imprint specimens have been used for FISH studies in solid organ malignancies such as carcinomas and neural tumors (5,6). In addition, in cases with a single good biopsy, unstained touch imprints can be processed immediately after evaluation at the time of onsite evaluation without waiting for the tissue block to be processed, and without the possibility of losing tissue in processing. This may help maximize the information obtained from a small specimen, given that processing issues may limit the amount of tissue in the tissue block for both immunohistochemical stains and FISH studies. Unstained TPs can also be a source of material for special stains in cases worrisome for infection that have only a few good passes of inflammatory debris, which may not be sufficient for a tissue block (7). This is especially true for necrotic inflammatory processes given that the core biopsy tissue is fragile and may not survive processing. However, multiple TPs may be needed for multiple special stains and the material may be thicker and more difficult to interpret. One of the biggest difficulties with unstained TPs is that high-quality slides need to be prepared at the time of onsite evaluation, which typically requires laboratory or cytology personnel to perform an immediate evaluation, prepare these unstained dedicated slides, and triage the specimen appropriately (e.g., to decide if additional unstained smears may be needed). Furthermore, these slides need to be stored in containers with individual slots for the slides, as they are not coverslipped and cannot be placed back-to-back with other slides. Laboratories should have a procedure for the preparation, storage, use, and retrieval of these unstained touch preparations and smears.

TABLE 13.1 Specimens Suitable for Ancillary Testing in Cases With CNB

- Touch imprint slides—unstained
- Touch imprint slides—destained
- Scrape from a touch imprint into a FFPE tissue block
- Cell transfer from a touch imprint onto separate slides
- FFPE tissue block of a core needle biopsy
- Alternative and/or concurrent specimens (e.g., FNA smears, FNA cell block)

CNB, core needle biopsy; FFPE, formalin-fixed paraffin embedded; FNA, fine-needle aspiration.

Destained Touch Preparations

Touch imprint slides, in addition to cytology scrapings or aspirates, can be destained and utilized for ancillary studies, particularly immunohistochemical stains. Immunostains have been successfully performed on destained Diff-Quik or Papanicolaou slides, even with multiple antibodies on the same slide in a sequential fashion or together with double stains (e.g., typically utilizing the combination of a nuclear stain and a membranous or cytoplasmic stain) (8,9). In a comparison of unstained smears that underwent alcohol fixation or air-drying, versus destained, alcohol-fixed Papanicolaou-stained smears, the results were comparable with no significant differences (9). The disadvantage of this approach is the fact that diagnostic slides would be sacrificed, and thus may need to be scanned (digitized) and archived prior to use. This also requires more time and labor to produce results, thereby increasing turnaround time. In addition, the use of alternative fixation and processing from routine surgical cases mandates separate validation of immunostains.

Scrape From Touch Preparation Into a Formalin-Fixed Paraffin Embedded Cell Block or Cell Transfer of Material From a Touch Preparation

Occasionally, touch preparations will contain abundant lesional cells whereas the subsequent histological sections of the core biopsy show insufficient tissue or the small tissue fragments are lost in processing. In these scenarios, material on the touch imprint slides can be scraped off with a scalpel blade and put into formalin for processing, after decoverslipping in xylene (Figure 13.1). This scraping technique tends to affect the morphology of the cells with distortion and crush, as has been described in the literature (Figure 13.1) (10,11). However, this can provide valuable material for immunohistochemical stains or other studies, if there is no alternative diagnostic material.

In addition, a cell transfer technique has been described whereby a cellular smear or touch imprint is sacrificed for multiple immunostains when alternative core biopsy or cell block material is unavailable or not representative of the lesional cells (12–16). This cell transfer technique has been shown in the literature to work best with stained and coverslipped slides that are soaked in xylene, and then the material is cut into small fragments to be transferred to multiple individual slides for an immunohistochemical panel. Alternatively, in cases that are difficult to formally transfer, the material in one touch imprint can be divided into subsections with a hydrophobic barrier pen (e.g., ImmEdge Pen, Vector Laboratories, Burlingame, CA) with multiple different antibodies being applied to different sections (Figure 13.2).

The drawback of this technique is that diagnostic material is sacrificed and therefore the slides should be converted to virtual slides beforehand. In addition, there is a delay in turnaround time, given that there is extended processing before the material can be lifted off the slides. However, if this can be done on acquired material to avoid a repeat biopsy, the rewards may outweigh the disadvantages.

Formalin-Fixed Paraffin Embedded Core Needle Biopsy

Histological sections of a CNB are the most commonly utilized material for ancillary studies, particularly immunohistochemical stains. The reason is that many validation tests performed on surgical specimens use formalin-fixed paraffin embedded tissue, and thus application to small FFPE biopsies is seamless and does not require a separate validation (1). However, if small biopsies or cytology specimens are sent in alternative media, then this should be indicated in the gross description, and a separate validation should be done for alternative fixatives. One of the most difficult issues with ancillary studies performed on a CNB is that the qualitative and quantitative nature of the specimen varies from level to level given the limited tissue. Thus, it is imperative to avoid excessive trimming of a tissue block by ordering all necessary slides upfront with the initial slide that is hematoxylin and eosin (H&E) stained, which may involve simply ordering blank slides for use later, or ordering a preliminary limited immunopanel based on the immediate assessment of the touch imprint (Figure 13.3) (1). This initial assessment of the imprint cytology can be very informative in providing a preliminary differential diagnosis, leading to the appropriate allocation and triage of the specimen, and thereby decreasing the turnaround time for a final diagnosis. Alternatively, some hospitals have a small biopsy protocol whereby two levels are cut for routine H&E-stains, and the intervening levels are saved as blanks for potential immunostains or molecular studies.

When processing small biopsies, it is essential for the laboratory personnel to describe the number of biopsy pieces and the size of the individual pieces in the gross description. This is important so that one can compare the amount of tissue seen on the initial H&E section to what was identified grossly, in order to determine if the block was adequately sectioned. Sometimes histology technicians are reluctant to cut into a small tissue block if multiple slides are requested, and so the initial slides may not have enough tissue. It is also helpful to number sectioned slides sequentially, so that ancillary studies of highest importance can be performed on those levels with the most tissue (Figure 13.4).

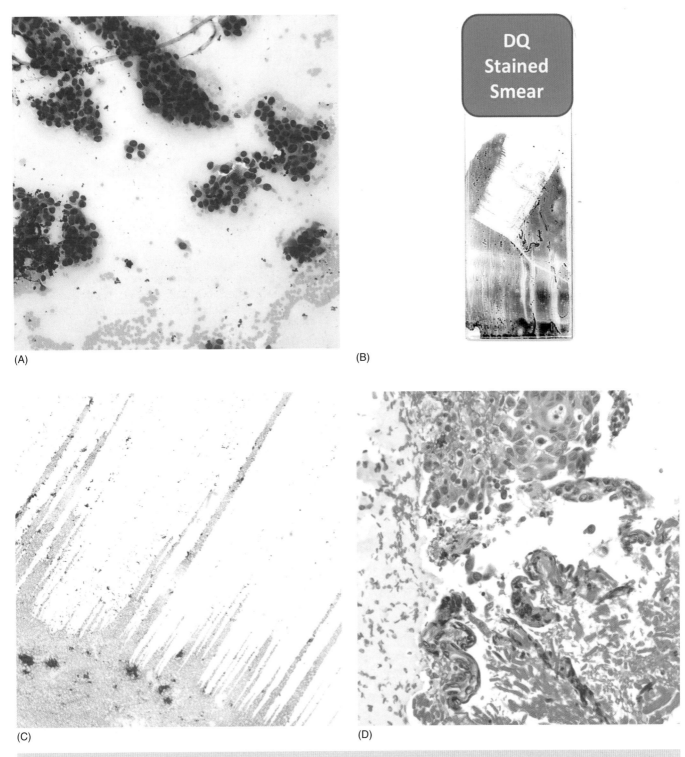

(A)

(B)

(C)

(D)

FIGURE 13.1 Scrape from TP for ancillary studies. (A) A cellular TP or aspirate smear can be sacrificed for ancillary studies if there is insufficient lesional material in the core biopsy. (B and C) This can be performed by removing the cover slip carefully after soaking in xylene, then using a scalpel blade to scrape the cellular areas of lesional cells, which are then transferred to formalin. (D) The material will appear as small, crushed, stained fragments within the formalin that can be spun down into a formalin-fixed cell block. The morphology of the cells will be altered given the distortion during the scrape process, but is usually suitable for immunostains as a last resort for characterization ((A) DQ-stained TP, high power; (B and C) DQ-stained TP, low power; (D) H&E-stained, high power). DQ, Diff-Quik; H&E, hematoxylin and eosin; TP, touch preparation.

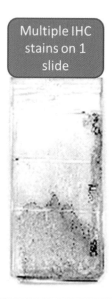

FIGURE 13.2 Multiple immunostains on a single slide. A cytology smear or touch imprint can be divided using a hydrophobic pen and each section can be stained with a different antibody, in order to maximize results in limited specimens.

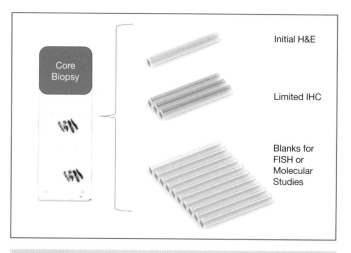

FIGURE 13.3 Processing of small core biopsies. It can be helpful to order a limited immunopanel and/or blank slides upfront when a touch imprint is reviewed for immediate assessment or as a routine protocol on all small biopsies. This helps avoid tissue loss when returning to a tissue block to cut slides after the original H&E has been reviewed. FISH, fluorescence in-situ hybridization; H&E, hematoxylin and eosin; IHC, immunohistochemistry.

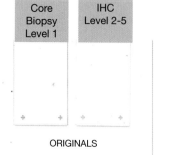 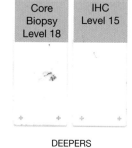

ORIGINALS   DEEPERS

FIGURE 13.4 Tissue on core biopsy sections utilized for ancillary studies. The different levels of a CNB can have drastically different amounts of tissue, thus correlation with the measurements of the tissue fragments in the gross description can be critical, in order to ensure that all of the tissue is represented on the slide and that the histology lab has cut far enough into the block. In the case shown tissue only starts to show up on sections for level 18. CNB, core needle biopsy. IHC, immunohistochemistry.

TYPES OF ANCILLARY TESTING

Special Stains

Special histochemical stains were utilized more in the past, prior to the availability of multiple immunohistochemical stains. Now, immunostains have largely replaced these special stains for the characterization and localization of malignancies. However, special stains can be helpful to confirm the presence of mucin or other secretory products in cells (7). In addition, the most widely utilized role for special stains in a CNB is to confirm or exclude infectious etiologies, especially bacteria with a Gram stain, fungal elements with a Gomori methenamine silver (GMS) stain, and mycobacteria with an acid-fast (e.g., acid-fast bacilli [AFB]) stain (Figure 13.5). Imprint cytology can be helpful to immediately assess a core biopsy, trigger the appropriate triage of the specimen (e.g., culture, special stains), and provide a preliminary diagnosis for treatment. The presence of granulomas should prompt fungal and mycobacterial stains. In some cases of granulomatous inflammation with hyalinization, where the imprint is limited by scant cellularity and no definitive granulomas are seen, the presence of a few multinucleated giant cells may provide enough of a clue that there is an infection or granulomatous inflammation (Figure 13.6). Another helpful feature is negative images on a Diff-Quik stained touch preparation of mycobacteria.

Immunohistochemical Stains

Immunostains are typically performed on FFPE CNB sections, and given that antibodies are often validated using FFPE surgical tissue a separate validation for cytology is not needed. In addition, multiple blank slides can be cut from a single block to perform a panel of immunostains, making it easier to locate cells of interest for characterization. However, it is also possible to perform intraoperative immunostaining on touch imprints (17,18). This has been reported to be particularly helpful for sentinel lymph node evaluations in breast cancer patients, whereby a modified immunostaining protocol can provide results within 30 minutes (17). Immunohistochemical stains are particularly helpful to subclassify neoplastic processes and to provide grading information (Figures 13.7 and 13.8). Furthermore, sequential sections of a tissue block stained with different immunostains can help characterize the cells present, such as separating tumor cells from background benign cells (Figure 13.9). When performing immunostains, the use of alternative chromagens should be considered in cases with inherent pigment in the lesional cells or in the background. The best example is in cases of pigmented melanoma where melanin pigment may be erroneously interpreted as a positive brown chromagen. Such cases are best stained utilizing antibodies with a red chromagen (Figure 13.10).

Fluorescence In Situ Hybridization

FISH studies can be successfully applied to unstained touch imprints or smears, and do not have the artifacts associated with formalin fixation or nuclear truncation that can be seen with a cell block or core biopsy tissue section (3). Another effect that can occur in a small CNB is crush artifact due to cell fragility, especially with lymphoid proliferations. Thus, in cases suspicious for lymphoma, a touch imprint can be particularly helpful to run FISH. However, even if touch imprints are not prepared or cytopathology services are not available onsite, a CNB can be submitted for FISH studies (2). One caveat to keep in mind is that preanalytical factors can impact the ability to do FISH testing on CNB specimens. Bone CNB cases undergoing decalcification or cases fixed in certain fixatives (e.g., Bouin's fixative) may fail FISH testing. Therefore, soft tissue and bone fragments in osseous lesions can be separated into different tissue blocks so that decalcification agents are not applied to all of the tissue. Onsite evaluation of a touch imprint from a bone CNB can be helpful to look for metastatic tumor, lymphoma, or a small round blue cell tumor to see if FISH studies could potentially be required in order to withhold decalcification in these cases. In addition, if erythrosine is used to help visualize small tissue fragments in processing, this can create a granular precipitate that makes enumeration of FISH signals difficult or impossible. Thus, for small biopsy processing, toluidine blue to track such samples is preferable.

Molecular Genetic Testing

Molecular diagnostic testing has been successfully performed on CNBs with similar success rates as FNA specimens (1,2,19). In most cases, a cancer patient may have multiple different specimens available, and thus, comparison of the tumor cellularity and other features is important in selecting the best specimen for molecular testing (Figure 13.11). CNBs are typically superior in providing a larger fragment of tissue for testing. However, there is no reliable way to determine how much tumor tissue is available at the time of the biopsy procedure. Thus, there are situations where a touch imprint may be highly cellular, while the tissue block has insufficient tumor cells for testing. In some cases, this may be explained by forceful touch imprints that can be more disruptive to the CNB. Therefore, excessive force should be avoided when preparing touch imprints (20). Another potential problem is that the CNB may have abundant desmoplastic stroma or normal tissue, which lowers the tumor cellularity in the CNB (Figure 13.11). These cases may benefit from microdissection to optimize the results of molecular testing, but this is more laborious. In addition, a concurrent aspiration cytology specimen may be able to avoid this issue, as the FNA needle is believed to microdissect during aspiration and decrease the benign background, thereby optimizing the tumor cellularity on aspirate smears and cell block sections (1).

Flow Cytometry

Flow cytometry is typically a crucial ancillary study for CNB cases suspicious for lymphoma. As mentioned before, touch imprints can be particularly helpful in these cases to confirm the clinical suspicion of lymphoma and to triage a case for necessary ancillary studies. One of the issues with using a CNB for flow cytometry is that the tissue must be made into a cellular suspension prior to processing. This is typically done by disaggregation with mechanical or enzymatic methods, which may in turn damage the cells resulting in low viability or nondiagnostic specimens. In contrast, FNA specimens provide a cellular suspension that does not require extensive processing prior to analysis and is accordingly more optimal for flow cytometry (21). The advantage of CNB over FNA is that usually there are less indeterminate or nondiagnostic cases given that architectural information can be evaluated, which the FNA typically lacks. In addition, it has been shown that as you increase the needle gauge of the CNB and thus the tissue volume, the percentage of cases with a definitive diagnosis increases (22). Flow cytometry should be performed in all cases worrisome for a lymphoma. Besides FNA, obtaining CNBs for histological evaluation and other ancillary studies is encouraged given the modern, multidisciplinary approach to lymphoproliferative disorders.

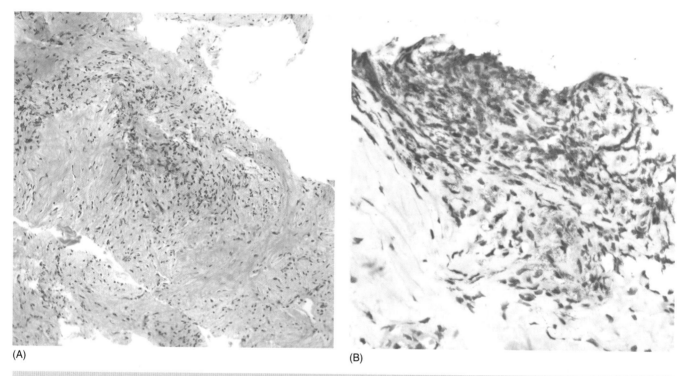

(A)

(B)

FIGURE 13.5 Special stains on core needle biopsies. A CNB can provide material for special stains such as an AFB stain in cases of nonnecrotizing granulomatous inflammation worrisome for mycobacterial infection. ((A) H&E-stained, high power; (B) AFB stain, high power.) AFB, acid-fast bacilli; CNB, core needle biopsy; H&E, hematoxylin and eosin.

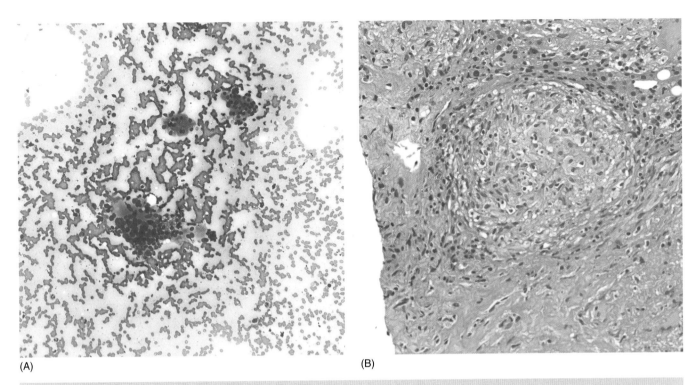

(A)

(B)

FIGURE 13.6 Granulomatous inflammation with hyalinization in a liver core biopsy. When looking for granulomas or organisms on TPs, some cases of hyalinized granulomas may yield scant TPs. A few multinucleated giant cells may be a clue that there are granulomas in the core biopsy and can be helpful to thoroughly investigate for organisms with special stains. ((A) DQ-stained TP, medium power; (B) H&E-stained, high power.) DQ, DIff-Quik; H&E, hematoxylin and eosin; TP, touch preparation.

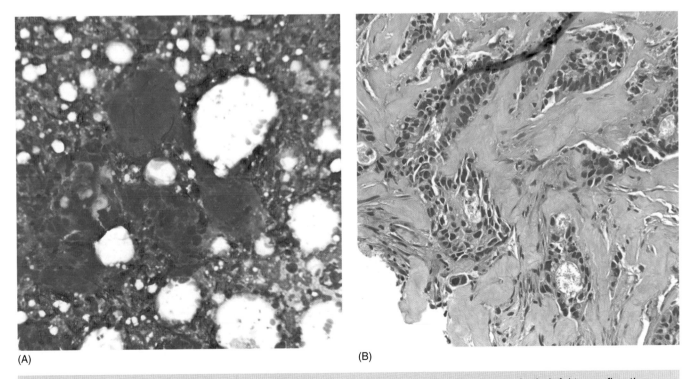

(A)

(B)

FIGURE 13.7 TP and core biopsy with immunostains for subclassification. TP evaluation can be helpful to confirm the presence of tumor and to provide a preliminary diagnosis that can guide the immunostains to order and expedite the turn-around of the final results. In the example shown, (A and B) this moderately differentiated colon adenocarcinoma is immunoreactive for (C) CK20 and (D) CDX2. ((A) DQ-stained TP, high power; (B) H&E-stained, high power; (C) CK20 immunostain, high power; (D) CDX2 immunostain, high power.) DQ, Diff-Quik; H&E, hematoxylin and eosin; TP, touch preparation. (*continued*)

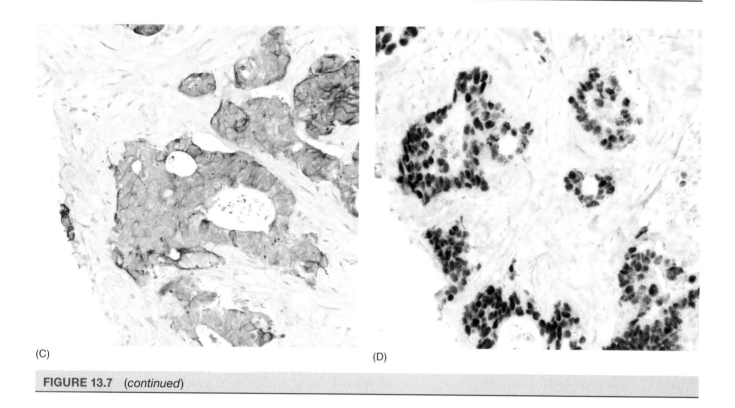

(C)

(D)

FIGURE 13.7 (*continued*)

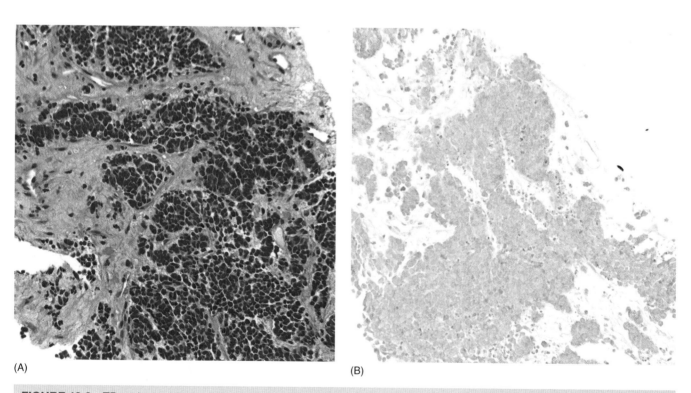

(A)

(B)

FIGURE 13.8 TP and core biopsy with immunostains for grading. (A) In this core biopsy of a lung neuroendocrine tumor (B) that stains with synaptophysin, (C) the Ki67 stain is helpful to confirm that this is a high-grade neuroendocrine tumor with a high proliferation index, compatible with small cell carcinoma. ((A) H&E-stained, medium power; (B) synaptophysin immunostain, medium power; (C) Ki67 immunostain, medium power.) H&E, hematoxylin and eosin. (*continued*)

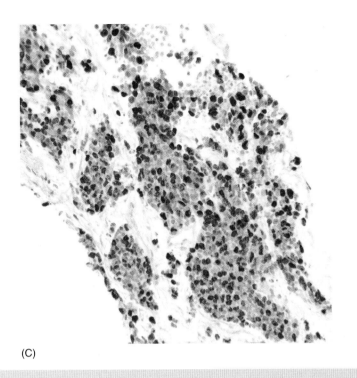

(C)

FIGURE 13.8 *(continued)*

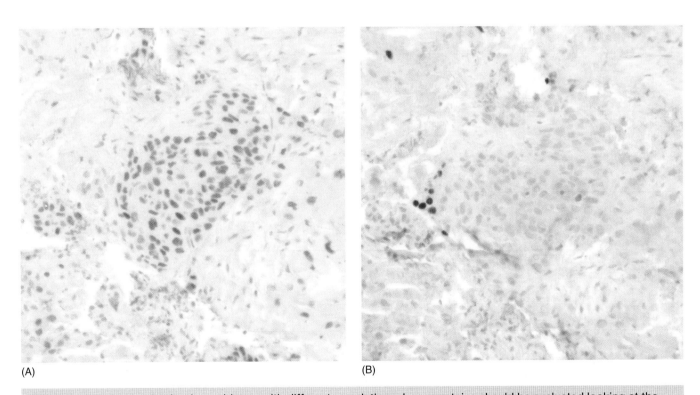

(A)

(B)

FIGURE 13.9 Immunostained core biopsy with different populations. Immunostains should be evaluated looking at the cells of interest, not simply stating if they are positive or negative. In this lung biopsy of a squamous cell carcinoma (see also Figure 5.20), the tumor cells (A) show positive nuclear staining for p40, (B) while the scant background bronchial epithelial cells surrounding the tumor show nuclear staining for TTF1. ((A) p40 immunostain, high power; (B) TTF1 immunostain, high power.) H&E, hematoxylin and eosin; TTF1, thyroid transcription factor 1.

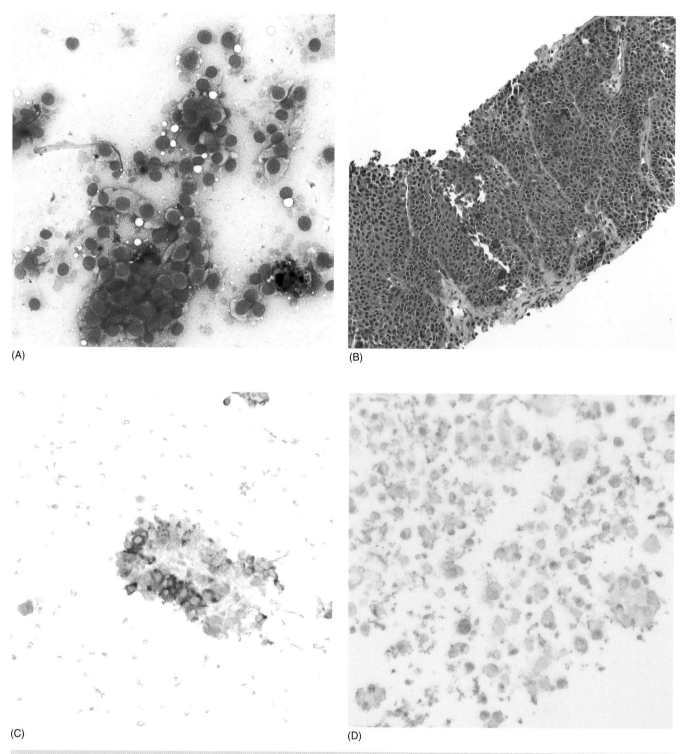

(A)

(B)

(C)

(D)

FIGURE 13.10 Use of different chromagens. In tumors containing pigment, alternative chromagens are preferred to avoid falsely interpreting pigment as positive staining. A TP can help in making this determination. For example, in this case of a pigmented melanoma (A and B), a MelanA immunostain (C) with a red chromagen was utilized to highlight the tumor cells making it easy to distinguish from brown melanin pigment. In contrast, another case of a pigmented melanoma stained with S100 (D) using a brown chromagen is very difficult to interpret. ((A) DQ-stained TP, high power; (B) H&E-stained, medium power; (C) MelanA immunostain (red chromagen), high power; (D) S100 immunostain (brown chromagen), high power.) DQ, Diff-Quik; H&E, hematoxylin and eosin; TP, touch preparation.

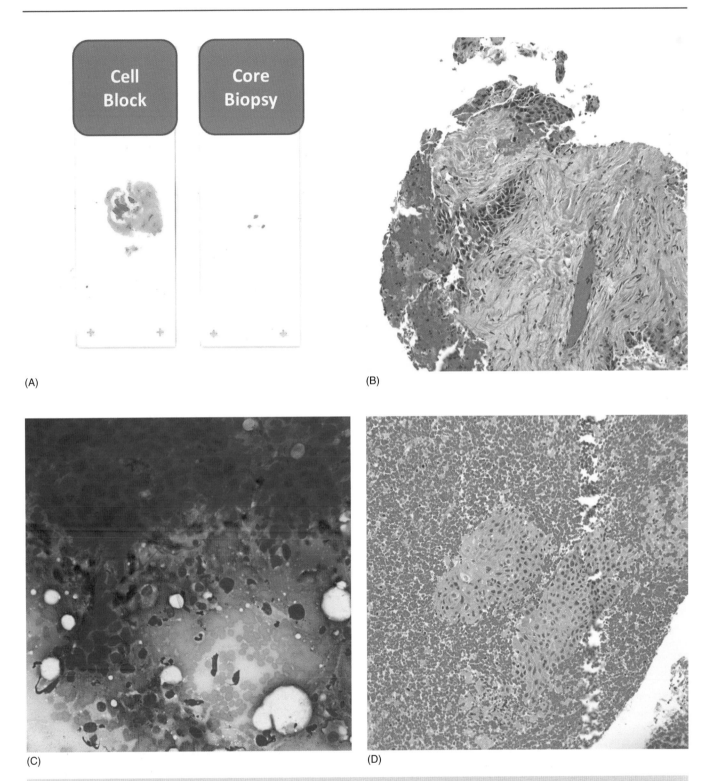

FIGURE 13.11 Molecular testing in core biopsy samples and alternative specimens. (A) The cellularity of a core biopsy should be compared to other specimens from the same patient to determine which specimen is optimal for molecular studies. Molecular testing on core biopsies (B) such as this lung carcinoma usually require microdissection of tumor cells from the background stroma. If the core biopsy contains insufficient tumor volume, then additional specimens can be used, particularly if a concurrent TP or FNA were performed with the core biopsy. TPs or smears can be sacrificed for molecular testing, and cell blocks from the FNA can also be used. For this non-small cell carcinoma case (C) FNA smears and (D) cell blocks are enriched with tumor cells with minimal background stroma, which makes such cases easier to process and maximizes the percent tumor cellularity. ((A) H&E-stained, low power; (B) H&E-stained, high power; (C) DQ-stained TP, high power; (D) H&E-stained, high power.) DQ, Diff-Quik; FNA, fine-needle aspiration; H&E, hematoxylin and eosin; TP, touch preparation.

PITFALLS OF ANCILLARY TESTING

In small biopsies utilized for ancillary studies, there can be prominent edge artifact, which may reflect differences in fixation. This is important to recognize and to avoid overcalling positive staining in these cases if the cells within the center of the biopsy are negative or not showing the correct localization of the antibody (Figure 13.12). Another issue, particularly in small, fragmented specimens are folds or overlapped tissue sections, which can occur with thick or bony tissue that is difficult to cut, as well as floaters from processing, which can make interpretation difficult, impossible, or inaccurate (Figure 13.13). In these situations, focusing on the areas of lesional cells that correspond to the H&E-

stained slides is essential. In some scenarios, repeat immunostaining on another level may be warranted. When floaters are seen, these fragments should be circled and indicated as floaters on the slide. CNB cases from the mediastinum and lung can have prominent anthracotic pigment, which should not be misinterpreted as positive immunostaining (Figure 13.14). In addition, hemorrhagic lesions may have abundant brown, refractile hemosiderin, which similarly should not be interpreted as positive immunostaining. Alternate fixatives, particularly those with harsh acids (e.g., Bouin's fixative) can lead to artifactual changes in morphology (Figure 13.15). In these cases, molecular and FISH studies may also not be possible. Thus, harsh fixatives are best avoided if ancillary studies will be needed.

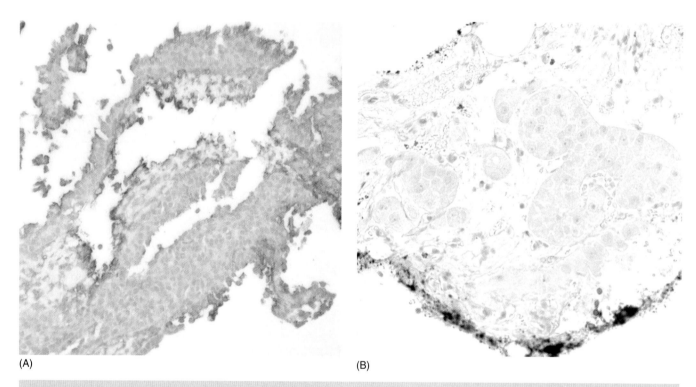

(A)   (B)

FIGURE 13.12   Immunostained core biopsy section with edge artifact. In small biopsies utilized for immunohistochemical stains, there can be pronounced artifactual staining on the edge of the biopsy, which should not be overinterpreted as positive staining in the absence of the correct localization of the antibody in more central areas of the tissue. This tends to be more common with cytoplasmic and membranous immunostains. (A) is an example of CD99 staining in a core biopsy of metastatic carcinoma, that is negative but shows nonspecific staining on the edge of the small tissue fragments. (B) shows CD10 staining on the periphery of a core biopsy of a renal oncocytoma. ((A) CD99 immunostain, medium power; (B) CD10 immunostain, high power.)

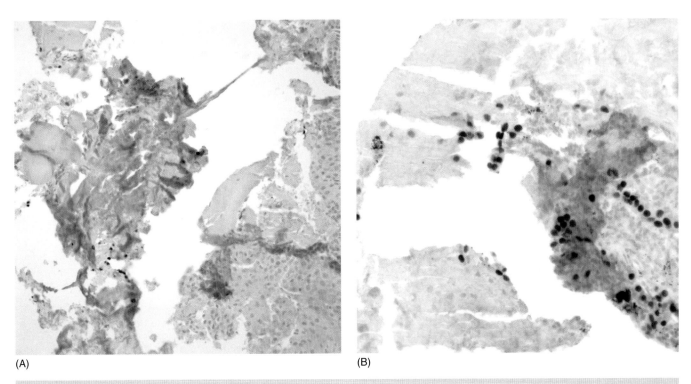

(A)

(B)

FIGURE 13.13 Immunostained core biopsy section with overlapping and tissue floaters. Small, fragmented biopsies may suffer from overlapping or folded small fragments, and may have small tissue floaters from processing. This is more common in cases from bone. ((A) TTF1 immunostain, medium power; (B) TTF1 immunostain, high power.) TTF1, thyroid transcription factor 1.

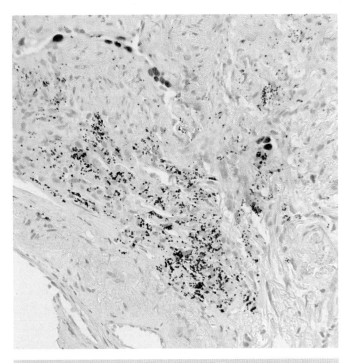

FIGURE 13.14 Immunostained core biopsy with anthracotic pigment. When core biopsies from the lung or mediastinum have anthracotic pigment, this black anthracotic pigment should not be misinterpreted as positive immunostaining with a brown chromagen (TTF1 immunostain, high power). TTF1, thyroid transcription factor 1.

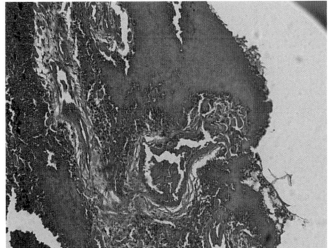

FIGURE 13.15 Bouin's fixative in a core biopsy. Bouin's fixative can lead to indeterminate molecular and FISH testing results due to acidic agents (picric acid and glacial acetic acid) that lead to poor DNA and RNA quality, as well as altered morphology in some cases (H&E-stained, medium power). DNA, deoxyribonucleic acid; FISH, fluorescence in situ hybridization; H&E, hematoxylin and eosin; RNA, ribonucleic acid.

REFERENCES

1. Aisner DL, Sams SB. The role of cytology specimens in molecular testing of solid tumors: techniques, limitations, and opportunities. *Diagn Cytopathol*. 2012;40:511-524.

2. Gibson J, Young S, Leng B, et al. Molecular diagnostic testing of cytology specimens: current applications and future considerations. *J Am Soc Cytopathol*. 2014;3:280-294.

3. Monaco SE, Teot LA, Felgar RE, et al. Fluorescence in situ hybridization studies on direct smears: an approach to enhance the fine-needle aspiration biopsy diagnosis of B-cell non-Hodgkin lymphomas. *Cancer*. 2009;117:338-348.

4. Khalbuss WE, Teot LA, Monaco SE. Diagnostic accuracy and limitations of fine-needle aspiration cytology of bone and soft tissue lesions: a review of 1114 cases with cytological-histological correlation. *Cancer Cytopathol*. 2010;118:24-32.

5. Proietti A, Alì G, Pelliccioni S, et al. Anaplastic lymphoma kinase gene rearrangements in cytological samples of non-small cell lung cancer: comparison with histological assessment. *Cancer Cytopathol*. 2014;122:445-453.

6. Tamiolakis D, Papadopoulos N, Venizelos I, et al. Loss of chromosome 1 in myxopapillary ependymoma suggests a region out of chromosome 22 as critical for tumour biology: a FISH analysis of four cases on touch imprint smears. *Cytopathology*. 2006;17:199-204.

7. Silowash R, Monaco SE, Pantanowitz L. Ancillary techniques on direct-smear aspirate slides: a significant evolution for cytopathology techniques. *Cancer Cytopathol*. 2013;121:670.

8. Dabbs DJ, Wang X. Immunocytochemistry on cytologic specimens of limited quantity. *Diagn Cytopathol*. 1998;18:166-169.

9. Dabbs DJ, Hafer L, Abendroth CS. Intraoperative immunocytochemistry of cytologic scrape specimens. A rapid immunoperoxidase method for triage and diagnosis. *Acta Cytol*. 1995;39:157-163.

10. Blumenfeld W, Hashmi N, Sagerman P. Comparison of aspiration, touch and scrape preparations simultaneously obtained from surgically excised specimens. Effect of different methods of smear preparation on interpretive cytologic features. *Acta Cytol*. 1998;42:1414-1418.

11. Doughty MJ. Comparison of morphology of bulbar conjunctival cells assessed by impression cytology versus scrape and smear methods. *Curr Eye Res*. 2014;39:973-981.

12. Sherman ME, Jimenez-Joseph D, Gangi MD, RojasCorona RR. Immunostaining of small cytologic specimens: facilitation with cell transfer. *Acta Cytol*.1994;38:18-22.

13. Gong Y, Joseph T, Sneige N. Validation of commonly used immunostains on cell-transferred cytologic specimens. *Cancer*. 2005;105:158-164.

14. Hunt JL, Van de Rijn M, Gupta PK. Immunohistochemical analysis of gel-transferred cells in cytologic preparations following smear division. *Diagn Cytopathol*. 1998;18:377-380.

15. Miller RT, Kubier P. Immunocytochemistry on cytologic specimens and previously stained slides (when no paraffin block is available). *J Histotech*. 2002;25:251-257.

16. Zu Y, Gangi MD, Yang GC. Ultrafast Papanicolaou stain and cell-transfer technique enhance cytologic diagnosis of Hodgkin lymphoma. *Diagn Cytopathol*. 2002;27:308-311.

17. Salem AA, Douglas-Jones AG, Sweetland HM, Mansel RE. Intraoperative evaluation of axillary sentinel lymph nodes using touch imprint cytology and immunohistochemistry. *Part II. Results. Eur J Surg Oncol*. 2006;32:484-487.

18. Salem AA, Douglas-Jones AG, Sweetland HM, Mansel RE. Intraoperative evaluation of axillary sentinel lymph nodes using touch imprint cytology and immunohistochemistry: I. Protocol of rapid immunostaining of touch imprints. *Eur J Surg Oncol*. 2003;29:25-28.

19. Lozano MD, Labiano T, Echeveste J, et al. Assessment of EGFR and KRAS mutation status from FNAs and core-needle biopsies of nonsmall cell lung cancer. *Cancer Cytopathol*. 2015;123(4):230-236.

20. Rekhtman N, Kazi S, Yao J, et al. Depletion of core needle biopsy cellularity and DNA content as a result of vigorous touch preparations. *Arch Pathol Lab Med*. 2015;139(7):907-912.

21. Boyd JD, Smith GD, Hong H, et al. Fine-needle aspiration is superior to needle core biopsy as a sample acquisition method for flow cytometric analysis in suspected hematologic neoplasms. *Cytometry B Clin Cytom*. 2015;88:64-68.

22. Hu Q, Naushad H, Xie Q, et al. Needle-core biopsy in the pathologic diagnosis of malignant lymphoma showing high reproducibility among pathologists. *Am J Clin Pathol*. 2013;140:238-247.

Index